DENTAL EDUCATION AT THE DISCARDED CROSSROADS

CHALLENGES AND CHANGE

Committee on the Future of Dental Education
Marilyn J. Field, Ph.D., Editor

Division of Health Care Services   JA20'95

INSTITUTE OF MEDICINE

NATIONAL ACADEMY PRESS
Washington, D.C. 1995

National Academy Press • 2101 Constitution Avenue, N.W. • Washington, D.C. 20418

NOTICE: The project that is the subject of this report was approved by the Governing Board of the National Research Council, whose members are drawn from the councils of the National Academy of Sciences, the National Academy of Engineering, and the Institute of Medicine. The members of the committee responsible for the report were chosen for their special competences and with regard for appropriate balance.

This report has been reviewed by a group other than the authors according to procedures approved by a Report Review Committee consisting of members of the National Academy of Sciences, the National Academy of Engineering, and the Institute of Medicine.

The Institute of Medicine was chartered in 1970 by the National Academy of Sciences to enlist distinguished members of the appropriate professions in the examination of policy matters pertaining to the health of the public. In this, the Institute acts under both the Academy's 1863 congressional charter responsibility to be an adviser to the federal government and its own initiative in identifying issues of medical care, research, and education. Dr. Kenneth I. Shine is president of the Institute of Medicine.

Support for this project was provided by the Robert Wood Johnson Foundation under Grant No. 19634, the American Fund for Dental Health, the National Institute of Dental Research under Contract No. NO1-DE-22594, the Health Resources Services Administration under Contract No. 240-91-0051, the Department of Veterans Affairs, the Department of Defense, the American Association of Retired Persons, and CIGNA Dental Health, Inc. The views presented are those of the Institute of Medicine Committee on the Future of Dental Education and are not necessarily those of the funding organizations.

Library of Congress Cataloging-in-Publication Data

Dental education at the crossroads : challenges and change / Committee
   on the Future of Dental Education, Division of Health Care Services,
   Institute of Medicine ; Marilyn J. Field, editor.
         p.   cm.
   Includes bibliographical references and index.
   ISBN 0-309-05195-9
   1. Dentistry—Study and teaching—United States. 2. Dental
policy—United States. I. Field, Marilyn J. (Marilyn Jane).
II. Institute of Medicine (U.S.). Committee on the Future of Dental
Education.
RK91.D39   1995   94-41301
617.6'0071'173—dc20   CIP

COMMITTEE ON THE FUTURE OF DENTAL EDUCATION

JOHN P. HOWE III (*Chair*), President, The University of Texas Health Science Center at San Antonio, San Antonio, Texas

MYRON ALLUKIAN, Jr.,* Assistant Deputy Commissioner and Director, Personal Health Services and Community Dental Programs, Department of Health and Hospitals, City of Boston, Boston, Massachusetts

HOWARD L. BAILIT,* Senior Vice President, Health Services Research, Aetna Life and Casualty, Hartford, Connecticut

EVA C. DAHL, Practice of Endodontics and Oral Pathology, Department of Dental Specialists, Gundersen Clinic, Ltd., La Crosse, Wisconsin

CHESTER DOUGLASS, Professor and Chairman, Department of Oral Health Policy and Epidemiology, Harvard School of Dental Medicine, and Professor of Epidemiology, Harvard School of Public Health, Boston, Massachusetts

RASHI FEIN,* Professor of the Economics of Medicine, Department of Social Medicine, Harvard Medical School, Boston, Massachusetts

JOEL F. GLOVER, Private Practice, Reno, Nevada

JOSEPH L. HENRY,* Associate Dean, Professor, and Chair, Department of Oral Diagnosis and Oral Radiology, Harvard School of Dental Medicine, Boston, Massachusetts

CARLOS MANUEL INTERIAN, JR., Private Practice, Miami, Florida

JAMES D. ISBISTER, President, Pharmavene, Inc., Gaithersburg, Maryland

MARJORIE K. JEFFCOAT, Rosen Professor and Chairman, Department of Periodontics, School of Dentistry, University of Alabama, Birmingham, Alabama

TERRELL E. JONES, Oral Surgery Resident, The University of Tennessee, College of Dentistry, Memphis, Tennessee

LINDA G. KRAEMER, Senior Associate Dean, College of Allied Health Services, Thomas Jefferson University, Philadelphia, Pennsylvania

J. BERNARD MACHEN, Dean, School of Dentistry, University of Michigan, Ann Arbor, Michigan

ELIZABETH F. NEUFELD,* Professor and Chairman, Department of Biological Chemistry, School of Medicine, University of California, Los Angeles, California

J. DENNIS O'CONNOR, Chancellor, University of Pittsburgh, Pittsburgh, Pennsylvania

NEAL A. VANSELOW,* Chancellor, Tulane University Medical Center, New Orleans, Louisiana

THERESA VARNER, Director, Public Policy Institute, American Association of Retired Persons, Washington, D.C.

---

*Institute of Medicine member

Preface

Early in 1990, a group of leaders in dental education asked whether the Institute of Medicine (IOM) would undertake an independent assessment of dental education. After the governing bodies of the IOM approved a preliminary proposal for such a project, the IOM convened a planning meeting in June 1990 that recommended a study to identify measures to strengthen dental education in the United States and stabilize its position within the university. The next step involved discussions with other leaders in dentistry to determine their interest in and receptivity to an IOM study. The study was not conceived as a follow-on project to any previous study but as an independent examination of dental education. It was overseen by an 18-member committee of experts in dental practice and education, oral health and health services research, other areas of health professions and higher education, health care delivery and financing, and public policy.

During its work, the committee faced a number of questions about the nature of the IOM. The IOM is part of the National Academy of Sciences, a private nonprofit organization chartered by Congress in 1863 to provide advice on scientific matters. IOM members include physicians, dentists, nurses, biomedical and health services researchers, and others. Despite its name, one-quarter of the Institute's members must by charter come from outside the health field. Funding for studies comes from both public and private organizations.

The work of the IOM has covered a broad range of health issues since its founding nearly 25 years ago. In recent years, it has issued reports on such disparate issues as the future of public health, measuring access to health care (including oral health services), the effects of mustard gas, preventing mental illness, career paths for clinical research (including dentistry), food and nutrition, employment and health benefits, health care data systems, and health care reform. Past or planned reports on health professions education and supply include studies of the allied health services (including dental hygiene), education for primary care, nursing education, health professions education and minorities, geriatric care in physician training, physician staffing for veterans' hospitals, and nurse staffing in community hospitals. In 1980, the IOM issued a report on financing dental care, and a 1994 report on career paths for clinical researchers includes oral health research. Elsewhere in the National Academy of Sciences, the Office of Scientific and Engineering Personnel issues periodic reports on national needs for such personnel. Its 1985 and 1994 reports cover oral health research workers. By way of historical note, within the National Academy of Sciences, the first committee to consider issues in dental science was formed in 1919 by the Division of Medical Sciences. This group later considered priorities for research grants awarded by the American Dental Association.

CHARGE TO THE COMMITTEE

The charge to the Committee on the Future of Dental Education, as revised by the committee, is as follows. The IOM committee will assess dental education in the United States and make recommendations regarding its future. It will

• examine the current status of dental education and oral health in the United States and consider future scientific, demographic, economic, organizational, and other developments that may affect oral health status and the system for educating dentists and other dental personnel;
• develop a statement of how, over the next 25 years, oral health and oral health services should be improved in the United States, and identify the short-term and long-term implications of this statement for dental education and public policy;
• describe strategies that will help dental education, research, and practice improve oral health by responding effectively to current problems and future developments in both science and society; and

• consider ways in which each dental school can better relate to the mission of its university and to the community at large.

COMMITTEE APPROACH

The committee engaged in a very broad-ranging effort to collect information and perspectives on dental education in the context of the broader systems of health professions education and health care delivery. Members made site visits to 11 of the 54 U.S. dental schools and in the process visited with approximately 600 faculty, students, administrators, alumni, and dental society leaders. (The committee chair and the study director participated in every site visit.) The committee also undertook a mail survey of all deans of dental schools (in cooperation with the American Association of Dental Schools) and a telephone survey of two dozen university presidents, chancellors, and other senior officials. A public hearing in September 1993 generated oral testimony from 25 groups and written testimony from nearly 30 more (out of more than 80 groups invited). In addition, the committee established and met with three liaison panels representing regional dental society leadership, specialty societies, and dental school faculty.

Members of the committee met with leaders of major dental organizations including the American Association for Dental Research, the American Association of Dental Schools, the American College of Dentists, the American Dental Association, the American Dental Assistants' Association, and the American Dental Hygienists' Association. Committee members and staff also discussed the project at annual meetings and other sessions organized by a number of dental groups.

To inform its analyses and provide additional background for this report, the committee commissioned seven papers that are being published separately by the *Journal of Dental Education*. In addition, committee and staff reviewed a wide variety of published and unpublished literature on topics related to the committee's charge. The committee also consulted the literature on medical education and sometimes cites it as a reference point but not necessarily a standard or ideal. The committee report was reviewed under the procedures of the National Research Council. This document constitutes the committee's final statement.

Acknowledgments

Many individuals and groups assisted the study committee and staff in the development of this report. Initial direction for this project was provided by a planning committee that met in June 1990. That meeting was chaired by John C. Greene, and the participants were Howard Bailit; Ben Barker; James Beck; Jack Brown; Teresa Dolan; Chester Douglass; Robert Ferris; Allan Formicola; James Gaines; Robert Genco; Robert Gerlach; Jay Gershen; Joel Glover; Albert Guay; Robert Heaney; Garland Hershey, Jr.; George Keller; Linda Kraemer; Warren Lesmeister; James Lipton; Preston Littleton; Kent Nash; Howard Oaks; Richard Ranney; Paul Schwab; Jeanne Sinkford; Paul Van Ostenberg; Neal Vanselow; and Richard Weaver. Many of those involved in this meeting continued to play a role in the study either as committee members or as sources of advice and information. Michael Millman, who was senior staff officer for the study before leaving for the Department of Health and Human Services, developed the project proposal and fund-raising strategy over a 2-year period. He left a valuable legacy to the committee and staff who came later. Karl Yordy, who was director of the Division of Health Care Services from the point at which this study was first discussed through September 1993, continued to take an active role in the study even after his departure from Washington, D.C. Samuel Thier, former president of the Institute, took a particular interest in launching this project.

The members of three liaison panels that met with committee members are listed in Appendix A. Members of these panels also assisted by reviewing background materials developed by the committee and by answering a variety of questions. Appendix B lists the organizations that prepared written testimony for the committee's public meeting in the fall of 1993.

The committee commissioned seven papers that provided useful background and insights for this report, as did two other papers drafted by committee members. These papers, which are being published in the January 1995 issue of the *Journal of Dental Education*, are listed with their authors in Appendix C. In addition to preparing background papers, James Bader, Eli Capilouto, William Clark, Lisa Tedesco, and Alex White contributed more generally to the study through their ideas and comments. During one of the committee meetings, Eli and Mary Lynne Capilouto also participated in a panel discussion of dental work force issues that also included James Bader, Gloria Bronstein, Norman Clark, Steven Eklund, Kent Nash, and Eric Solomon. Joseph Consani and Lindsay Hunt helped in sorting out the complexities of dental school financing by meeting with the committee and reviewing background materials.

The American Association of Dental Schools (AADS) and the American Dental Association (ADA) have been unfailingly helpful in providing information, answering our many questions, and giving us the opportunity to discuss the report during their annual meetings and board meetings and at other sessions. At the AADS, we particularly appreciate the assistance of Thomas Freeland, Carolyn Gray, Martha Liggett, and Preston Littleton. Without their help, the survey of dental school deans would not have been feasible. Of course, without the constructive responses received from all 54 deans, the survey also would not have been useful. Linda DeVore and Arthur Dugoni, while each was president of the AADS, also supported the committee's work in a variety of ways. The ADA provided extensive assistance including a wealth of statistical information on dental education, licensure, accreditation, and practice as well as help in sorting out the limits of the information's use. The committee particularly appreciates the perspectives and information provided by Thomas Berger, Tommi Cole, Clifford Miller, and John Zapp and by ADA Presidents James Gaines and Jack Harris.

The AADS also contributed to the American Fund for Dental Health, which helped fund this study; other major contributors to the Fund were Colgate-Palmolive and Warner-Lambert.

The committee and staff also met with representatives of the American Association for Dental Research (John Clarkson and Harold Slavkin), the American College of Dentists (Juliann Bluitt and Sherry Keramidas), the American Dental Assistants' Association (Judith Andrews and Kathy Zweig), the American Dental Hygienists' Association (Kathleen Alvarez, Gail Bemis, Elizabeth Brutvan, and Sarah Turner) to discuss issues of concern to the organizations and their members. John Clarkson, Jane Kendall, Karen Sealander, and Kathy Zweig also answered questions and provided information to the committee on a number of issues. In addition, staff and members of the American Board of Dental Examiners, American College of Dentists, American Academy of Oral Pathology, American Academy of Pediatric Dentistry, American Academy of Periodontology, American Association of Endodontists, American Association of Oral and Maxillofacial Surgeons, American Association of Orthodontists, American Board of Dental Public Health, American College of Prosthodontists, and the Academy of General Dentistry patiently answered our questions.

Many staff of the National Institute of Dental Research helped the committee in a variety of ways. James Corrigan, the project officer for this study, was an invaluable resource. Harold Löe and Dushanka Kleinman met with the committee to discuss research issues and directions and were supportive throughout the project. At the Department of Defense, Robert Augsburger, the project officer, helped answer a number of questions about dental issues for the military.

Although we agreed not to identify them individually, the chancellors and other senior officials of over 22 universities and academic health centers took time from their busy schedules to participate in telephone interviews or personal interviews with committee members and staff. Others provided time during the committee's site visits to 11 dental schools. The deans, faculty, and administrative staff at each of these schools made every effort to broaden and deepen our understanding of dental education and its environment, as evidenced by the meetings they arranged with some 800 people including students, faculty from inside and outside the dental schools, community practitioners, dental society leaders, and alumni. The committee particularly acknowledges the substantial effort required to arrange the site visits and thanks: Allen Formicola and Zoila Noguerole at Columbia University; Robert Knight and Ethel Newman at Howard University; Edward Kaufman and Joan Pano at New York University; Michael Heurer at Northwestern University; Arthur Dugoni and Edward Hayashida at the

University of the Pacific; Henry Cherrick, Jay Gershen, and Christy Kemp at the University of California, Los Angeles; Allen Anderson and Michael Valadez at the University of Illinois at Chicago; John Stamm at the University of North Carolina; John Greene and Anne Buchanan at the University of California at San Francisco; Howard Landesman and Janice Balin at the University of Southern California; and Kenneth Kalkwarf and Karen Fuller at the University of Texas at San Antonio. (In addition, the study director, whose dental emergency provided an unplanned opportunity to learn about an advanced general dentistry clinic, thanks John Greene, Terry Chin, and Ed Hayashida for their advice and assistance.)

Among the many others who contributed substantively to the committee's understanding of dental education and its environment were Brownell Anderson, Roger Bulger, Charles Cartwright, Kenneth Chance, Skip Collins, Stephen Corbin, Dominick De Paola, David Denton, Linda DeVore, Arthur Dugoni, Patrick Ferillo, Jay Gershen, James Kennedy, Sherry Keramidas, Rowland Hutchinson, Peter Lockhardt, Lawrence Meskin, Linda Niessen, David Nash, Spencer Redding, Henry Sazima, Aidan Stephens, and Barry Wogelman.

At the University of Texas Health Science Center at San Antonio, Sylvia Cantu helped coordinate work with the committee chairman. Frances Poillon was our most helpful copy editor, and Sally Stanfield at the National Academy Press was supportive, as always. Nina Spruill helped us keep our somewhat complicated financial accounts straight, and Claudia Carl managed the logistics of an extensive report review process. Although she participated in all aspects of the study, Lisa Chimento made particular contributions in literature review, data collection and analysis, and planning and analysis of the public meeting and site visits. During the final stages of report preparation, Helen Rogers provided assistance with references and fact checking, especially in the regulatory area. With her superb computer and logistical skills and unflappable good humor, Donna Thompson handled smoothly the preparation of the committee report, the revising of the commissioned papers, and the arrangements for an extensive array of meetings and other activities. The committee also benefited from the work of other committees and staff of the Institute of Medicine or the National Research Council that produced the reports noted in the reference list, in particular, the reports on national needs for biomedical and behavioral science researchers, careers in clinical research, and racial and ethnic diversity in the health professions.

Contents

TABLES AND FIGURES

TABLES

FIGURES

DENTAL
EDUCATION
AT THE
CROSSROADS

Summary

Dental education has arrived at a crossroads. During the last 150 years, it has evolved from a short prelude to apprenticeship into a comprehensive program of professional education. Advances in science, technology, and public health have greatly reduced tooth decay and tooth loss. In addition, dentists are now respected professionals, and dental schools are part of many of the nation's leading public and private universities.

This progress notwithstanding, questions persist about the position of dental education within the university and its relationship to medicine and the overall health care system. The dental profession is at odds with itself on a number of matters including work force policies, licensure, and health care restructuring. These and other issues create tensions between practitioners and educators that can undercut the profession's position within the university. Six dental schools—all private—have closed in the last decade, and enrollment reductions over the last decade and a half are equivalent to the closure of another 20 average-sized dental schools. Of the 54 remaining dental schools, several are vulnerable to closure.

The future of dental education will be shaped by scientific, technological, political, and economic factors that are in part beyond the profession's control. Nonetheless, dental educators—individually and collectively—have important choices to make.

They may attempt to preserve the status quo—in effect, a path toward stagnation and eventual decline. Alternatively, they could follow a more difficult path of reassessing and renewing their missions of education, research, and patient care so that they could contribute more—and more visibly—to the university and the community. Taking this latter path would require new vigor in implementing longstanding recommendations for educational reform as well as attention to new issues and objectives. For dental educators to pursue change successfully, they will need the active cooperation of the larger dental community as well as support from university officials and state, local, and national policymakers.

This Institute of Medicine (IOM) study was prompted by concerns that the challenges confronting dental education, although generally recognized, were not adequately understood or appreciated and that effective responses had yet to be identified or persuasively presented. The purpose of the study was "to assess dental education in the United States and make recommendations regarding its future." The study was overseen by an 18-member committee that was appointed after extensive consultation with dental and related organizations. The group included members with expertise and experience in dental practice and education, oral health and health services research, other areas of the health professions and higher education, health care delivery and financing, and public policy. The committee undertook a wide range of information-collecting activities including 11 site visits, 3 liaison panels, a public hearing, and meetings with leaders of many dental organizations. Eight background papers developed to assist the committee will be published separately in the January 1995 issue of the *Journal of Dental Education*. The committee's report was submitted for outside review in accordance with IOM and National Research Council procedures and policies.

In concluding its work, the committee proposed that the IOM convene a conference or workshop to bring interested parties together, within a year after this report's publication, to assess the report's initial impact. The agenda would include responses from relevant organizations, discussion of initial individual or collective steps to implement recommendations, and suggestions about follow-up strategies. If the spirit of cooperation among dental leaders that led to this study persists, that gathering should find that this study has begun to make a constructive contribution to the health of the profession and the public.

ENVISIONING THE FUTURE

To move successfully into a new century, dental educators and the larger dental community need greater agreement on common purposes and directions for the field. Formulating such agreement requires, in turn, an understanding of how well current modes of thought and operation equip dental education and dentistry in general to face a future that will be quite different from the past. Building understanding and agreement was the major objective of this report.

The IOM committee adopted a set of eight policy and strategic principles (Table 1) that it combined with an extensive analysis of dental education's present and future to form a broad picture of dental education in the twenty-first century. This picture is not a vision of an ideal world. Rather, it offers a distilled view of what the future will likely bring combined with the committee's conclusions about how dental educators and others can reasonably, if not easily, prepare the profession to play a constructive role in improving oral health for all Americans in the years ahead.

In the future envisioned in this report, five elements stand out. *First*, dentistry will and should become more closely integrated with medicine and the health care system on all levels: educa-

TABLE 1 Policy and Strategic Principles

1. Oral health is an integral part of total health, and oral health care is an integral part of comprehensive health care, including primary care.

2. The long-standing commitment of dentists and dental hygienists to prevention and primary care should remain vigorous.

3. A focus on health outcomes is essential for dental professionals and dental schools.

4. Dental education must be scientifically based and undertaken in an environment in which the creation and acquisition of new scientific and clinical knowledge are valued and actively pursued.

5. Learning is a lifelong enterprise for dental professionals that cannot stop with the awarding of a degree or the completion of a residency program.

6. A qualified dental work force is a valuable national resource, and support for the education of this work force must continue to come from both public and private sources.

7. In recruiting students and faculty, designing and implementing the curriculum, conducting research, and providing clinical services, dental schools have a responsibility to serve all Americans, not just those who are economically advantaged and relatively healthy.

8. Efforts to reduce the wide disparities in oral health status and access to care should be a high priority for policymakers, practitioners, and educators.

tion, research, and patient care. The march of science and technology in fields such as molecular biology, immunology, and genetics will continue to forge links between dentistry and medicine, as will the needs of an aging population with more complex health problems. The financial strains on universities and academic health centers will likewise encourage consolidation and coordination. Pressures from government and private purchasers of health services will maintain the movement toward integrated systems of care that stress cost containment, primary care, and services provided by teams of professional and allied personnel.

Second, to prepare their students and their schools for change, dental educators will need to teach and display desirable models of clinical practice. Using excellent practice in the community as a model, dental school clinics should seek to be more patient-friendly and efficient and to provide students with a greater volume and breadth of clinical experience. All dental graduates should have the opportunity for a year of postgraduate education with an emphasis on advanced education in general dentistry.

Third, securing the resources essential for educational improvement and, indeed, survival will require that dental schools demonstrate their contributions to their parent universities, academic health centers, and communities. These contributions include achievements not only in education but also in research, technology transfer, and community and patient service. Said differently, dentistry cannot afford isolation.

Fourth, dental leaders should cooperate to reform accreditation and licensing practices so that they support rather than obstruct the profession's evolution. Priorities include greater uniformity in licensing, reduced legal barriers to professional mobility, and revision of laws that limit dentists from working more productively with allied dental personnel. A uniform national clinical examination should be developed for acceptance by all states. Voluntary accreditation should focus on dental schools with significant deficiencies and reduce administrative burdens on other schools.

Fifth, continued testing of alternative models of education, practice, and performance assessment for dentists and allied dental professionals is necessary to prepare the dental community—educators, practitioners, regulators, and policymakers—for an uncertain future. In particular, experimentation and learning will help dentistry face one major uncertainty, namely, whether the future supply of dental practitioners and services will match, exceed, or fall below population requirements for dental care. The committee found no compelling evidence to predict with confidence a future under- or oversupply of dental services. Trends in supply and demand should, however, be monitored. Contingency planning is stressful—but essential—given the unpredictable nature of key developments in science, technology, social policy, and other areas. If a shortage in dental services should develop, responses should emphasize more productive use of allied dental personnel, continued elimination of ineffective or inefficient services, and, only if these steps prove inadequate, increased dental school enrollments.

Environmental change and dental education's efforts to respond constructively may exacerbate tensions with dental practitioners, for example, as dental schools experiment with new models of patient care and extend their outcomes research agenda. Thus, efforts to manage and resolve conflicts must also have a high priority. Still, compared to other health professions, dentistry may experience a less rapid restructuring of its place in health care, but any such respite should be used not as a time to reinforce resistance to change but as an opportunity to achieve a smoother transition for patients, practitioners, and educators.

FINDINGS AND RECOMMENDATIONS

In developing specific recommendations, the committee attempted to be both principled and pragmatic. That is, it tried to be neither so idealistic that its recommendations would be of little use to real-world decisionmakers nor so fixated on the practical difficulties of change that it would provide no direction, motivation, or benchmarks to help decisionmakers move through difficulties toward desired goals. The committee's recommendations individually or collectively may strike some as weighted toward the idealistic and others as weighted toward the status quo. If, however, a 10- to 20-year horizon is accepted as necessary and reasonable for the more demanding recommendations, then the possible and the ideal draw closer together. The recommendations are not a specific blueprint for the future of dental education. Such a blueprint would not fit the particular circumstances and needs of individual dental schools.

ORAL HEALTH STATUS AND SERVICES

The committee emphasized four broad objectives for the effective use of health resources to advance the nation's oral health. These objectives are to:

1. *improve our knowledge of what works and what does not work* to prevent or treat oral health problems;

2. *reduce disparities* in oral health status and services experienced by disadvantaged economic, racial, and other groups;

3. *encourage prevention* at both the *individual level* (e.g., feeding practices that prevent baby bottle tooth decay, reduced use of tobacco) and the *community level* (e.g., fluoridation of community water supplies and school-based prevention programs); and

4. *promote attention to oral health* (including the oral manifestations of other health problems) not just among dental practitioners but also *among primary care providers, geriatricians, educators, and public officials.*

Dental education can play a central role in each of these areas. In particular, dental educators should be involved in basic science, clinical, and health services research to distinguish effective and ineffective oral health services, to clarify oral disease patterns and trends and the factors affecting them, and to develop cost-effective strategies likely to help those with the poorest health status and those with limited access to oral health services. In their outreach activities, dental educators and practitioners should continue to encourage physicians, nursing home personnel, public officials, and others to be alert to oral health problems among those they serve and to provide information about good oral health habits.

Public support is critical if disparities in health status and access to oral health services are to be reduced. This committee therefore recommends that all parts of the dental community work together to secure more adequate public and private funding for personal dental services, public health and prevention programs, and community outreach activities, including those undertaken by dental school students and faculty.

The Mission of Education

The problem in reforming dental education is not so much achieving consensus on directions for change but difficulty in overcoming obstacles to change. Agreement on educational problems is widespread. The curriculum is crowded with redundant or marginally useful material and gives students too little time to consolidate concepts or to develop critical thinking skills. Comprehensive care is more an ideal than a reality in clinical education, and instruction still focuses too heavily on procedures rather than on patient care. Linkages between dentistry and medicine are insufficient to prepare students for a growing volume of patients with more medically complex problems and an increase in medically oriented strategies for prevention, diagnosis, and treatment. The basic and clinical sciences do not adequately relate the scientific basis of oral health to clinical practice. Lack of flexible tenure and promotion policies and of resources for faculty development limits efforts to match faculty resources to educational needs. Despite progress, an insensitivity to students' needs is still a concern.

In the hope of stimulating movement toward generally held goals, the committee proposes that each dental school develop a plan and timetable for curriculum reform. It urges closer integration of dental and medical education and more experimentation with new formats for such integration.

THE MISSION OF RESEARCH

Research is a fundamental mission of dental education, but too many dental schools and dental faculty are minimally involved in research and scholarship. A commitment to research in dental schools is important because research builds a knowledge base for improving the effectiveness and efficiency of oral health services; enriches the educational experience for students; reinforces the school's role as a disseminator of validated practice advice to dental practitioners; and strengthens the stature of dentistry within the university and the broader community.

The committee recognizes the problems facing schools that are trying to build or maintain a strong research program. These are, most notably, limited funding and a dearth of capable researchers. Expanding the oral health research work force is an important priority.

Dental schools will differ in how they define the specifics of their research priorities, but all schools need to formulate a program of faculty research and scholarly activity that meets or exceeds the expectations of their universities. To build research capacity and resources, as well as to foster relationships with other researchers, it is important for dental schools to pursue collaborative research opportunities that start with the academic health center or the university and extend to industry, government, dental societies, and other institutions able to support or assist basic science, clinical, and health services research. Throughout this report, the committee has tried to point out opportunities for dental school faculty to participate in clinical, behavioral, and health services research that will support the missions of education and patient care and will help improve voluntary and governmental oversight of the profession.

THE MISSION OF PATIENT CARE

The typical dental clinic, put simply, is not patient centered. A procedure-oriented model of care must give way to a model that is patient and community oriented, focused on outcomes, scientifically and technologically up to date, team based, and efficient.

Current trends in health care delivery and financing are requiring academic health centers to compete for patients and for inclusion in managed care plans of various sorts. Whether the patient care activities of the dental school add to or subtract from the overall institution's market position is likely to be an issue in its future. Over the long term, the committee believes that dental schools have no ethical or practical alternative but to make their programs more attentive to patients as well as more economically viable and to develop the programs and the data needed to document and assess the quality and efficiency of care. They will have to ensure that their activities and objectives are compatible with those of their parent institutions.

THE DENTAL SCHOOL IN THE UNIVERSITY

To fulfill their missions of education, research, and patient care, dental schools need the intellectual vitality, support, and discipline of universities and academic health centers. In return, dental educators must contribute to university life, especially through research, scholarship, and efficient management of educational and patient care programs.

Overall, the world of higher education is likely to become less stable and thus more unpredictable and stressful for its constituent parts. Universities and government policymakers will continue to reevaluate their programs—adding, deleting, and restructuring them. The closure of several dental schools has made the vulnerability of their relationship to the university clear. Reducing the factors that put dental schools at risk in the university is not an overnight task, and some factors are less subject to a school's influence than others. This makes it all the more important that each school assess its own position and develop a specific plan for analyzing and reinforcing that position within the university.

Although education at all levels faces financial constraints ranging in severity from routine to critical, dental education faces particular challenges given its relatively high costs and specialized needs. For most schools, financial health will not be achieved through a single grand solution. Rather, some combination of more modest and difficult steps will be necessary. Schools will need to develop better cost and revenue data if they are to design steps that match their particular problems and characteristics and minimize potential harm to their educational, research, and patient care missions.

ACCREDITATION AND LICENSURE

Accreditation and licensure are components of a broad social strategy to ensure the quality of dental care by protecting the public from poorly trained, incompetent, or unethical dental practitioners. They also account for much of the tension between dental schools and the profession. The dental community has taken important actions to improve licensure and accreditation processes, but further work is needed.

The accreditation process remains too focused on process and too inhospitable to educational innovation. The committee believes that the process tolerates some inferior educational programs, although data to document this are not publicly accessible. Accreditation reform should focus on dental schools with significant deficiencies and reduce the administrative burden on other schools. Improved methods of assessing educational outcomes are as central to achieving accreditation reform as they are to improving predoctoral education, entry-level licensure, and assessment of continued competency. Thus, cooperation and coordination among responsible organizations in each of these arenas should be established to avoid conflicting strategies and costly duplication of effort.

The major deficiencies of dental licensure are concentrated in a few areas: the use of live patients in clinical licensure examinations; variations in the content and relevance of clinical examinations; unreasonable barriers to the movement of dentists and dental hygienists across state lines; practice acts that unreasonably restrict the use of appropriately trained allied dental personnel; and inadequate means of assessing competency after initial licensure. The committee concluded that it is neither practical nor necessary to construct new national systems for licensure and accreditation. A uniform national clinical examination (one that does not include real patients) should, however, be developed for acceptance by each state.

THE DENTAL WORK FORCE

The dental community is characterized by much anxiety and disagreement about whether the nation faces a future shortage or oversupply of dental services. The committee found no compelling evidence that would allow it to predict either outcome with sufficient confidence to warrant recommendations that dental school enrollments be increased or decreased. On the one hand, the ratio of dentists to the general population is declining, and the coverage of dental services under expanded public or private health insurance could substantially increase the demand for such services, especially if additional efforts are made to reach people with significant unmet needs. On the other hand, scientific and technological developments could increase or reduce overall need and demand for dental services depending on whether they promoted prevention or expensive treatments. In addition, the current dental work force appears to have reserve capacity that could be mobilized through better use of allied dental personnel, improved identification and elimination of care with little or no demonstrated health benefit, and more efficient delivery systems.

In the face of uncertainty, the committee believes it is prudent to continue monitoring trends in the supply of dental personnel and developing a better understanding of their productivity, of the appropriateness of dental services, and of the factors that impede access to dental care. This course will require a more sustained investment in a comprehensive oral health data infrastructure than has been evident over the last decade.

Two persistent work force problems involve (1) parts of the country in which dental services are in short supply and (2) minority representation in the future. The National Health Service Corps (NHSC) and other federal or state programs link the provision of financial assistance to a commitment to practice in an underserved area for a specific period, and thus help both to overcome service shortages and the serious problem of high student debt. The shrinkage in dental positions in the NHSC should be reversed. Efforts to increase the cultural and ethnic representativeness of the dental work force encounter a limited pool of candidates for admission, stiff competition from other professional schools for those candidates, and disproportionate attrition among minority predoctoral students. Building a dental work force that reflects the nation's diversity will require broad-based efforts to reduce attrition and to enlarge the pool of candidates for admission through information, counseling, and financial aid programs; improved precollegiate education in science and mathematics; and other supportive arrangements for precollegiate and collegiate students.

The committee's individual recommendations are listed below. The list generally follows the order in which the items appear in the report; they are not listed in order of priority. The recommendations underscore that the future of dental education is necessarily linked to its contributions to improving the effectiveness and efficiency of oral health services through education, research, and patient care. It must not only contribute but also be perceived as contributing—by the dental profession, the university, and society generally. For dental education to meet the challenges that lie ahead will require the support and involvement of the practitioner community as well as researchers and policymakers. The intent of this report is to provide guidance for each of these important groups.

RECOMMENDATION 1

To support effective and efficient oral health services that improve individual and community health, the committee recommends that dental educators work with public and private organizations to

- **maintain a standardized process in the U.S. Department of Health and Human Services to regularly assess the oral health status of the population and identify changing disease patterns at the community and national levels;**
- **develop and implement a systematic research agenda to evaluate the outcomes of alternative methods of preventing, diagnosing, and treating oral health problems; and**
- **make use of scientific evidence, outcomes research, and formal consensus processes in devising practice guidelines.**

RECOMMENDATION 2

To increase access to care and improve the oral health status of underserved populations, dental educators, practitioners, researchers, and public health officials should work together to

- **secure more adequate public and private funding for per-**

sonal dental services, public health and prevention programs, and community outreach activities, including those undertaken by dental school students and faculty, and

• address the special needs of underserved populations through health services research, curriculum content, and patient services, including more productive use of allied dental personnel.

RECOMMENDATION 3

To improve the availability of dental care in underserved areas and to limit the negative effects of high student debt, Congress and the states should act to increase the number of dentists serving in the National Health Service Corps and other federal or state programs that link financial assistance to work in underserved areas.

RECOMMENDATION 4

To stimulate progress toward curriculum goals long endorsed in dental education, the committee recommends that dental schools set explicit targets, procedures, and timetables for modernizing courses, eliminating marginally useful and redundant course content, and reducing excessive course loads. The process should include steps to

• design an integrated basic and clinical science curriculum that provides clinically relevant education in the basic sciences and scientifically based education in clinical care;

• incorporate in all educational activities a focus on outcomes and an emphasis on the relevance of scientific knowledge and thinking to clinical choices;

• shift more curriculum hours from lectures to guided seminars and other active learning strategies that develop critical thinking and problem-solving skills;

• identify and decrease the hours spent in low priority preclinical technique, laboratory work, and lectures; and

• complement clinic hours with scheduled time for discussion of specific diagnosis, planning, and treatment-completion issues that arise in clinic sessions.

RECOMMENDATION 5

To prepare future practitioners for more medically based modes of oral health care and more medically complicated patients, dental educators should work with their colleagues in medical schools and academic health centers to

• move toward integrated basic science education for dental and medical students;

• require and provide for dental students at least one rotation, clerkship, or equivalent experience in relevant areas of medicine, and offer opportunities for additional elective experience in hospitals, nursing homes, ambulatory care clinics, and other settings;

• continue and expand experiments with combined M.D.-D.D.S. programs and similar programs for interested students and residents; and

• increase the experience of dental faculty in clinical medicine so that they—and not just physicians—can impart medical knowledge to dental students and serve as role models for them.

RECOMMENDATION 6

To prepare students and faculty for an environment that will demand increasing efficiency, accountability, and evidence of effectiveness, the committee recommends that dental students and faculty participate in efficiently managed clinics and faculty practices in which

• patient-centered, comprehensive care is the norm;

• patients' preferences and their social, economic, and emotional circumstances are sensitively considered;

• teamwork and cost-effective use of well-trained allied dental personnel are stressed;

• evaluations of practice patterns and of the outcomes of care guide actions to improve both the quality and the efficiency of such care;

• general dentists serve as role models in the appropriate treatment and referral of patients needing advanced therapies; and

• larger numbers of patients, including those with more diverse characteristics and clinical problems, are served.

RECOMMENDATION 7

The committee recommends that postdoctoral education in a general dentistry or specialty program be available for every dental graduate, that the goal be to achieve this within five to ten years, and that the emphasis be on creating new positions in advanced general dentistry and discouraging additional specialty residencies unless warranted by shortages of services that cannot be provided effectively by other personnel.

RECOMMENDATION 8

To permit faculty hiring and promotion practices that better reflect educational objectives and changing needs, the committee recommends that dental schools and their universities supplement tenure-track positions with other full-time nontenured clinical or research positions that provide greater flexibility in achieving teaching, research, and patient care objectives.

RECOMMENDATION 9

To expand oral health knowledge and to affirm the importance of research and scholarship, each dental school should

• support a research program that includes clinical research, evaluation and dissemination of new scientific and clinical findings, and research on outcomes, health services, and behavior related to oral health;

• extend its research program, when feasible, to the basic sciences and to the transformation of new scientific knowledge into clinically useful applications;

• meet or exceed the standard for research and scholarship expected by its parent university or academic health center;

• expect all faculty to be critically knowledgeable about scientific advances in their fields and to stay current in their teaching and practice; and

• encourage all faculty to participate in research and scholarship.

RECOMMENDATION 10

To build research capacity and resources, as well as foster relationships with other researchers, all dental schools should develop and pursue collaborative research strategies that start with the academic health center or the university and extend to industry, government, dental societies, and other institutions able to support or assist basic science, clinical, or health services research.

RECOMMENDATION 11

To strengthen the research capacity of dental schools and faculty, the committee recommends that the National Institute of Dental Research

• continue to evaluate and improve its extramural training and development programs;
• focus more resources on those extramural programs with greater demonstrated productivity in strengthening the oral health research capacity of dental schools and faculties; and
• preserve some funding for short-term training programs intended primarily to increase research understanding and appreciation among clinical teaching faculty and future practitioners.

RECOMMENDATION 12

To affirm that patient care is a distinct mission, each dental school should support a strategic planning process to

• develop objectives for patient-centered care in areas such as appointment scheduling, completeness and timeliness of treatment, and definition of faculty and student responsibilities;
• identify current deficiencies in patient care processes and outcomes, along with physical, financial, legal, and other barriers to their correction; and
• design specific actions—including demonstration projects or experiments—to improve the quality, efficiency, and attractiveness of its patient services.

RECOMMENDATION 13

To ensure that dental education and services are considered when academic institutions evaluate their role in a changing health care system, the committee recommends that dental schools coordinate their strategic planning processes with those of their academic health centers and universities.

RECOMMENDATION 14

To respond to changes in roles and expectations for providers of outpatient health services including dental school clinics, the Commission on Dental Accreditation and the American Association of Dental Schools should

• reexamine processes for assessing patient care activities in dental schools and ensuring the quality of care, and
• begin to evaluate new options such as eventual participation by dental schools in separate accreditation programs for their ambulatory care facilities.

RECOMMENDATION 15

To consolidate and strengthen the mutual benefits arising from the relationship between universities and dental schools, each dental school should work with its parent institution to

• prepare an explicit analysis of its position within the university and the academic health center;
• evaluate its assets and deficits in key areas including financing, teaching, university service and visibility, research and scholarly productivity, patient and community services, and internal management of change; and
• identify specific objectives, actions, procedures, and timetables to sustain its strengths and correct its weaknesses.

RECOMMENDATION 16

To provide a sound basis for financial management and policy decisions, each dental school should develop accurate cost and revenue data for its educational, research, and patient care programs.

RECOMMENDATION 17

Because no single financing strategy exists, the committee recommends that dental schools individually and, when appropriate, collectively evaluate and implement a mix of actions to reduce costs and increase revenues. Potential strategies, each of which needs to be guided by solid financial information and projections as well as educational and other considerations, include the following:

- increasing the productivity, quality, efficiency, and profitability of faculty practice plans, student clinics, and other patient care activities;
- pursuing financial support at the federal, state, and local levels for patient-centered predoctoral and postdoctoral dental education, including adequate reimbursement of services for Medicaid and indigent populations and contractual or other arrangements for states without dental schools to support the education of some of their students in states with dental schools;
- rethinking basic models of dental education and experimenting with less costly alternatives;
- raising tuition for in- or out-of-state students if current tuition and fees are low compared to similar schools;
- developing high quality, competitive research and continuing education programs; and
- consolidating or merging courses, departments, programs, and even entire schools.

RECOMMENDATION 18

To protect students and the public from inferior educational programs and to reduce administrative burdens and costs, the committee recommends that the Commission on Dental Accreditation involve concerned constituencies in a sustained effort to

- expand the resources and assistance devoted to schools with significant deficiencies, and decrease the burden imposed on schools that meet or exceed standards;
- increase the emphasis on educational outcomes rather than on detailed procedural requirements; and
- develop more valid and consistent methods for assess-

ing clinical performance for purposes of student evaluation, licensure, and accreditation.

RECOMMENDATION 19

To improve the current system of state regulation of dental professionals, the committee recommends that the American Association of Dental Examiners, American Association of Dental Schools, professional associations, state and regions boards, and specialty organizations work closely and intensively to

• develop valid, reliable, and uniform clinical examinations and secure acceptance of the examinations by all state licensing boards as replacements for state or regional clinical examinations and as complements to current National Dental Board Examinations;

• accelerate steps to eliminate examinations using live patients and replace them with other assessment methods, such as the use of "standardized patients" for evaluating diagnosis and treatment planning skills and simulations for evaluating technical proficiency;

• strengthen and extend efforts by state boards and specialty organizations to maintain and periodically evaluate the competency of dentists and dental hygienists through recertification and other methods;

• remove barriers to the movement of dental personnel among states by developing uniform criteria for state licensure except in areas where variation is legitimate (e.g., dental jurisprudence); and

• eliminate statutes and regulations that restrict dentists from working with allied dental personnel in ways that are productive and consistent with their education and training.

RECOMMENDATION 20

Because the prospects for a future oversupply or undersupply of dental personnel are uncertain and subject to unpredictable scientific, public policy, or other developments, the committee recommends that public and private agencies

• avoid policies to increase or decrease overall dental school enrollments; and

• maintain and strengthen programs to forecast and monitor trends in the supply of dental personnel and to analyze information on factors affecting the need and demand for oral health care.

RECOMMENDATION 21

To respond to any future shortage of dental services and to improve the effectiveness, efficiency, and availability of dental care generally, educators and policymakers should

• continue efforts to increase the productivity of the dental work force, including appropriately credentialed and trained allied dental personnel;
• support research to identify and eliminate unnecessary or inappropriate dental services; and
• exercise restraint in increasing dental school enrollments unless other, less costly, strategies fail to meet demands for oral health care.

RECOMMENDATION 22

To build a dental work force that reflects the nation's diversity, dental schools should initiate or participate in efforts to expand the recruitment of underrepresented minority students, faculty and staff, including

• broad-based efforts to enlarge the pool of candidates through information, counseling, financial aid, and other supportive programs for precollegiate, collegiate, predoctoral, and advanced students and
• national and community programs to improve precollegiate education in science and mathematics, especially for underrepresented minorities.

1

Background and Introduction

Dental education has arrived at a crossroads. During the last 150 years, it has evolved from a prelude to apprenticeship into a comprehensive program of professional education. Advances in science, technology, and public health programs have greatly reduced tooth decay and tooth loss. Dentists are respected professionals, and dental schools are part of many of the nation's leading public and private universities.

This progress notwithstanding, the position of dental education within the university is being questioned as is its relationship to medicine and the larger health care system. Six dental schools—all private—have closed in the last decade (Table 1.1), and others among the 54 remaining schools are in jeopardy. The dental profession is at odds with itself on a number of issues including work force policies, licensure, and health care restructuring. Tensions between practitioners and educators can undercut the profession's position within the university.

The future of dental education will be shaped, in part, by scientific, technological, political, and economic factors that are largely beyond the profession's control. Nonetheless, dental educators—individually and collectively—have important choices to make. They may attempt to preserve the status quo—in effect, a path toward stagnation and eventual decline. Alternatively, they can choose a more difficult path of reassessing and renewing their missions of education, research, and patient care so that they

TABLE 1.1   Number of U.S. Dental Schools, 1970-1993

Dental Schools	1970	1975	1985	1993
Public	28	35	35	35
Private	25	24	25	19

NOTE: The universities that have closed dental schools since 1985 are Oral Roberts University, Tulsa, Oklahoma (1986); Emory University, Atlanta, Georgia (1988); Georgetown University, Washington, D.C. (1990); Fairleigh Dickinson University, Rutherford, New Jersey (1990); Washington University, St. Louis, Missouri (1991); and Loyola University, Chicago, Illinois (1993).

SOURCE: American Association of Dental Schools.

contribute more—and more visibly—to the university and the community. Taking this latter path will require more vigor in implementing long-standing recommendations for educational reform as well as attention to new issues and objectives. For dental educators to pursue change successfully, they will need the active cooperation of the larger dental community as well as support from university officials and state and national policymakers.

This Institute of Medicine (IOM) study was prompted by concerns that the challenges confronting dental education, although generally recognized, were not understood or appreciated adequately and that effective responses had yet to be identified or presented in a persuasive manner. The purpose of the study was "to assess dental education in the United States and make recommendations regarding its future." It was overseen by an 18-member committee that was appointed after extensive consultation with dental and related organizations. The group included members with expertise and experience in dental practice and education, oral health and health services research, other areas of health professions and higher education, health care delivery and financing, and public policy. The committee as a whole met six times between February 1993 and May 1994. As described in the Preface and summarized in Appendix 1.A, it undertook a wide range of activities to collect information and perspectives from all segments of the dental community and other relevant, interested groups. (The papers commissioned by the committee will be published in the *Journal of Dental Education*; they are listed in Appendix C.) This document, which was submitted for outside review in accordance with

IOM and National Research Council procedures and policies,* constitutes the committee's final report.

DENTAL EDUCATION IN CONTEXT

THE BROADER ENVIRONMENT

The achievements of dental education and its current problems must be set against a larger societal backdrop. For the United States through most of this and the last century, that backdrop was generally one of growth and innovation. The nation's economy expanded and became vastly more complex. Scientific and technological development proceeded at a remarkable pace. The forms and purposes of government were reshaped and enlarged. The infrastructures of higher education and the health professions were greatly elaborated. Major improvements in personal health, wealth, and education accompanied these social and economic changes.

Today, growth and innovation continue, but they occur in an environment more generally characterized by reevaluation, reorganization, and retrenchment. Public confidence in government, education, and other basic social institutions has diminished. The aging of the population is reshaping the country's view of itself and stimulating debates about generational equity in social policies. Fiscal stress seems an almost routine state of affairs from the governmental to the individual level, and the gap between the more and the less advantaged segments of society threatens to become a gulf in some areas.

As this committee was deliberating, health care reforms that would extend health insurance to all or most Americans were once again on the national political agenda, but the prospect for meaningful action was in doubt. Even without federal legislation, concern about health care costs has already prompted major and sometimes traumatic restructuring in the way health care is delivered and financed. Increasingly, providers and consumers are finding their options limited by the growth of health plans characterized by capitated provider payment systems, closed panels of health care practitioners, limited access to specialists, and various other constraints.

---

*The National Research Council is the administrative arm of the National Academy of Sciences, the National Academy of Engineering, and the Institute of Medicine.

Universities and their constituent parts are likewise under stress. Their stewardship in managing research funds has been questioned, and political controversies have raised public questions about the scholarly objectivity and merit on which such institutions pride themselves. Like private organizations, some have "downsized" by eliminating uneconomic or marginal programs. One consequence of the pressures on public and private institutions alike is an increased emphasis on accountability, performance measurement, and quality improvement.

CHALLENGES FOR DENTAL EDUCATION

Developments in dentistry and dental education reflect the larger societal patterns of growth and realignment just discussed. In the decades after the founding of the first school in 1840, dozens of dental schools were established. Many eventually disappeared, but more than 50 schools became established within public and private universities. The fixtures of a profession also accumulated: associations, journals, licensure laws, educational standards, and specialization. Technical improvements in procedures and materials made dental services more effective and less painful and, thus, more acceptable to the public.

In addition to broader social, economic, and scientific changes that have altered expectations and opportunities, recent decades have brought pressures for change that are more specific to oral services and that will continue to reshape the profession in the next century. First, the oral health of the American people has improved substantially, thereby affecting the demand for many traditional dental services such as extractions, dentures, and restorations. As recently as World War II, the primary physical reason for rejection of military recruits and draftees was dental defects; nearly 9 percent of those examined were rejected because they did not meet the requirement for six opposing teeth in each jaw. Such rejections are now rare. Preventive strategies at the individual and community levels have reduced tooth decay dramatically in children, and the number of older Americans with no teeth has declined significantly in recent decades. Still, oral disease remains commonplace, although it is concentrated in a subset of the population. For example, one-quarter of U.S. children experience three-quarters of the tooth decay or caries found in children. In general, minority groups and families with low levels of income and education and with limited access to dental services suffer disproportionately from oral health problems.

Second, demographic changes are affecting dental practice. In the future, the number and proportion of elderly patients, who tend to have more complicating medical conditions and are retaining more of their teeth, will grow (Figure 1.1). In addition, the oral health care needs of other patients with complex medical problems such as cancer and AIDS are becoming better appreciated.

Third, scientific and technological advances are reinforcing the medical aspects of dental practice as new or improved preventive, diagnostic, and pharmacological interventions challenge procedure-oriented dental education. Computer-based technologies are changing the nature of dental practice and providing new opportunities for evaluating and improving the outcomes of care.

Fourth, health plans that restrict patient access to a selected panel of dentists are moving beyond their historically small base. However, because more than half the population is not insured for dental services compared to less than one-fifth with no health insurance, the impact of health care restructuring has, so far, been relatively limited for many practitioners and patients. Overall, about 6 percent of all expenditures for personal health services

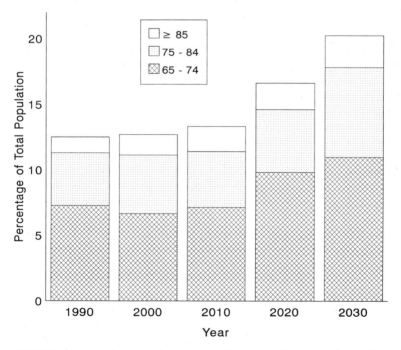

FIGURE 1.1 Trends in age distribution of U.S. population aged 65 and over, 1990-2030. SOURCE: U.S. Department of Commerce, 1993.

are accounted for by dental services, but the majority of this expense is not covered by insurance.

Fifth, although the number of dentists is still growing, projections suggest that the number will drop gradually after the turn of the century (Figure 1.2). This drop will reflect the decrease in dental school enrollments in the last decade, which has been *equivalent to the closure of 20 average-sized dental schools*. Because the U.S. population almost certainly will continue to grow, the ratio of dentists to the general population is expected to drop even more sharply—almost as sharply as it increased in the 1970s. How this downturn will affect future access to dental services and priorities for dental education depends on a number of economic, social, technological, and other factors. For example, the inclusion of dental benefits in a health care reform package would likely increase the demand for care because insured persons use more services than do those who are uninsured.

Sixth, dental education faces serious financial problems that, in many respects, constrain its ability to respond to the changes identified above. Within the university, dental education is viewed as relatively expensive, and as dental schools have reduced enrollments, many essentially fixed costs remain to be spread over a smaller number of students. During site visits and other discussions, the committee learned that discontinuation of several schools (in addition to the six that have already closed) is a serious—although not necessarily publicly acknowledged—possibility.

Dental education and dentistry are made vulnerable by their relative isolation from the broader university, from other health professions, and from the restructuring of health care delivery and financing that characterizes most of the health care system. This vulnerability is further increased by tensions between the practitioner and education communities. These tensions are most visible in the two areas, professional licensure and work force policy, both of which involve professional economic interest in the supply of dentists and allied dental practitioners and the conditions for entry into the profession. Other tensions have arisen from dental school efforts to increase revenues by creating faculty practice plans, to restructure departments, and to conduct research on such issues as access to dental care and the effectiveness of specific dental treatments. Failure to resolve or reduce these tensions will undermine the efforts of dental educators to improve their performance and solidify their positions within their parent universities and communities. This could jeopardize the future of the profession.

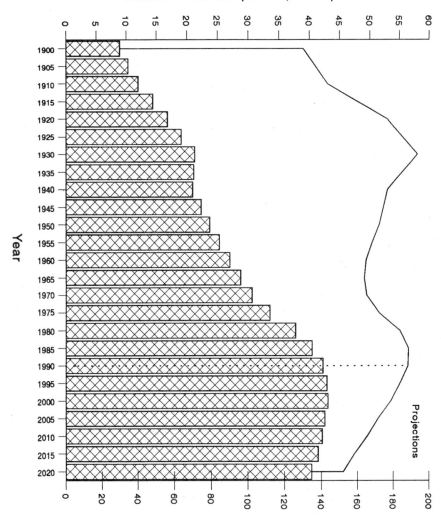

FIGURE 1.2 Trends in the supply of dentists. SOURCE: American Association of Dental Schools, 1993b.

ENVISIONING THE FUTURE

To respond to the challenges just outlined and to move successfully into a new century, dental educators and the larger dental community need some agreement on common purposes and directions. Formulating such agreement, in turn, requires an understanding of how well current modes of thinking and operation equip dental education and dentistry in general to face a future that is likely to be quite different from the past.

This report is intended to help build understanding and agreement. It combines a set of policy and strategic principles with an extensive analysis of dental education's present and future to form a broad picture of dental education in the twenty-first century. This picture is not a vision of an ideal world. Rather, it distills the committee's general view of what the future will bring, combined with its conclusions about how dental educators and others can reasonably, if not easily, prepare the profession for a constructive role in improving oral health in the twenty-first century.

PRINCIPLES

To guide its deliberations about the future of dental education and practice, the committee adopted eight general policy and strategic principles. These principles, which are woven throughout the text of this report, include those that follow.

Oral health is an integral part of total health, and oral health care is an integral part of comprehensive health care, including primary care. For oral health problems to be appropriately addressed, these connections need to be better understood and strengthened by dentists and other health professionals, educators, policymakers, and the public in general.

The long-standing commitment of dentists and dental hygienists to prevention and primary care should remain vigorous. This commitment has served the public well in the past and is consistent with demands that the broader health system—including health professions education—focus more on primary care in the future.

A focus on health outcomes is essential for dental professionals and dental schools. The effectiveness of dental services in achieving desired health outcomes for individuals and communities cannot simply be assumed but must be demonstrated to patients, other purchasers of dental services, and policymakers.

Dental education must be scientifically based and undertaken in an environment in which the creation and acquisition of new scientific and clinical knowledge are valued and actively pursued. Research and scholarship are essential elements of university-based education and are critical to continued improvements in oral health.

Learning is a lifelong enterprise for dental professionals that cannot stop with the awarding of a degree or the completion of a residency program. Preparing dental professionals to continue to learn and to critically appraise new and traditional technologies is a critical function of dental education.

A qualified dental work force is a valuable national resource, and support for the education of this work force must continue to come from both public and private sources. Although industry, alumni, and students each have a contribution to make, government must play a strong role because a well-prepared oral health work force is a public good. Further, its future is too important to be determined solely by the isolated decisions of individual universities and states.

In recruiting students and faculty, designing and implementing the curriculum, conducting research, and providing clinical services, dental schools have a responsibility to serve all Americans, not just those who are economically advantaged and relatively healthy. Efforts by some dental schools to serve disadvantaged individuals and communities—and to provide students and faculty with direct understanding of their needs—are challenged by reductions in public support for both education and patient care. The creation of a dental work force and faculty that reflect the nation's diversity is a goal only partially achieved at this time.

More generally, *efforts to reduce the wide disparities in oral health status and access to care should be a high priority for policymakers, practitioners, and educators.* With its traditional emphasis on prevention and primary care at the individual and the community levels, dentistry has a good foundation on which to build.

PROSPECTS

As the twentieth century ends, dental education faces many challenges—financial, intellectual, organizational, and technological. In the future as envisioned in this report, four elements stand out.

First, dentistry will and should become more closely integrated with medicine and the health care system on all levels: research, education, and patient care. The march of science and technology in fields such as molecular biology, immunology, and genetics will, in particular, continue to forge links between dentistry and medicine as will the needs of an aging population with more complex health problems. These links combined with the financial strains on the university and academic health center will encourage these institutions to consolidate or otherwise link programs in related areas such as dentistry and medicine. Government and private purchasers of health services can be expected to maintain and indeed increase the pressure on health care practitioners and institutions to develop more highly integrated and constrained systems of care that stress cost containment, primary rather than specialty care, and services provided by teams of professional and other personnel. Although dentistry may experience a less rapid restructuring of its place in health care compared to other health professions, any such respite should be used not as a time to reinforce resistance to these developments but as an opportunity to achieve a smoother transition for patients, practitioners, and educators.

Second, to prepare both their students and their schools for change, dental educators will need to teach and display desirable models of clinical practice. Such education will be scientifically and technologically up to date, focused on outcomes, interdisciplinary, efficient, patient and community oriented, and team based. For most schools, this will require substantial departures from current practices. These practices fall short for various reasons including incomplete implementation of long-standing and still valid proposals for reforming the curriculum, relatively slow recognition of new emphases on health outcomes and sophisticated information capabilities, and increasingly constrained resources.

Third, securing the resources essential for educational improvement and, indeed, survival will require that dental schools demonstrate their contributions to their parent universities, academic health centers, and communities through achievements not only in education but also in research, technology transfer, and community and patient service. Said differently, dentistry cannot pursue isolation. The process of change may exacerbate tensions with dental practitioners, for example, as dental schools experiment with new models of patient care and extend their outcomes research agenda. Thus, efforts to manage and resolve conflicts must have a high priority.

Fourth, the dental community—educators, practitioners, regulators, and policymakers—will benefit from continued testing of alternative models of education, practice, and performance assessment for both dentists and allied dental professionals. Experimentation and learning will also help dentistry face one its major uncertainties, namely, whether the future supply of dental practitioners and services will match, exceed, or fall below population requirements for dental care. That uncertainty is, in large measure, a function of the unpredictability of scientific and technological advances and of social policies affecting access to oral health services. Under these circumstances, contingency planning is stressful but essential.

The committee's specific recommendations are not, in general, highly prescriptive statements about what individual schools should do and how they should do it. Likewise, although concerned about the sources and some of the consequences of the variation across schools, the committee views variation as inevitable and often desirable. Recommendations are not directed at dental educators alone but call upon the entire dental community to work collectively toward improved oral health through more effective education, research, and practice.

MISSIONS OF DENTAL EDUCATION AND ORGANIZATION OF REPORT

The central chapters of this report are organized around the three basic missions of dental education: educating practitioners (Chapter 4), conducting research (Chapter 5), and providing patient care (Chapter 6). This organization reflects both the development of the American university and the emergence of the academic health center as a major part of the university.

The European university historically emphasized two missions—education and scholarship. The twentieth century vision of American universities as centers for scientific and technological progress has led the second mission to be widely relabeled—and in some ways profoundly redefined—as research. Service was incorporated as a third mission as the nation successfully harnessed higher education in the service of economic and social development, most visibly through the system of land-grant institutions initiated in the 1860s. With the post-World War II increase in university-based medical research, private and public health insurance, and demand for sophisticated hospital care, the position of the academic health center and the health professions schools rose relative to the rest of the university. Patient care became a distinct mission, one without a clear equivalent in other professional schools such as law and architecture. Thus, although universities speak of the missions of education, research, and service, many academic health centers summarize their missions as education, research, and patient care.

By organizing central chapters around the missions of education, research, and patient care, this report highlights the purposes that justify the existence of dental schools. This structure, however, inevitably sharpens distinctions that frequently—and usefully—blur in the operating reality of any given school. The missions of dental schools and academic health centers are clearly intertwined. Patient care is essential in predoctoral and postdoctoral clinical education, and patients also serve as subjects in clinical trials and other research activities. Education itself provides the focus for faculty research on the effectiveness of different instructional strategies. Ideally, both clinical and educational research, in turn, provide findings that help improve patient care and instruction. For many institutions, patient care includes provision of care for the disadvantaged, a crucial community service.

Although this report focuses on education, research, and patient care, it also considers activities more conventionally described as part of the service mission of the university. These include continuing education, support for public health services, and participation in mentoring, tutoring, and other programs for precollegiate minority youths that benefit the community as well as the young people themselves.

To understand dental education today and put current issues in perspective, the committee believed that it needed to understand something of dentistry's past. Chapter 2, therefore, presents a brief review of the evolution of dental practice and dental education. This history underscores issues that dentistry has wrestled with for a very long time such as standard setting, work force size and composition, and scientific foundations.

Chapter 3 examines oral health status and services, suggests basic objectives and directions for oral health, and discusses their implications for dental education. Chapters 7, 8, and 9 examine in more detail how dental education relates to the university, the profession, and the larger society. These chapters consider such controversial topics as dental school closures, educational financing, licensure, accreditation, and size of the dental work force. Several chapters, in particular Chapter 7, discuss leadership challenges and skills. In Chapter 10, the committee reconsiders the challenges facing dental education, presents its views on the strengths and weaknesses of dental education in facing these challenges, and recapitulates its findings and recommendations.

Although the discussion that follows includes many references to the relationship between the dental school and its parent university or academic health center, this overstates reality. Some dental schools are not part of academic health centers, and some are part of academic health center campuses that are not part of a university (although they may be part of a state university system). Some schools are formally part of a university or academic health center but are physically isolated and, in some cases, fairly independent organizationally. For the sake of simplicity and emphasis, this report's discussion of the dental school within the university or academic health center is generally not accompanied by references to the special circumstances just cited.

SUMMARY

The future of dental education is inextricably linked to its contributions to improving the effectiveness and efficiency of oral health services through education, research, and patient care. It must not only contribute but also be perceived as contributing— by society generally, by the dental profession, and by other relevant social institutions, in particular, the university. For dental education to meet the challenges ahead will require the support and involvement of the practitioner community as well as researchers and policymakers. The intent of this report is to provide guidance for each of these important groups.

APPENDIX 1.A Information Collection Activities of the Committee on the Future of Dental Education

Dental School Visits
11 schools—May to November 1993
6 states—California, District of Columbia, Illinois, New York, North Carolina, Texas
>600 participants—students, faculty, administrators, alumni, dental society leaders

Liaison Panels
Regional practitioner-leader panel, 16 members, met June 1993
Faculty panel, 17 members, met September 1993
Specialty panel, 9 members, met November 1993

Public Hearing and Panels at Committee Meetings
Testimony invited from more than 80 organizations
Oral testimony from 24 organizations, September 1993
Written testimony submitted by 30 additional organizations
Panel on Predicting Supply, Demand, and Need for Dental Personnel and Services (May 1993)
Panel on Financing Dental Education (September 1993)
Leaders of Dental and Allied Dental Organizations (various meetings)

Commissioned Papers, Surveys, Other
    Oral health status*
    Effectiveness and outcomes for dental care*
    Issues in dental curriculum development and change*
    Research, technology transfer, and the dental school*
    Research frontiers in oral health*
    Projecting supply, demand, and need for dental services and practitioners*
    Financing dental education*
    Licensure and accreditation*
    Telephone survey of officials at 12 universities
    Mail survey of 54 deans of dental schools
    Literature reviews

---

*These papers will be published in the January 1995 issue of the *Journal of Dental Education.*

2

Evolution of Dental Education

The history of dental education is marked by both change and continuity. As dental science and technology have advanced, instruction in dental practice has become more sophisticated both in substance and in method. During the last century and a half, training through apprenticeship—and purely self-taught and self-proclaimed competency—have been replaced by a lengthy period of formal instruction. Free-standing, profit-making schools have given way to university-based schools of dentistry, and postgraduate education in general and specialized fields of practice has become widespread.

Despite convergence in many areas, differences in opinion about dental practice and education persist. One fundamental disagreement involves the relationship between medicine and dentistry. Another involves the relative importance of instruction in technique versus education in scientific and critical thinking. The question of who should assess dental practice and education—and in what fashion—has provoked controversy for more than a century.

The following brief account of the evolution of dental education provides context for the rest of this report. Table 2.1 summarizes key dates in dentistry and dental education with an emphasis on developments *before* 1970. Additional historical information is also found in later chapters of this report and in the background papers.

TABLE 2.1 Time Line of Selected Dates in Dentistry and Dental Education

1530	First textbook on dentistry published in Leipzig
1683	Van Leeuwenhoek identified microorganisms in material scraped from teeth
1728	Fauchard's comprehensive dental textbook published in France, noted need for school of surgery to include dentistry
1765	First U.S. medical school founded in Philadelphia (later became the University of Pennsylvania)
1801	First American book on dentistry published
1839	*Journal of Dental Science* initiated, first national dental journal (discontinued in 1860)
1840	First American dental school founded in Baltimore by four physicians
1840	First national dental organization founded (disbanded in 1850s following split over safety of mercury in amalgams, the so-called amalgam wars)
1844	Effectiveness of nitrous oxide as dental anesthetic demonstrated
1859	American Dental Association (ADA) created
1860	Four U.S. dental schools in existence
1867	Harvard started first university-based dental department in close association with medical department
1868	Kentucky, New York, and Ohio passed first effective dental licensing laws and created first dental examiner boards with power to license graduates of reputable schools
1870	Fifteen percent of dentists held dental school diplomas
1872	Practical dental drilling engine invented
1882	ADA offered prize for paper on etiology of caries
1884	National Association of Dental Faculties established to encourage standardization of curricula
1884	Dental school established at Howard University
1891	Data published indicating infectious basis of tooth decay
1891	Two-year dental school curriculum required by dental faculties association
1894	University of Michigan offered first graduate courses in dentistry
1896	Use of X rays (discovered in 1895) first promoted in dentistry
1899	Dental licensure requirements adopted by all states
1902	U.S. Public Health Service (PHS) published its first article on dentistry (observations linking mottled teeth to drinking water)
1905	National Board of Dental Examiners published percentage of graduates of schools who failed licensing examinations
1906	First dental hygienist trained
1906	First public school-based dental assessment funded in Rochester, New York
1909	Dental Educational Council of America established by national organizations of dental examiners, dental faculties, and dental practitioners
1910	Novocaine introduced in the United States
1910	Publication of Abraham Flexner's report on medical education
1910	Graduation from high school established as prerequisite for dental school admission
1911	Army Dental Corps established

1913   Tri-State Dental Association of Negro dentists founded (predecessor of present-day National Dental Association)

1913   First school of dental hygiene founded in Connecticut

1913   Scientific Foundation and Research Commission created by ADA

1916   First university-based dental hygiene program established at Columbia University

1916   Virginia became first state to include dentist on Board of Health

1917   Requirement for three-year dental curriculum adopted

1918   First rating of dental schools published by Dental Educational Council (at the request of the Army Surgeon-General)

1919   Committee on dental investigation appointed by National Research Council (NRC) of National Academy of Sciences (disbanded 1924, reappointed 1928)

1919   National Bureau of Standards created dental research unit (prompted by Army interest in dental filling materials)

1919   PHS commissioned first dental officer

1920   International Association for Dental Research established

1923   American Association of Dental Schools established (by merger of several organizations)

1923   American Dental Hygiene Association established

1924   University of California Dental School funded by Carnegie Foundation and NRC for study of pyorrhea

1925   NRC appointed committee to investigate mottled teeth

1926   Publication of William Gies' report on dental education

1931   Link between fluoride and mottled teeth established, potential for caries protection reinforced

1931   NRC dental advisory committee recommended creation of dental research bureau

1933   First national written board examinations administered

1941   Dental school accreditation standards published by ADA council

1944   Dental problems identified as major reason for rejecting recruits during World War II

1945   First controlled water fluoridation projects initiated by PHS in Grand Rapids, Michigan to test effect on decay

1948   National Institute for Dental Research (NIDR) established

1951   U.S. Surgeon General and NRC encouraged fluoridation

1956   NIDR initiated funding of extramural training centers at several universities

1959   First National Health and Nutrition Examination Survey conducted

1961   Hollinshead survey of dental education published

1963   Health Professions Educational Assistance Act passed

1970   National Health Service Corps established for medically and dentally underserved areas

1971   Comprehensive Health Manpower Act passed to increase health work force

1980   Kellogg report on advanced dental education published

1984   Pew Foundation National Dental Education Program initiated

---

SOURCES: Guerini, 1909; Gies, 1926; Prinz, 1945; McCluggage, 1959; Sissman, 1971; Ward, 1972; Kidd, 1979; Hoffman-Axhelm, 1981; Starr, 1982; Harris, 1989; Burt and Eklund, 1992.

ORIGINS OF DENTAL INSTRUCTION

In a very broad sense, the origins of dental education lie in the works of the ancient Middle Eastern and Asian writers who recorded explanations, descriptions, and advice—that is, instruction—about an array of health problems including oral health problems.[1] These writers often mixed myths with potentially helpful prescriptions for herbal and other compounds to treat pain, clean teeth, and combat foul breath. A 5,000-year-old Sumerian clay tablet, for example, refers to the legend of the "tooth worm" as the source of tooth decay ("let me [the tooth worm] drink among the teeth, and set me on the gums") (Prinz, 1945, p. 15). The tablet recommends treatment with pulverized henbane, gum mastic, and a thrice-repeated incantation. (The attribution of tooth decay to worms was not put finally to rest until the eighteenth century.)

The most famous early discussion of dental problems is found in the Ebers papyrus, which has been dated to 1550 B.C. and may include segments from much older sources. It prescribes several herbal and other compounds to treat pain and swelling but makes no reference to dental restorations, extractions, or appliances. Later Greek and Roman medical texts by authorities such as Hippocrates (ca. 460-377 B.C.) and Galen (A.D. 129-201) routinely discussed oral health problems and advised pharmacological and mechanical strategies for managing and sometimes preventing pain, tooth decay, tooth loosening, bad breath, gum swelling, and abscesses.

After the fall of Rome in the fifth century A.D., medical and scientific progress suffered throughout Western Europe for a millennium. In the Arabic-Persian world, however, advances continued despite religious limits on anatomical research and surgery. Once medical science begin to revive in the West during the Renaissance, few medical experts considered oral health interesting or challenging. Many kinds of surgery were likewise viewed as uninteresting and mechanical, but dental problems and services became, in particular, more isolated from medicine. Elite physicians and surgeons might minister to the teeth of princes and bishops, but dental services in Europe became largely the preserve of barber-surgeons and other nonphysicians. Other factors may

---

[1]Sources for this discussion include Guerini, 1909; Gies, 1926; Prinz, 1945; Hoffman-Axhelm, 1981; and Harris, 1989. These texts occasionally disagree about facts and interpretations of early texts; the most generally plausible account was used. No significant independent effort to resolve disputes was attempted.

also have contributed to occupational segregation. One early twentieth century history of dentistry suggests that from Hippocrates onward, physicians tended to favor a very slow—and painful—process of tooth extraction (Guerini, 1909). In contrast, "lay" practitioners such as barbers got the job done quickly. Such dispatch presumably would have encouraged people with this common problem to seek attention from nonphysicians and would, thus, have contributed to the separation of dental from medical care.

During the 1500s, advances in anatomy, microbiology, and other areas laid the foundations for specialized treatises on dentistry and for a theoretical—not just mechanical and empirical—approach to oral health. These advances included detailed anatomical descriptions of teeth and related structures, as well as van Leeuwenhoek's identification of microscopic organisms in tooth scrapings.

In 1728, Fauchard (1678-1761), who is widely described as the father of modern dentistry, published a two-volume text on the practice of dentistry, the first comprehensive treatment of the subject. This text has been called "a milestone" in the "separation of dentistry from the discipline of surgery, not medicine" (Bánóczy, 1993, p. 634). Fauchard saw the need for schools of surgery that would include instruction in dentistry, but he conceded that there was a dearth of written materials available to guide such instruction. Although a few medical schools included lectures on dentistry, the practice of dentistry was the province of either those who learned their "trade" through some kind of apprenticeship (or, later and more formally, a preceptorship) or those who simply offered their services without even this kind of training.

FORMAL EDUCATION: EARLY DEVELOPMENTS

A SLOW START

Formal or institutional dental education began in the United States in 1840 when the state of Maryland chartered the Baltimore College of Dental Surgery, possibly after the medical department of the University of Maryland refused a request that it include dental education in its curriculum.[2,3] Regardless of its origins,

---

[2]Interestingly, in his 1910 report on medical education, Abraham Flexner refers to this institution as the "so-called medical department of the so-called University of Maryland," one that established early in the nineteenth century the "harmful precedent" of proprietary institutions that "were not a branch

the college was eventually incorporated into the University of Maryland in 1923.

The nineteenth century saw a continuing debate about whether dental education was best organized within a medical school or in independent schools. Some groups viewed the establishment of independent schools as more practical on grounds that medical schools would be unwilling to supply the requisite physical space and expensive equipment, to support the greater technical or mechanical training needed by dentists, or to maintain truly collegial relationships with dental faculty (Sissman, 1971). Nonetheless, when the medical community sought out dentists, the latter could be skeptical and even hostile. For instance, "dentistry [is] altogether too large to be made the tail end of the kite of medical practice" and "the majority of the medical schools . . . are not so enviable in their reputation as to offer inducements for entering into relations with them" (quoted in McCluggage, 1959, p. 171). An alternative view was that "if we are not medical specialists we are a set of carpenters" (quoted in McCluggage, p. 169).

Whether or not the independent strategy was relatively easier than incorporation within a medical school, only four dental schools were in place by 1865. All were freestanding. The slow growth of dental schools reflected resistance on the part of both students and practitioners. Prospective dentists often found it less disruptive and expensive to serve an apprenticeship with an established local dentist rather than enroll in a formal program in a distant city.[4] For their part, established dentists profited financially by acting as preceptors. Arguing that the preceptor concept was inadequate amounted to arguing that the majority of existing practitioners were ill-trained. This was a politically unappealing position given that perhaps 15 percent of the nation's nearly 8,000 dentists were dental school graduates by 1870; the remainder had been trained under preceptor arrangements or were simply self-proclaimed as dentists.

---

growing out of the living university trunk" and that had, at best, "makeshift" connections with a university's core, its school of arts and sciences (p. 5). Flexner contrasted the Maryland example with the university-based medical departments or schools founded in the 1700s in Philadelphia (now the University of Pennsylvania), New York (now Columbia University), Cambridge (Harvard University), and Dartmouth.

[3]This discussion relies primarily on McCluggage, 1959, and also on Gies, 1926; Sissman, 1971; and Hoffman-Axhelm, 1981.

[4]"We live in a busy age; it takes but a little while to become a grandfather in dentistry, that is, to send out a student who in a short time will have sent out his student" (quoted in McCluggage, 1959, p. 163).

In gradually formalizing dental education, dentistry followed a path trod by other professions in response to dual concerns about the prevalence of outright quackery on the one hand and the large number of reputable but poorly trained practitioners on the other hand. Other responses included the establishment of professional societies, the creation of journals and other vehicles for professional communication of new information and ideas, the adoption of organizational certificates of competency and other forms of self-regulation, and the quest for statutory protection (e.g., licensure). Initial steps in each of these directions occurred in the late 1830s and early 1840s.

In 1860, the newly organized American Dental Association (ADA)[5] charged one of its committees with preparing an annual report on the state of dental education (McCluggage, 1959). This activity provided a forum for collective discussion and debate about dental education when the initial efforts of dental schools to organize an association dissolved amidst disputes about criteria for granting degrees, in particular, unearned degrees.

Between 1865 and 1870, five new dental schools were founded. This group included the first university-based dental program, which was established at Harvard in 1867—in "affiliation" with the medical school—following appeals by the president of the Massachusetts Dental Society (Gies, 1926). The other four schools were freestanding. By 1884, twelve additional schools had been founded— nine university-based programs and three freestanding schools.

In Europe, the origins of formal dental education were more diverse (Bánóczy, 1993). Several dental schools, primarily in northern Europe, were founded on the U.S. model of independent or at least separate schools. In southern Europe, dental education was more likely to develop as a discipline (labeled stomatology from the Greek word, *stoma*, for mouth) within a medical school, and graduates received a medical degree. As a result of changes in the 1980s spurred in part by directives of the European Economic Community, only Austria still links dental licensure to a medical degree. (For additional discussion, see the background paper by Guarino.)

---

[5]The ADA was renamed the National Dental Association in 1897 following a merger with the Southern Dental Association, which had been created after the Civil War. The ADA then resumed its original name in 1922 and later relinquished its right to the other name. In 1932, what had been first the Tri-State and then the Interstate Dental Association became the National Dental Association (Kidd, 1979). As early as the 1890s, however, African-American dentists had met as a dental section of the National Medical Association (Dummett, 1952).

PROPRIETARY SCHOOLS: ADVANCE AND RETREAT

During the 1880s and 1890s, dozens of freestanding proprietary (for-profit) schools were founded in the United States. In Illinois alone, 28 dental schools were chartered between 1883 and 1902 (Gies, 1926). Illinois was also known as "the prolific mother of thirty-nine medical colleges" (Flexner, 1910, p. 6). By 1900, the nation had 57 dental schools.

The major impetus for the rapid growth in proprietary dental schools was the adoption of state laws regulating dental practice. These laws often granted graduates of dental schools license to practice, without requiring that they take any qualifying examination. By 1900, about 60 percent of dentists were dental school graduates. By the mid-1920s, it was estimated that less than 3 percent of active dentists had trained under preceptor arrangements (Gies, 1926).

The regulatory stimulus for the creation of dental schools was not initially matched by corresponding standards of quality for those schools. The result was the creation of a number of dubious educational enterprises. More colorfully put, "Some of the dental schools of this period were busy diploma mills, which [were] created under the sanction of indifferent state laws, conducted with the collusion of unworthy dentists, and protected by unfaithful practitioners in posts of public responsibility, freely sold the degree of doctor of dental surgery at home and abroad, [and led] to the disgrace of the profession and to the dishonor of dental education. Many of the dental schools that were chartered since 1884 have been . . . completely worthless" (Gies, 1926, p. 28) .

Eventually, the proliferation of proprietary schools prompted a reaction. State practice acts began to require that graduates of dental schools take licensure examinations and that only graduates of "reputable" schools be permitted to take such examinations. (The term "reputable" was not defined but was essentially a code word for nonproprietary schools.) Not only did the founding of new schools drop off, but the charters of many schools were withdrawn. For example, between 1902 and 1905, 22 of the Illinois schools lost their charters. Also, as a result of "increasing requirements in equipment, supplies, teaching, and research," dental education ceased being a "profitable business" (Gies, 1926, p. 49).

DENTAL HYGIENE EDUCATION

The first short-lived dental hygiene school was established in 1910 and graduated one class before local dentists succeeded in closing it (Motley, 1986). In 1913, a second program, the Fones School of Dental Hygiene, was created in Bridgeport, Connecticut; it emphasized school- rather than office-based services. Two years later, Connecticut became the first state to authorize hygienists to provide services under a dentist's supervision. In 1916, the same year that a New York court found no law preventing the provision of care by hygienists, Columbia University founded the first university-based hygiene program, a step that shortly thereafter stimulated the founding of the dental school itself (Orland, 1992). The American Dental Hygienists' Association (ADHA) was founded in 1923, the same year as the American Association of Dental Schools (AADS). In 1947, the ADHA and the ADA set forth the first accreditation standards for dental hygiene programs. Today, accredited programs range in length from two to four years and lead to either an associate or a baccalaureate degree.

EDUCATION REFORM

THE FLEXNER REPORT

Early in this century, the Carnegie Foundation for the Advancement of Teaching funded a series of reports on professional education in the United States. The publication of the fourth report, Abraham Flexner's 1910 study of medical education, was a landmark event (Flexner, 1910; Vevier, 1987; Wheatley, 1988). More than 80 years later, the Flexner report still shapes medical—and dental—school curricula. The report reflected and reinforced several themes or innovations in medical education including the mobilization against proprietary medical schools; the rationalization of the relationship between universities and professional schools; the creation of higher standards for medical school admissions and for better-qualified, full-time faculty; and the movement toward education grounded in scientific research and thinking.[6]

---

[6]Flexner's promotion of full-time research-oriented medical faculty was attacked by many respected physicians. For example, William Osler foresaw "the evolution throughout the country of a set of clinical prigs, the boundary of whose horizon would be the laboratory . . . forgetful of the wider claims of a clinical professor as a trainer, a leader in the multiform activities of the profession, an interpreter of science to his generation, and a counsellor in public and in private of the people, in whose interests after all the school exists" (quoted in Wheatley, 1988, p. 69).

The Gies Report

The tenth in the series of Carnegie reports, which was published in 1926, focused on dental education. Its author, William Gies was a Columbia University biochemistry professor with a particular interest in dental research. The report, which took five years to research and write, consisted of 250 pages of text plus more than 400 pages of appendixes, including lengthy descriptions and evaluations of the existing dental schools, each of which was visited by Gies.

Table 2.2 presents Gies' basic conclusions. His commentary on his five conclusions was essentially as follows. *First*, dental schools deserved earnest attention by universities. They should not be regarded as trade schools and profit centers, whose profits were to be funneled to the medical schools. Dentistry can be appropriately regarded as the oral specialty of medicine, albeit an autonomous rather than a conventional specialty because of its mechanical emphasis. Indifference to research or graduate study as avenues to productive scholarship and leadership should not be acceptable. Libraries should be upgraded as a sign of credibility.

TABLE 2.2 Conclusions of the Gies Report on Dental Education, 1926

1. In universities, dentistry, an independent division of health service and, in effect, the oral specialty of the healing art, should receive the quality of consideration and support now deservedly accorded to medicine.

2. In dental schools, teaching and research should be as effectual as the best in a good university, and the status of dental teachers should be raised accordingly.

3. The preparatory education of dentists should be equivalent, in general character, to that of physicians, which now includes at least two years of approved work in an accredited academic college after graduation from a four-year high school.

4. The undergraduate curriculum in dentistry should be devised for intensive preparation for the duties of general practice only, and should be so organized that earnest and competent students could complete the training in three years.

5. An optional full-year graduate curriculum, separate or combined, including dispensary and hospital experience as well as opportunity and encouragement in research, should be provided for all types of specialization in oral science and art, especially those of practice, public health administration, teaching, and investigation.

SOURCE: Gies, 1926, p. 179.

Second, the sincere commitment of the university to dental education would be demonstrated most meaningfully by elevating the status of the dental teacher and supplying sufficient remuneration to attract full-time committed educators. Schools should not be allowed to retain successful practitioners whose teaching is "uninstructive or even farcical" and who subordinate their teaching duties to practice. Endowments should be established as further evidence of university commitment. Such endowments would discourage schools from maintaining programs that were "intended in many cases primarily to keep themselves alive and to prolong the residence of students" (Gies, 1926, p. 206).

Third, to underscore that dentistry is not a trade, predental and premedical collegiate education should be comparable, and predoctoral medical and dental curricula should be similar and shared insofar as possible. A liberal preprofessional education stimulates the spirit of inquiry and scientific thinking and helps prepare dental students to be the intellectual peers and colleagues of medical students. Better predental education would allow transfer of some courses from the predoctoral to the predental level and encourage better teaching of the basic sciences at the predoctoral level. Gies and the president of the Carnegie Foundation also urged that medical students be better trained in oral health.

Fourth, if some coursework could be transferred to the preprofessional level, if the great amount of both duplication and minutiae in classes could be eliminated, and if instruction in the mechanical aspects of dentistry could be reduced, then a three-year rather than a four-year program (nine to ten months per year) should be sufficient for training general practitioners. The curriculum could still be expanded to achieve greater "correlation" with clinical medicine. Given the continuing advancements in technique and knowledge, schools should concentrate on helping students "to teach themselves" and to be able "to learn and grow in proficiency" (Gies, 1926, pp. 190, 191). Specialization should be reserved for postdoctoral education.

Gies tersely condemned the shortfall between these aspirations and the reality as follows. "Although most of the schools are integral parts of universities, few enjoy income from endowment or the equivalent, and . . . a majority subsist on fees, pay small salaries for instruction, have few whole-time teachers, are deficient in library facilities, offer no opportunity for graduate work, ignore research, are not intimately associated educationally with medical schools or hospitals, give no financial assistance to students, and make no systematic effort to guide their graduates into communities in need of dental service" (Gies, 1926, p. 246).

IMPACT OF THE FLEXNER AND GIES REPORTS

Many of Flexner's and Gies's conclusions reflected existing—if not yet uniformly accepted—arguments and movements in professional education (Flexner, 1910; Rosebury, 1955; McCluggage, 1959; Starr, 1982). For example, a backlash against the proliferation of proprietary medical and dental schools predated the reports by several years. By 1926 when Gies's criticism of these schools was published, only three proprietary dental schools remained.[7]

Also, as already mentioned, the economic realities of bringing proprietary schools up to standards implied by state licensing laws or defined by the Council on Medical Education had a major effect. In Paul Starr's characterization, "these changing economic realities, rather than the [Flexner] report, were what killed so many medical schools in the years after 1906. . . . At most, Flexner hastened the schools to their graves and deprived them of mourners" (Starr, 1982, pp. 118, 120). It is also worth noting that Flexner proposed that no more than 31 medical schools were needed, but over 70 still survived in 1925, many due to special protection from state legislatures.

The economic realities just cited made affiliation with universities one of the few survival strategies for many schools. In 1908, six university-related schools (California, Michigan, Minnesota, Pennsylvania, Harvard, and Iowa) formed the Dental Faculties Association of American Universities to lobby for the principle of university affiliation. When the Gies report was published in 1926, only five unaffiliated schools remained.

Gies, like Flexner, forcefully supported a strong basic science education and almost certainly encouraged dental schools to strengthen this aspect of their curriculum. Dental schools, however, did not have the added impetus toward restructuring that was provided to medical schools after Abraham Flexner moved to the Rockefeller Foundation's General Education Board and mobilized its philanthropic resources to promote change (Wheatley, 1988). In general, the earlier advance of research within medical schools was not due to government funding or to internally generated revenues but to an infusion of such philanthropic funds (Starr, 1982).

Some of Gies's recommendations fared poorly. His recommendation for a two-year predental and three-year predoctoral model

---

[7]Gies' initial negative views of at least two proprietary schools, both in Cincinnati, may have helped speed their demise (see Gies, 1926, pp. 490-491, 494, 639-640, and 646).

of dental education was attempted by only five schools (Ward, 1972). In 1934, the ADA recommended a four-year curriculum, as did the AADS a year later. (An initiative in the 1970s to revive the three-year concept was also relatively unsuccessful, as described later in this chapter.)

Gies's conclusion that predoctoral education should emphasize general practice and avoid early specialization remains largely in place today, and predental educational requirements at most dental schools have become more or less equivalent to those for medical schools. Gies's support for hospital internships and a broad array of graduate specialty programs also had some influence. Although the University of Michigan dental school had established the first such program in 1894, only five such programs existed in 1925. Neither the AADS nor the ADA specified standards for such programs until the 1940s (AADS and Kellogg Foundation, 1980), and accreditation did not begin until the 1960s. The recognized specialties (dates of recognition in parentheses) include dental public health (1950), endodontics (1963), oral and maxillofacial surgery (1947), oral pathology (1949), orthodontics (1947), pediatric dentistry (1947), periodontics (1947), and prosthodontics (1947). (By the time this report is published, another specialty, dental anesthesiology, may be recognized.)

Finally, the Gies report surely provided some inspiration for university-based research. Gies may, however, have done more to encourage such research by founding the *Journal for Dental Research* in 1918 (first published in 1919) and, then, in 1920 helping to organize the International Association for Dental Research in 1920. A more powerful stimulus lay more than a quarter-century ahead in the founding and work of the National Institute for Dental Research (NIDR).

SUBSEQUENT STUDIES OF DENTAL EDUCATION

The Gies report was followed by (and to some extent it prompted) a succession of later studies. The most important of these studies are reviewed in the background paper by Tedesco. They include a 1935 study sponsored by the AADS (Blauch, 1935); a 1940 report by the Council on Dental Education (CDE) of the ADA (CDE, 1941), which also included accreditation standards for dental schools; a 1947 report by the Secretary of the CDE reviewing schools against these standards (Horner, 1947); a 1961 survey and recommendations, funded by the W.K. Kellogg Foundation (Hollinshead, 1961); a 1976 report (ADA, CDE, 1977) developed by the CDE with the assistance of the AADS; an ADA critique of the preceding report (ADA, 1980); and, in the 1980s, a series of conference proceedings published in the AADS *Journal of Dental Education.* Other relevant studies include the 1980 study of Advanced Dental Education sponsored by the W.K. Kellogg Foundation (AADS and W.K. Kellogg Foundation, 1980) and the 1993 report of the Pew Health Professions Commission. These reports document the development of the dental curriculum and the continuation or emergence of many of the problems discussed further in Chapter 4 of this report. Their sponsorship reflects the important role that private foundations have played and continue to play in encouraging critical thinking and change in dental education.

THE STRUGGLES OVER EDUCATIONAL STANDARD SETTING

The development of professions, in which the establishment of membership standards is a central element, has its roots in St. Benedict's sixth century description of the "profession" of adherence to the standards of the monastic community. Today, professional standards reflect both community interest and self-interest, and the professions' interest in the education of their prospective members derives from these sometimes, but not always, compatible objectives. The drive by many educators and practitioners to institute more stringent admission and graduation requirements, eliminate proprietary schools, develop formal assessment mechanisms, and set other standards for dental schools reflected triple desires: to protect the public from ill-trained practitioners, to discourage some competitors, and to improve the stature of the profession. The various objectives behind the drive for professionalization in general and educational standards in particular are sources of both tension and harmony between the practice and the education communities.

The National Association of Dental Examiners (NADE), organized in 1883, put pressure on the dental schools to improve standards for accepting students and granting degrees, and it criticized the weakness of the major association of dental educators, the National Association of Dental Faculties (NADF).[8] The latter organization, which was created in 1884, took most of the propri-

---

[8]Unless otherwise indicated, this discussion relies primarily on McCluggage, 1959.

etary schools as members. Their strength within the organization kept it from developing rigorous standards for schools, although it did lengthen the dental curriculum to three years in 1891 and four years in 1917. (A high school diploma was not required for dental school admission until 1916 [Ward, 1972].) Echoing the split between institutional and preceptor models of dental education in the late nineteenth century, the American Dental Association (then called the National Dental Association) split in the early part of this century between the supporters of university-based education and those who supported and typically were products of proprietary schools. Debates over educational standards and sponsorship were occasionally ill-tempered.

In 1909, in an effort at cooperation, the NADE and the NADF proposed that a council on dental education be created somewhat along the lines of the Council on Medical Education, an organization established in 1904 as a standing committee of the American Medical Association. The Dental Educational Council was, however, set up as an independent body composed of representatives of the NADE, the NADF, and the ADA (with the university-based faculty organization left out). The Dental Educational Council initially focused on surveys of dental education, inspection of schools, and advice on policy and curricula, but within its first decade it also began rating dental schools, using a highly controversial rating system. Gies criticized it for allowing schools not affiliated with universities to get "A" ratings, a practice that the council dropped in 1924 (McCluggage, 1959).

The 1920s and 1930s saw substantial changes in dental education. These included the formation in 1923 of the American Association of Dental Schools (a consolidation of four separate groups that William Gies helped negotiate) and the 1926 Gies report. The AADS, which was not troubled by a strong proprietary school contingent in its membership, received Carnegie Foundation support in 1930 for a curriculum study (Sissman, 1971), and the ADA undertook a major curriculum study at about the same time (McCluggage, 1959).

During this period, the leadership of the American Dental Association (as the National Dental Association renamed itself in 1922) became increasingly restive about the independence of the Dental Educational Council, and it sought to bring educational standard setting under ADA control. In 1938, the council became the Council on Dental Education), "the agency of the ADA" in dental education (McCluggage, 1959, p. 385). The council's board provided equal representation for the ADA, the AADS, and the

NADE. In 1948, the CDE took on the role of accrediting dental schools and approving specialty boards, internships, and residencies. In 1974, the council was succeeded by the Commission on Dental Accreditation, which is technically independent but is funded, staffed, and housed by the ADA.

The ADA was also interested in national educational standards as a step toward reciprocity in state licensure. Reciprocity has been described as a "treaty" between two states to accept each other's licensing procedures (McCluggage, 1959, p. 388). The issue of uniform licensing standards raised—and still raises—potent political controversies over states' rights and freedom of movement that spill over to the educational realm.

Initially, the battle over uniform standards focused on the development of a uniform written national examination that dealt with knowledge of the basic sciences and certain clinical matters. The National Board of Dental Examiners was created in 1928 amidst intense controversy over the initiation and control of such a uniform examination.[9] It administered the first nationwide written examinations in 1933 and 1934, but by 1958, only 32 states accepted the national examination certificates as a full or partial substitute for a state written examination (Damiano et al., 1992). Today, all states do.

Controversy now focuses on continued testing of clinical competency through a varied set of state and regional examinations. Regional cooperation in clinical examinations began in 1967 when New York and the District of Columbia administered a single examination, a step that led to the creation of the first regional board, the Northeast Regional Board. Three other regional boards have since been developed, and more than half the states participate in one or more of these boards. Dentistry and dental hygiene are among the very few health professions requiring direct assessment of clinical skills using real patients. Chapter 8 discusses more recent developments and issues in standard setting.

---

[9]The depth of feeling was illustrated by one dentist's claim that "Cleopatra had her asp; Hamilton had his Aaron Burr; Caesar had his Brutus; and Christ, his Judas Iscariot. Dentistry has its National Board of Dental Examiners" (McCluggage, 1959, p. 392)

BUILDING A RESEARCH BASE IN THE UNIVERSITY

BEFORE 1948

Dental research—inside and outside university-based dental schools—was relatively slow to establish itself. In the 1930s, William Gies, at the behest of several prominent New York dentists, suggested that "various biological researches be conducted at different dental schools," but the responses indicated that "neither inclination, facilities or abilities were available" (quoted in Orland, 1992, p. 207).

Like early dental education, early dental research, at least in its applied aspects, was troubled by disputes about commercialism. Particularly fierce battles pitted organized dentistry against practitioners seeking patents on dental crowns and inlays (McCluggage, 1959). On a related front, just as he criticized proprietary dental schools, Gies criticized commercial writing about innovations in dentistry. In introducing the *Journal of Dental Research* in 1919, he cited the "dominant trade journalism . . . for commercial efficiency, professional obtundity, and unlimited superficiality . . . [that] demoralized the spirit and impoverished the imagination of dentistry" (Gies, 1919, reprinted in Orland, 1992, p. 73).

According to Harris (1989), university-based research in the 1920s was concentrated in 10 dental schools—California, Louisville, Harvard (with the Forsyth Infirmary cooperating), Illinois, Michigan, Minnesota, Northwestern, Pennsylvania, Rochester, and Western Reserve. During this period, the ADA encouraged university research with grants administered through a committee of the National Research Council (McCluggage, 1959).[10] In the early decades of this century, the ADA also promoted research initiatives by various agencies of the federal government including the Public Health Service and the Bureau of Standards. These agencies, in turn, supported dental research in some universities, although they con-

---

[10]In her discussion of the National Research Council (NRC), the administrative arm of the National Academy of Sciences, Harris (1989) notes the low esteem in which dental research was held by medicine at the time Gies conducted his study. Although the NRC was one of the first federally supported bodies to support dental research, its division of medical sciences was relatively hostile. The chair of the division is recorded in 1920 with these comments: "Of course, they [dentists] can't do any real investigating . . . on their own, but in a cooperative thing I think we can make use of them . . . [and] eventually . . . [gain] control of the whole thing" (Christian quoted in Harris, 1989, p. 29).

ducted much research in their own laboratories. By 1948, however, only 18 institutions—not all dental schools—were conducting dental research with newly available National Institutes of Health (NIH) funds (Harris, 1989). Even though the 1941 standards of the ADA's Council on Dental Education (created in 1938) required that dental schools conduct research, only 21 of the 40 dental schools even applied for the new funds.

SINCE 1948

With the creation of the National Institute for Dental Research in 1948, the federal government initiated a focused—albeit still modest—effort to promote research in oral health problems. In addition to organizing NIDR's own research laboratories, the first director, H. Trendley Dean, proposed to promote dental research by "(1) [expanding] the training of dental researchers, (2) [encouraging] all the country's forty dental schools and certain graduate schools to expand dental research through research grants-in-aid, and (3) [establishing] some small research studies in universities coordinated and administered by NIDR" (Harris, 1989, p. 96). The emphasis on research training by NIDR reflected the conclusion that a shortage of qualified dental researchers hampered serious applied and basic research.[11]

A similar conclusion is reflected in a 1955 tribute to Gies that argued that many of the advances in dental practice had come not from dental schools but from medical schools and private industry (Rosebury, 1955, reprinted in Orland, 1992). In 1954, after finding a paucity of "good" dental research applications, members of an NIDR planning committee attempted to assess the research potential of the dental schools, and their site visits to schools may have acted as an additional stimulus for dental research (Harris, 1989).

Since its founding in 1948, NIDR has undertaken a number of more formal initiatives to encourage dental research and research training (Harris, 1989). Some of the programs are aimed at schools, others at individuals. They include the following:

• The extramural research program continued and built on the small preexisting base of NIH dental research grants. From 1956

---

[11]Federal government support for the training of health scientists began in 1937 with programs authorized by the National Cancer Act (IOM, 1990d).

to 1959, the percentage of dental schools participating increased from 50 to 94. The extramural program established special sections for training and research grants in 1962.

• The fellowship program also built on existing Public Health Service (PHS) and other programs for training researchers at government facilities. One, funded by the ADA, started in 1941 and continued until 1970.

• The research centers program, initiated elsewhere at NIH in 1959 and in dentistry in 1962, provided support for comprehensive investigation of specific oral health problems or general disease conditions. The first support went to the University of Pittsburgh Cleft Palate Center. The NIDR created a Dental Research Institutes and Centers program in 1965 that awarded grants for five regional centers in 1967.

• The NIDR contracted with the ADA in 1964 for an information center to collect and make available dental research data that could be used in designing and developing research and training programs.

• In 1974, the National Research Service Award Act created a separate congressional authorization for research training, after the Nixon administration had impounded all NIH training funds and proposed elimination of all federally supported research training (IOM, 1990d). The act restricted student support to those pursuing research careers and included a service or payback obligation for those receiving training.

• The Dentist Scientist Award, created in 1984, supported individuals in a five-year program of dental specialty training and research training leading to a Ph.D., generally in a basic science.

HEALTH STATUS AND
EPIDEMIOLOGICAL RESEARCH

Until the 1950s, when the National Health and Nutrition Examination Survey (NHANES) was launched, data on oral health status were limited largely to community and special surveys undertaken by a variety of public health, educational, and professional groups (Harris, 1989). The historical importance of even small-scale dental epidemiological research should be noted. Although dental practitioners individually were all too aware of the prevalence of tooth decay and other problems, their testimony did not provide the compelling evidence needed to achieve broad public recognition and action to attack the problems. One starting point was data amassed from the physical examinations of military draftees and recruits beginning as early as the Civil War and from the records that the Marine Hospital Service began to collect in the 1870s. Limited though these data were, the widespread problems of decay, tooth loss, and poor function that they identified did stimulate incremental steps to improve oral health services, training, and research (Harris, 1989).

At the community level, the first dental inspection of schoolchildren began in 1906 in Rochester, New York. These inspections were undertaken primarily as part of an oral hygiene movement. This movement also included the founding of children's dental clinics with funding from George Eastman in Rochester and the Forsyths in Boston (McCluggage, 1959). Both clinics evolved into leading centers of dental research and postgraduate education.

The data collected from inspections of school children in dozens of cities helped build understanding of the high prevalence of tooth decay. States also began school-based service programs and data collection efforts. As of 1936, 14 states provided by statute that "Vincent's infection" (trench mouth) be reported to the state health department (U.S. Department of the Treasury, 1936). In the 1920s, surveys conducted by the Division of Child Hygiene in the PHS focused on dental fluorosis (permanent discoloration of teeth) and the possible influence of diet and climate on caries. Fluorosis was first viewed purely as a dental defect. Its role in caries prevention was only later suspected.

In the 1930s, the PHS in cooperation with the ADA sponsored two national surveys, one polling state health departments and institutions and the other examining 1.5 million children aged 6 to 14 in 26 states (McCluggage, 1959; Harris, 1989). Nothing comparable was done again until the first NHANES study. Unfortunately, variability in examiners' recording of caries led to a probable underestimate of caries prevalence. Nonetheless, the geographical variation in caries experience was regarded as one piece of evidence linking fluorosis with the control of tooth decay (Harris, 1989).

Data on oral health status began to improve substantially in the 1960s and 1970s. As discussed further in Chapter 3, these data are still limited in important respects.

In light of their generally limited involvement in research at midcentury, it is not surprising that dental schools figure little in the most important oral health research of that period, that is, investigation of the oral health effects of fluoride (Rosebury, 1955, reprinted in Orland, 1992; McNeil, 1957; McClure, 1970; Harris,

1989). That research was the culmination of a process that began in the early 1900s with the observations and persistence of a Colorado dentist, Dr. Frederick McKay, who was fascinated by the problem of mottled enamel. He caught the attention of Dean G.V. Black of the Northwestern University Dental School, who collaborated in some studies to understand the problem. Another dental school dean, H.E. Friesell of the University of Pittsburgh, tried unsuccessfully to get federal funding to study the same problem, which had been noted by a Pittsburgh graduate practicing in Arizona. Instead, researchers at the University of Arizona Agricultural Experiment Station linked mottled enamel to drinking water containing fluoride.

In 1931, the PHS agreed to investigate mottled enamel and brought in Dr. H. Trendley Dean to lead the work. The eventual result was the major trial of artificial fluoridation in Grand Rapids, Michigan. (Dean was later named the first director of NIDR.) The effectiveness of this and later trials in reducing caries led to strong public health support of community fluoridation. This support, however, was soon countered by fierce opposition from an unusual combination of forces including Christian Scientists, skeptical scientists and clinicians, chiropractors, health food advocates, and right-wing groups that viewed fluoridation as a Communist conspiracy to usurp individual rights and impose socialized medicine (McNeil, 1957; McClure, 1970). Chapter 3 examines the current status of fluoridation.

OTHER CONTROVERSIES

Clinic Services

In addition to disagreements about the process and substance of accreditation and licensure, other bones of contention between educators and practitioners should be noted. From time to time, for example, controversy has focused on dental school clinics as a source of competition for practitioners and a form of "corporate dental practice," akin to the prepaid group practices that provoked the opposition of physicians from their earliest days. When the dean of the dental school at Columbia University proposed early in this century to offer dental services "at a moderate charge to persons in moderate circumstances," rather than only low-cost preventive and medical services, he was strongly criticized (Orland, 1992, p. 102). The committee's site visits and other meetings indicated that initiatives by dental schools to establish faculty practices or otherwise to expand clinical services can still provoke resistance by area practitioners.

More generally, the financing of dental services has incited bitter debate since at least the 1920s. One starting point was the work of the private Committee on the Costs of Medical Care. With funding from several foundations, the committee set out to collect data on the cost and availability of health services. Its five-year investigation generated 27 field studies and a controversial final report (Anderson, 1968; Starr, 1982; IOM, 1993b). One part of this investigation was a survey of the incidence of dental disease and of the cost and availability of dental services (McCluggage, 1959). These studies found that 12 percent of health care spending went to dental services versus 30 percent to physician services and 24 percent to hospitals. The proportion of dentists to population varied from 1:500 to 1:4,000 for the population generally, but it was 1:8,500 among the segregated black population. The committee's proposals for change, which included group practice and voluntary private insurance, were strongly opposed by both the medical and the dental professions. The controversy discouraged the Roosevelt administration from including health coverage as part of its social security proposals.

In the 1940s, a series of government actions almost inadvertently encouraged employers to expand nonwage compensation to their employees (Somers and Somers, 1963; Starr, 1982). Substantial growth in private, employment-based health insurance was one major consequence, although dental insurance specifically did not really begin to grow until the 1970s. Less than 2 percent of the population was covered by private dental insurance in 1965 compared to over 25 percent in 1978 (IOM, 1980). When the Medicare program was established in 1965, it excluded dental services—and that exclusion remains in place. Although required to cover some services for children, most state Medicaid programs pay relatively little for dental care, especially for adults (OTA, 1990). Today, not quite half the U.S. population has some form of public or private coverage for dental services (Keefe, 1994).

Controversy has also surrounded other steps to extend access to dental services. In 1970, Congress established the National Health Service Corps (NHSC; P.L. 91-623) to improve health services in underserved areas. Although the focus was on areas with shortages of health personnel, the legislation also included provisions for partly or fully subsidized care to those who could not afford to pay. In most cases, local medical or dental societies as well as local governments had to agree to designations of shortage areas. Opposition by dental groups was apparently more frequent than medical society opposition (Carnegie Council on Policy Studies in Higher Education, 1976). Later legislation established a scholarship program for selected health professions students. In return, the recipient was required to provide one year of service in the NHSC or the Public Health Service for each year of scholarship support. The current status of this program is discussed in Chapters 4 and 9.

DENTAL SCHOOL ENROLLMENTS

Yet another source of controversy involves the fundamental questions of how many dental schools are needed and how many students they should enroll. The 1950s and 1960s saw a growing—but not undisputed—sentiment that there was a shortage of physicians and some other health professionals (Somers and Somers, 1963; Coggeshall, 1965; Fein, 1987). One early response came in the Health Professions Educational Assistance Act of 1963 (P.L. 88-129), which provided for construction and expansion grants to schools and for loans to students.

In 1970, the report of the Carnegie Commission on Higher Education, *Higher Education and the Nation's Health,* reflected widespread agreement that the nation had a shortage of physicians, dentists, and certain other health professionals. It encouraged expansion in health professions education, warned against overspecialization, supported training of physician and dentist assistants, and proposed creation of a national health service corps.

The Comprehensive Health Manpower Act (P.L. 92-157) of 1971, like its 1963 predecessor, provided loan and scholarship money as well as funds for both new and expansion construction and operating costs. It provided an even more powerful incentive for growth by linking schools' eligibility for funds to increases in first-year enrollments—10 percent for schools with 100 or fewer first-year students and 5 percent (or 10 students, whichever was greater) for larger institutions. Funding for dental schools (excluding research and postgraduate programs) increased from $64 million in 1970-1971 to $80 million in 1971-1972 but dropped back to $57.8 million in 1974-1975 (Carnegie Council on Policy Studies in Higher Education, 1976). Between 1971 and 1975, six new dental schools were established.[12] Then, just six years after the 1970 Carnegie

---

[12]Other provisions in the 1971 legislation encouraged medical and dental schools to move from a four- to a three-year curriculum. Sixteen schools made the change, but when funding ended, all but the University of the Pacific returned to

report, a report by a successor organization warned that too many medical schools were being established and that the increased supply of physicians was not eliminating geographic disparities (Carnegie Council on Policy Studies in Higher Education, 1976). The report suggested, however, that enrollments in some *dental* schools should be expanded and that new schools were needed in Arizona and probably in Florida. Today, Arizona still has no dental school, and Florida continues to have a single school as it did in 1976. Congress reacted to the changing view of the health care supply question (particularly the view that there was a "physician glut") by reducing direct support for health professions education, including dental schools.

The whipsaw effect of adopting and then removing a significant stimulus for enrollment growth had disruptive effects on both educators and practitioners that still persist in debates about the size, distribution, and composition of the dental work force and the appropriate number and size of dental schools. As noted in Chapter 1, six schools have closed since 1985, and the overall enrollment drop is equivalent to closing about 20 average-sized schools (Consani, 1993). Chapter 9 examines the dental work force today.

SUMMARY

The twentieth century opened for dental education with an abundance of proprietary schools, a trade not fully transformed into a profession, and a primitive regulatory structure. The population was beset by serious dental disease, resigned to tooth loss, and limited in the treatments available to it. The science and research base was minuscule. During the twentieth century, dental practice, education, and regulation have been transformed. Proprietary schools have vanished amidst a series of educational reforms, and a significant—albeit still limited—research capacity has emerged. The next chapter focuses on the trends in oral health that have greatly diminished the incidence and severity of dental disease.

---

the four-year schedule. Earlier, most dental schools had adopted year-round three-year programs during World War II but only the University of Tennessee continued that pattern after the war (Santangelo, 1981).

3

Oral Health Objectives and Dental Education

A fundamental purpose of dental education is to develop health professionals who will maintain and improve the oral health status of individuals and populations. One task, then, for this committee as it evaluated future directions for dental education was to examine the status of oral health in this country and the ramifications for dental education in both the short and the long term.

In undertaking this task, the committee reviewed information on the health status of the U.S. population, including data on trends and differences across population subgroups, and evaluated the recommendations of other groups whose primary task was to articulate goals for oral health. A background paper on oral health status by White et al. includes a more extensive and detailed presentation and analysis of trend data than found by the committee in any other single published source. This chapter briefly reviews key indicators of oral health status and recommendations of other groups; it then presents the committee's views on oral health status goals and their implications for dental education.

DATA SOURCES

The data on oral health status and services reviewed by this committee came from three primary sources. The first was the National Health and Nutrition Examination Survey (NHANES) of the National Center for Health Statistics (NCHS). The first survey (then called the Health Examination Survey), which took place between 1959 and 1962, included some measures of oral health status as did the second survey conducted from 1971 to 1974. Unfortunately, the measures, particularly the measure of periodontal disease, in the first survey are considered sufficiently imperfect that they are rarely cited in trend analyses (Spolsky et al., 1983), and debates about measurement continue. Recently, Caplan and Weintraub (1993, p. 856) stated that "until there is a reliable diagnostic tool for measuring active periodontal disease on a one-time basis, methods of evaluating periodontal health in cross-sectional studies will be inconsistent." The third NHANES (which took place from 1976 to 1980) did not include measures of oral health. The latest survey, which began in 1988 and does include oral health measures, is to be analyzed by the National Institute for Dental Research (NIDR) rather than NCHS, and results are yet to be published. No preliminary data from this survey were available to the committee.

The second source of data was the NIDR Examination Survey. The NIDR surveyed dental caries in children in 1979-1980 and in 1986-1987, and it surveyed employed adults and seniors attending senior centers in 1985-1986. Unfortunately, because the surveys differed in many of their measures or categories, the 1971-1974 NHANES and the three NIDR surveys permit only limited assessments of trends in health status for adults and children.

The third source of data was the National Health Interview Survey (NHIS), also conducted by the NCHS. The NHIS collected dental data in 1969, 1970, 1973, and 1975 through 1977, but it eliminated dental utilization data from the core survey in 1982 (NRC and IOM, 1992). It now collects such data irregularly for special supplements.

The committee also consulted various other sources. These included the RAND Health Insurance Experiment report on dental health status (Spolsky et al., 1983), some state surveys, a recent National Institute on Aging (NIA) study of elders in New England (Douglass et al., 1993), and selected historical sources (see Chapter 2). The background paper by White et al. provides a more extensive discussion of oral health status and trends.

As suggested in this review of sources, the collection of data on oral health status has been somewhat less regular and frequent than the collection of information about many other health problems. This oversight reflects the tendency noted elsewhere in this report for the health of the mouth to be considered an isolated category rather than an integral part of overall health. In addition, measurement inconsistencies limit comparisons across studies and across time (Spolsky et al., 1983; Burt and Eklund, 1992; Caplan and Weintraub, 1993; see also the background paper by White et al.). Measures often change as knowledge related to the diagnosis and progression of oral disease advances. Treatment changes can also affect measurement. For example, fluoridation and certain kinds of restorations have complicated accurate classification of carious and noncarious surfaces (Edelstein, 1994). Another limitation of national population surveys is that they cannot be expected to reach certain vulnerable populations, for example, the homeless and illegal immigrants.

ORAL HEALTH STATUS

Their limitations notwithstanding, data on oral health status in the United States point to three broad conclusions. First, the oral health status of Americans has improved substantially in recent decades. Second, despite overall improvements in health status, oral health problems remain very common. Third, significant disparities in oral health status characterize the less-well-off and better-off segments of the population.

IMPROVED HEALTH STATUS

The last 50 years have seen significant improvements in oral health status (see, for example, NIDR, 1990; Burt and Eklund, 1992; Brown, 1994; and the background paper by White et al.). A few examples illustrate that progress is not limited to the reduction of dental caries, although that is the best-known achievement of preventive dentistry.

• During World War II, the primary physical reason for rejection of military recruits and draftees was "dental defects" (Harris, 1989, p. 78). Nearly 9 percent of those examined were rejected because they did not meet the requirement for six opposing teeth in each jaw. By way of contrast, in 1992, the Navy did not even list this among the five dental reasons for rejection, and the head of oral diagnosis at the major naval recruiting center could remember only one recruit rejected for dental problems in the previous three years (cited in J.W. Hutter, personal communication, February 9, 1994).

• Trench mouth (now known as acute necrotizing ulcerative

gingivitis), which includes infections of the soft tissues in the mouth and throat, was the first dental disease to be regularly recorded and reported by government hospitals. It was a serious enough problem—especially for the military—to prompt the National Institutes of Health to negotiate with the American Dental Association for a fellowship to support research into the disease starting in 1941 (Harris, 1989). This research established an infectious cause of the disease in 1949. Treatment by local debridement and, when necessary, antibiotics has made the disease a minor problem in the United States, although it remains a serious and common infection in many less developed areas (NIDR, 1990).

• The 1985-1986 NIDR survey of seniors found that 41 percent of those aged 65-74 were edentulous—that is, missing all their teeth—compared to 55 percent in the 1957-1958 NHIS and 46 percent in the 1971-1974 NHANES. For those aged 65 and over, the average number of missing teeth was 15 in the first survey and 10 in the second. Three state surveys by the North Carolina Division of Dental Health from 1960 to 1986-1987 show a considerable drop in the mean number of missing teeth in children— from 0.60 to 0.04 (Caplan et al., 1992).[1]

• From the 1971-1974 NHANES through the 1979-1980 and the 1986-1987 NIDR surveys, the average number of decayed, missing, or filled surfaces on permanent teeth declined for children at all ages, especially those aged 12 or older. The reduction of caries in children following the widespread addition of fluorides to community drinking water is one of the major public health achievements of this century.

• For cleft palate and other dentofacial deformities, major advances in surgical, imaging, and other techniques and better understanding of tissue growth, healing, and regeneration have allowed the full or partial correction of defects that impair social and physical functioning (e.g., breathing, eating, speaking). Trend data on the prevalence of these problems are, however, relatively limited.

As noted earlier, tracking changes in periodontal disease is difficult because of measurement problems (Spolsky et al., 1983; Caplan and Weintraub, 1993). Periodontal disease includes gingivitis (in-

---

[1]The number of missing teeth is no longer regarded as a strong indicator of caries experience. Children, for example, may have more teeth removed to correct orthodontic problems than are lost to decay.

flammation confined to the gingiva or gum tissue) and periodontitis (inflammation leading to bone loss and destruction of soft tissue attachment to the tooth, a process that frequently results in "pockets," the depths of which can be measured by a periodontal probe during an examination). According to RAND analysts, data from the NCHS surveys of 1960-1962 and 1971-1974 "do not reflect any change in the prevalence of periodontal disease" (Spolsky et al., 1983, p. 21). However, the 1985-1986 NIDR survey of adults "gives the impression that the severity and extent of periodontal disease among middle-aged, working Americans is less than previously thought" (NIDR, 1990, p. 49). In contrast, the NIA study found a higher level of periodontal disease in older adults compared to NIDR findings for that group (Douglass et al., 1993). Thus, the picture for periodontal disease is not clear.

CONTINUED PREVALENCE OF ORAL HEALTH PROBLEMS

Despite the trends cited above and a general acceptance that most oral health problems are preventable, dental disease remains one of the most common—if not the most common—human health problems. By age 17, more than 8 out of 10 children have experienced dental caries in their permanent teeth (NIDR, 1989). Few data on caries in children's primary or deciduous teeth are published, but caries experience during preschool years is an indicator of subsequent risk for caries in permanent teeth (Newbrun and Leverett, 1990; Kaste et al., 1992; O'Sullivan and Tinanoff, 1993). Nursing caries or "baby bottle" tooth decay is an underrecognized health problem and preventive priority (USDHHS, 1990).

Virtually all employed adults have experienced caries, and nearly half of those between 18 and 64 are affected by gingivitis and adult-onset periodontitis (NIDR, 1989). The 1989 NHIS suggested that about one in five Americans had experienced some kind of orofacial pain (Lipton et al., 1993).

Today, more than one-third of persons aged 65 and above are missing all their teeth (NCHS, 1992a; Douglass et al., 1993). Nonetheless, because the elderly are retaining more teeth than in the past, they have a larger number of teeth at risk for caries and other diseases. Caries on the root surfaces of teeth become more common as people age, and more than half of those aged 65 and over have one or more filled or untreated root caries. The elderly and middle-aged also have invested in more dental work than their predecessors, and that work itself predisposes its beneficiaries to future problems. A recent report suggested that between

60 and 70 percent of restorations replace failed restorations or treat secondary caries adjacent to past restorations (Corbin and Kohn, 1994). One estimate is that while the population aged 65 and over will increase by 104 percent from 1990 to 2030, the number of teeth at risk in this age group will increase by 153 percent (Reinhardt and Douglass, 1989).

Further, because older individuals are more likely to have other health problems and because the proportion of the population that is aged 65 and over is growing, dental practitioners are seeing more individuals with oral health problems that complicate or are complicated by other medical conditions. For example, individuals who have had hip, knee, or other joints replaced and who suffer from untreated oral disease are susceptible to infections in these joints that may be severe enough to require replacement. Dental treatment is itself a risk factor for persons with replacement joints. To cite a more general example, the NIA study found that more than 70 percent of elderly persons living in the community (not in institutions) are taking prescription medications that may affect both the diagnosis and the treatment of oral health problems.

In addition, the number of individuals with AIDS, who appear more susceptible to a number of relatively uncommon oral health problems, has increased. Their complex and sometimes life-threatening oral health problems include fungal infections, oral candidiasis, herpes, Kaposi's sarcoma, and aggressive periodontal disease.

Cancers of the oral cavity and pharynx are less common and less likely to be fatal than the four most common cancers (breast, lung, colon/rectal, and prostate) (NCI, 1989). They are, however, roughly as common as melanoma and leukemia, although less likely to be fatal than the latter. Oral and pharyngeal cancers are the sixth and twelfth most common types of cancer among men and women, respectively.

DISPARITIES IN ORAL HEALTH STATUS

Although oral health status has improved generally across the U.S. population, important disparities in status persist. Twenty-five percent of children account for three-quarters of the caries found in national surveys (unless otherwise indicated, data are from the NIDR 1986-1987 survey). These children are disproportionately found among minority groups (particularly Native Americans and Alaska Natives) and families with low levels of income and education. For example, 4 percent of African-American children have had teeth extracted for caries compared to only 1 percent of white children. Among children and adults, African-Americans have a larger percentage of untreated dental problems. Table 3.1 shows changes in survey findings for decayed, missing, and filled teeth for children from the early 1960s to the late 1980s.

Tooth loss is substantially higher for lower-income groups. For example, among those aged 65-74 years living in noninstitutional settings, 46 percent of those with incomes of less than $10,000 have lost all their teeth, compared to 12 percent of those with incomes of $35,000 and higher (NCHS, 1992a). Hispanic and non-Hispanic Americans and black and white Americans differ little in rates of total tooth loss for those under age 65. Among blacks aged 75 and older, however, 53 percent are edentulous compared to 42 percent of whites in the same age group.

Figure 3.1 shows that African-American males have considerably higher rates of oral cancers than white males, and men in general have a higher incidence than women. Mortality from oral cancers is likewise considerably higher among African-American males than in other groups. In 1988, only 31 percent of African-Americans with oral cancers reached the five-year survival point compared to 53 percent of white Americans. This difference in survival rates exceeds that for all other major cancers.

Visible disparities in health status may translate into other problems

TABLE 3.1 Mean Number and Percentage Component of Decayed, Missing, and Filled Permanent Teeth (DMFT) Among Children by Age Group and Race, United States 1963-1987

Race	Age Group (years)	Mean DMFT	Percentage D of DMFT	Percentage M of DMFT	Percentage F of DMFT
White Americans					
1963-1965	6-11	1.4	28.6	7.1	64.3
1966-1970	12-17	6.3	23.8	9.5	66.7
1986-1987	5-17	1.97	11.7	0.8	87.5
African-Americans					
1963-1965	6-11	1.1	70	10	20.0
1966-1970	12-17	5.6	57.1	23.2	319.7
1986-1987	5-17	1.99	27.2	3.2	69.6

SOURCE: Excerpted from White et al., 1994.

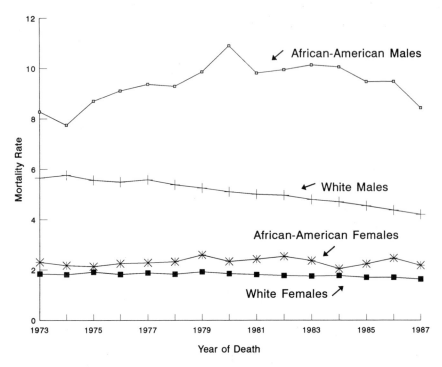

FIGURE 3.1 Age-adjusted mortality rates for oral and pharyngeal cancers by race, gender, and year of death, 1973-1987. SOURCE: White et al., 1994.

if they affect individual performance at school or work or if they prompt negative assessments by teachers and employers. The impact of such assessments on obese individuals is beginning to be understood, but little if any systematic research has been undertaken to document the effects of visible dental defects (e.g., missing, discolored, or maloccluded teeth) on hiring or promotion decisions. A 1993 overview by Hollister and Weintraub cited only one such study.

Data from the NHIS indicate that the number of days lost from work due to acute dental conditions differed considerably between whites and blacks and between higher- and lower-income workers. Overall, the work-loss days for dental problems were "similar or larger than the rate for eye conditions, acute ear infections, indigestion, and headache (excluding migraine)" (Hollister and Weintraub, 1993, p. 908).

UTILIZATION AND COVERAGE OF DENTAL SERVICES

The average American adult or child visits the dentist twice a year.[2] This figure has increased since the 1950s and 1960s when the average was about 1.5 visits. In 1989, some 58 percent of nonelderly adults and 62 percent of children had at least one dental visit. Although the elderly are more likely than other adults to have a medical visit, the percentage of the elderly with at least one dental visit (43 percent) is lower than for other adults (Burt and Eklund, 1992). This contrast presumably reflects the higher rate of edentulism among older people (34 percent for those aged 65 and over versus less than 5 percent for other adults).

Disparities in the use of dental services are related to both income and race. For example, 4 percent of poor children (family income less than $10,000) have had dental sealants applied compared to more than 17 percent of children from families with income of $35,000 or higher. (A sealant is a plastic film painted onto tooth surfaces to prevent tooth decay.) For poor families, slightly more than 20 percent have not seen a dentist in more than five years; for better-off families, the figure is less than 6 percent (NCHS, 1992a). Sixty percent of whites have seen a dentist in the last year compared with 43 percent of blacks (NCHS, 1992a). In the recent Institute of Medicine report *Access to Health Care in America* (IOM, 1993a), statistics on dental utilization were highlighted as a frequently neglected indicator of disparities in access to health care.

Differences in dental care utilization are also linked to insurance coverage. In 1989, those with private insurance averaged 2.8 dental visits per year compared to 1.7 for those without. In the same year, 41 percent of the population reported some form of private dental insurance, much of it quite limited. In contrast, over 70 percent of nonelderly Americans have private medical insurance, and virtually all elderly Americans have medical coverage under Medicare, which does not cover dental services. For physician services, consumer out-of-pocket expenses accounted for only 19 percent of spending in 1990; for dental services, the corresponding figure was 53 percent (Burner et al., 1992). For the

---

[2]Unless otherwise indicated, utilization data are from the 1989 National Health Interview Survey (NCHS, 1992a) and cover persons 2 years of age and older. Trend data are from Burt and Eklund, 1992.

nation overall, the percentage of total personal health care expenditures devoted to dentistry was 5.8, down from 6.5 in 1980 (Burner et al., 1992). The figure is projected to drop to 3 percent by 2010.

Most private coverage for health services, including dental services, is obtained through employers. Those employers that cover dental services generally do so under a freestanding dental plan (Bradford, 1992; Keefe, 1994). Coverage of dental services by health maintenance organizations is very limited, although the number of freestanding dental plans that limit coverage to a defined network of dental providers is growing.

As noted earlier, Medicare has essentially no dental coverage, and Medicaid coverage for dental services is quite limited, especially for adults. In 1989, only 20 percent of all children eligible for Medicaid received such care (USPHS, 1993). A 1990 study by the congressional Office of Technology Assessment reported that among seven states surveyed, none adequately covered "basic" dental services for children eligible for the Early and Periodic Screening, Diagnosis, and Treatment program (reported in USPHS, 1993). For the Medicaid program, dental services accounted for only 1 percent of program expenditures in 1990.

For a subset of low-income adults, the Department of Veterans Affairs (usually abbreviated as the VA) provides a source of dental services for veterans who meet eligibility requirements, which are more restrictive than those for medical services. The VA operates the country's largest hospital-based system of dental care. In FY 1992, nearly 400,000 veterans made almost 1,300,000 dental visits, an average of 3.3 per user (Jones et al., 1993).

PROSPECTS FOR THE FUTURE

A statement of how oral health status and services should be improved over the next 25 years must consider both the factors that contribute to dental diseases and to their prevention or successful treatment and the prospects for change in those factors (Bailit, 1987). What developments might substantially affect oral health status? Four likely sources of change merit brief review: expanded use of existing technologies, new scientific and technological discoveries, more patient outcomes research and guidelines for dental practice, and improved access to oral health services. The following discussion draws in particular on the background papers by Bader and Shugars, Jeffcoat and Clarke, and Greenspan.

EXPANDED APPLICATION AND REFINEMENT OF EXISTING INTERVENTIONS

Fluoridation of Community Water Supplies

Water fluoridation is a simple, inexpensive, and effective method of preventing caries in all populations. In 1992, however, only 62 percent of the population that was supplied by public water systems received water with recommended levels of fluoridation (natural or added). By state, this percentage ranged from 2.1 in Nevada to 100 percent in South Dakota (CDC, 1993). As described in Chapter 2, political controversies have blocked fluoridation in many communities and continue to do so today (McNeil, 1957; McClure, 1970; USDHHS, 1991).

Sealants

In the 1980s, only 14 percent of children had sealants applied whereas public health experts have set a target of 50 percent by the year 2000 (Appendix 3A). Unlike water fluoridation, the application of sealants requires positive action by parents. Some, however, will not be able to afford this care for their children, and some will be unaware of its advantages. In addition, acceptance of sealants by dentists has been relatively slow (Gift and Frew, 1986; NIDR, 1990). School-based programs are attractive, but legal restrictions on the use of allied personnel to apply sealants may reduce the scope of school-based sealant initiatives until simpler techniques are developed or licensure restrictions are eased. If health care reforms were enacted to cover childhood preventive services, financial obstacles to broader use of this technology would be much reduced.

Oral Hygiene and Personal Responsibility

The toothbrush and dental floss are, despite the latest rounds of innovations by manufacturers, at the low end of the technology scale. Nonetheless, when used regularly and correctly, they are remarkably effective (Mandel, 1994). Regular use of dental floss is, however, far less common than brushing. To the extent that good oral hygiene habits are related to income and education, health maintenance strategies that depend on these habits are less likely to affect those most in need. This explains the emphasis on population-oriented actions such as fluoridation, which does not require individual behavior to change, and application of dental sealants, which involves a single episode of care rather than maintenance of certain behaviors over long periods and which can be organized as a public health program. Nonetheless, the message of personal responsibility for one's health remains a valid one.

Biomaterials

Developments in dental biomaterials tend to attract considerable attention, in part because of the aesthetic benefits of many new materials and in part because material-based interventions are more consistent with established practice and reimbursement patterns than are pharmacological strategies. Because many of these innovations are most accessible to the more affluent—and healthier—populations and because they often emphasize aesthetic benefits, their potential impact on population health status appears more limited than interventions that affect the high-risk groups that have limited access to dental care.

Nonetheless, refinements in existing bonding, implant, and other interventions and better appreciation of their overall benefits for many patients will expand their application (NIDR, 1990; Leinfelder, 1993). New materials and related processes now under development, such as restorative products incorporating fluorides and antimicrobials, are likely to continue to improve the life of restorations and to reduce the incidence of secondary caries, endodontic problems, and other conditions associated with restoration failures and replacements.

Dental schools have been criticized for slow introduction of some biomaterial innovations into the curriculum (see, for example, ADA, 1992c). Educators can contribute to the appropriate use of biomaterials to improve oral health status in two ways. First, they can educate students in new—and established—techniques. Second, they can educate students and faculty to critically evaluate the appropriateness of a particular intervention or material for an individual patient's specific clinical problem. In an area where technical innovation is common and voluminous, continuing education that stresses both technique and decision making will be particularly important.

SCIENTIFIC AND TECHNOLOGICAL BREAKTHROUGHS

Medical Management

In coming decades, advances in medical management have substantial potential to improve oral health status, particularly for higher-risk individuals. Medical advances are occurring on two broad (but not unrelated) fronts. The first involves preventive, diagnostic, and therapeutic strategies for patients with uncommon oral health problems (e.g., disorders of the salivary glands) or problems complicated by other medical conditions (e.g., AIDS, cancers that require radiation treatment). The second front involves relatively common problems (e.g., caries and periodontitis). On both fronts, research on nontactile diagnosis of caries, molecular probes for identifying a variety of oral problems, antibacterial and anti-inflammatory agents, tissue regeneration products, and genetically engineered saliva substitutes may fundamentally realign the emphasis on medical versus mechanical interventions (see, for example, Baum et al., 1989; Taubman et al., 1989; NIDR, 1990; and the background papers by Greenspan and by Jeffcoat and Clark). The *Journal of the American Dental Association* recently devoted an entire special issue to the emerging field of oral pharmaceuticals, a key component of the medical management of diverse oral health problems (Douglass and Fox, 1994). Practitioners' understanding of the systemic and biological bases for oral health care is becoming ever more important, as is clear and timely communication among dentists, dental hygienists, physicians, nurses, and other health professionals involved in the care of individuals with complex health problems.

CAD/CAM Technology

The computer-assisted design (CAD) and manufacture (CAM) of dental restorations has the potential to reduce substantially the total time required to fabricate restorations such as crowns and bridges. Currently available systems are expensive, limited in practical utility, and not widely used. Whether design breakthroughs will increase the technical acceptability, convenience, and cost-effectiveness of the technology is uncertain. Thus, how widely it will diffuse into everyday dental practice remains a question.

Caries and Periodontal Vaccines

Despite the impact of fluorides in reducing caries, a vaccine for caries has the potential to achieve substantial further reductions, particularly among older children and adults. Investigators are studying strategies that include vaccines aimed primarily at high-risk individuals, polyvalent vaccines to cover several common childhood diseases as well as caries, and vaccines developed or administered in traditional ways. Although the knowledge base has advanced substantially, the time demands of clinical trials, worries about product liability, and declining public compliance with immunization recommendations make it relatively unlikely that oral health status, dental practice, or dental education will be changed significantly by the availability of a caries vaccine within the next 5 to 15 years (Taubman and Smith, 1993; Edelstein, 1994; see also background papers by Greenspan and Jeffcoat and Clark).

The prospects for effective and feasible periodontal vaccines are cloudier than those for caries for several reasons. Periodontal disease is not a single disease but several diseases that are associated with a fairly large number of pathogens. Important questions of disease causation remain to be answered (NIDR, 1990; Genco, 1994). Although unexpected breakthroughs are certainly possible, no generally effective vaccine is expected within the foreseeable future. Furthermore, in light of the nation's difficulties in achieving widely accepted goals for childhood immunization against a variety of diseases, widespread adult immunization against periodontal disease may be difficult to achieve.

OUTCOMES RESEARCH AND GUIDELINES FOR PRACTICE

The last decade has seen an explosion of interest in the effectiveness of health services, the extent and sources of variation in clinical practice patterns, and the formulation of evidence-based guidelines for clinical decisionmaking (see, for example, Eddy, 1984, 1990, 1991; Wennberg, 1984, 1990; IOM, 1985, 1989b, 1989c, 1992; Brook, 1989; Audet et al., 1990). As defined by the Institute of Medicine (IOM), clinical practice guidelines are "systematically developed statements to assist practitioner and patient decisions about appropriate health care for specific clinical circumstances" (IOM, 1990a, p. 38).[3]

The background paper prepared for this study by Bader and Shugars is the most comprehensive analysis to date of these issues in the context of oral health services. This paper describes efforts to analyze dental practice variations, measure outcomes of dental interventions, and develop guidelines for dental practice. The

---

[3]The American Dental Association and some other dental organizations have followed the conventions of the American Medical Association (AMA) in using the term "practice parameters" rather than guidelines. The AMA has had an active program to guide the development and dissemination of practice parameters (AMA, 1990a,b, 1991).

relevant literature is not, however, voluminous. Many clinical interventions in dentistry—as well as in medicine—have never been subjected to rigorous scientific investigation. Their effectiveness has been assumed on the basis of experience, indirect scientific evidence, and judgment.

Policymakers, insurers, and consumers are, however, demanding that more be done to document what works and what does not work in health care, and dentistry is not immune from these demands (Bader, 1992; Kantor, 1992; Pew Health Professions Commissions, 1992; Antczak-Bouckoms, 1993). Several dental organizations have developed practice guidelines, but the efforts of the American Dental Association to do so have been troubled by disagreements about purposes, procedures, and content (Berry, 1991; Spaeth, 1993). A new project to develop guidelines was approved in 1993 and began work in January 1994 (Spaeth, 1994). To the extent that better evidence of the effectiveness of dental interventions is accumulated and transformed into guidelines that, in turn, shape dental practice, the result should be further improvements in dental care and oral health status.

Practice guidelines are not, however, self-implementing. Some of the problems in implementation can be traced to deficiencies in the guidelines themselves including vagueness, bias, inconsistency, poor documentation of the evidence behind recommendations, unhelpful formats, and limited dissemination or availability (IOM, 1992). Other problems lie on the user side—organizational constraints, economic counterpressures, habit, psychological resistance to change, and failure to stay abreast of new knowledge (see, for example, Eisenberg, 1986; Lomas, 1991; Kibbe et al., 1994). Given the relatively cool reception of dentistry to initial guidelines development efforts, considerable persistence will likely be required before guidelines become a vehicle for change in dental practice. Nonetheless, as the pressures for accountability for both patient outcomes and costs increase in dentistry as they are elsewhere in health care, they will encourage clinicians to welcome guidelines that are clear, specific, and grounded in science. Researchers in dental schools have an important role to play in developing the clinical research base for guidelines and in assessing the factors that influence their acceptance and use by clinicians.

IMPROVED ACCESS TO CARE

Access to dental care could be improved by reducing economic, geographic, cultural, and other obstacles to access. For example, dental insurance, which is associated with better financial access to care and higher use of services, could be extended through public or private action or both. As this report was being drafted, a number of legislative proposals for health care reform were being considered that would extend coverage of some dental services to some of the population. Three dimensions of potential health care reform are particularly important: the definition and administration of a standard or basic benefit package; the tax treatment of private insurance coverage beyond a basic or standard benefit package; and the provisions for the elderly and the poor. At issue in decisions about the benefit package are: What would be covered (e.g., primarily preventive services or restorative care as well); who would the package cover (e.g., only children or adults also); and when would coverage take effect? The major issue in the taxation of health benefits is whether all or some employer-paid coverage of services in excess of a standard plan would be taxed (e.g., counted as taxable income for individuals or treated as nondeductible expenses for employers). Such benefits are not now taxed. Were dental benefits to be excluded from a standard benefit package *and* also subject to taxation, then coverage might actually decrease from current levels.

Although dental insurance helps transform the need for care into effective demand, geographic, cultural, and other barriers to care may remain (IOM, 1993a). Some of these barriers may be offset by community-wide prevention programs (e.g., fluoridation of water supplies), but local, state, and federal programs designed to make personal oral health services more accessible to special populations will continue to be important. School-based programs, as described earlier, focus on underserved children who account for a disproportionate share of untreated caries, and the Community and Migrant Health Centers program and the National Health Service Corps (NCHS) target underserved rural and urban areas. The dental component of the latter program, however, declined substantially in the 1980s as the number of NHSC dental field positions dropped from about 500 in 1982 to 50 in 1989. (See Chapters 4 and 9 for further discussion of this program.) Since the 1970s, the oral health activities of the U.S. Department of Health and Human Services have, according to a 1989 report, been "disaggregated, dispersed, reduced drastically, or altogether eliminated" (USDHHS, p. 9). The same report was unable to identify a "discernable oral health policy" or a focal point of administrative responsibility for dental activities within the department.

In addition, as the number and proportion of elderly individuals grow dramatically in coming years, the need for programs aimed at nursing home patients and homebound individuals will also grow. Medicare's lack of dental benefits (which most reform proposals would not change) and state restrictions on services provided by allied dental personnel will likely become more significant policy issues.

It now seems unlikely that public policymakers will undertake either major or incremental steps to extend covverage for oral health care. Thus, the prospects for improved access to oral health care are uncertain, particularly for those most in need.

RECOMMENDATIONS OF OTHER GROUPS

ORAL HEALTH STATUS AND SERVICES

The most common dental diseases—caries and periodontal disease—are largely preventable through a combination of community, professional, and personal practices. Thus, most proposals to improve oral health status of individuals and populations over the long run focus on preventive rather than curative strategies. However, disparities in treatment across socioeconomic groups make effective access to basic dental care a major objective of some proposals.

As part of the Healthy People 2000 initiative, the federal government published in 1990 a set of comprehensive and specific objectives for improving the health of Americans (USDHHS, 1990). Oral health was one of the 22 defined priority areas for which more than 300 objectives were set. The project defined 16 primary goals for oral health, most of which included subgoals for groups with poorer than average health. (Appendix 3A lists the 16 Oral Health 2000 goals and associated data and research needs.) The 16 goals have been endorsed by most major dental groups including the American Dental Association.

A major initiative on behalf of the Healthy People 2000 objectives is Oral Health 2000, which was launched by the American Fund for Dental Health with funding from NIDR and support from an array of public and private organizations. The three broad goals of this initiative are "to reduce the occurrence and severity of oral diseases in the U.S. population; to prevent the unnecessary loss of teeth, whether resulting from oral diseases, neglect or trauma; [and] to alleviate the physical, cultural, racial, ethnic, social, educational, health care delivery system and environmental barriers that prevent individuals from achieving healthy oral functioning" (American Fund for Dental Health, 1992, p. 1).

A generally similar set of goals guides the NIDR program focused on the oral health of higher-risk individuals. These goals are "to eliminate toothlessness in America in future generations; to prevent further deterioration of the oral health of those with already compromised dentition; [and] to ensure that adults already in good health maintain that state as they advance to the retirement years" (NIDR, 1990, p. 6).

The 1989 report of the U.S. Preventive Services Task Force noted the importance of good oral health status. Appendix 3B presents an excerpt from the guidelines developed by that group to advise physicians on oral health counseling. The task force noted that little evidence exists about the impact of physician counseling and that the efficacy of some oral health interventions or the appropriate interval for some services is unclear.

A 1980 IOM study focused on national health insurance, not goals for oral health status or oral health services per se. Nonetheless, its priorities for coverage reflect judgments about the most cost-effective, long-range strategies for improving oral health (IOM, 1980, p. 6). The priorities targeted, in order,

- preventive services for children and adolescents,
- other services for children and adolescents (beginning with diagnostic services),
- preventive services for adults, and
- other services for adults.

Appendix 3C includes the more detailed priorities described in the IOM report. Although it recommended coverage priorities for a national health plan, the study observed that national insurance coverage was not, overall, the most cost-effective strategy to improve oral health. Rather, because oral problems are concentrated among the poor, an expansion of Medicaid dental coverage and, in particular, school-based programs might very well accomplish more. Thus, the 1980 committee recommended, "that at a minimum, and even if national health insurance is not enacted, steps should be taken to assure that the children of low-income families have access to . . . basic dental services" (IOM, 1980, p. 8).

PRACTICE GUIDELINES

The Institute of Medicine has issued two major reports on guidelines for clinical practice with recommendations about their development and implementation (IOM, 1990a, 1992). Appendix 3D lists attributes for sound clinical practice guidelines set forth in these studies.[4]   Each attribute affects the probability that guidelines will be perceived as credible and usable or that they will, if used, help achieve desired health outcomes. As described in the 1992 IOM report (pp. 29, 31), "these attributes imply a challenging analytic strategy for developers of practice guidelines that, in summary, involves the following steps:

- formulation of the problem (for example, the clinical condition to be considered, the key issues to be addressed, and the relevant alternative courses of care to be examined, which may include 'watchful waiting');
- identification and assessment of the evidence from clinical trials, case-control studies, and other sources to determine where evidence is weak, missing, or in dispute;
- projection and comparison of health benefits and harms (including how they are perceived by patients) associated with alternative courses of care;
- projection of net costs associated with achieving the benefits of alternative courses of care;
- judgment of the strength of the evidence (considering key areas of scientific uncertainty and theoretical dispute), the relative importance of the projected benefits and risks (again with patient perspectives considered), and—overall—how compelling is the case for particular interventions;
- formulation of clear statements about alternative courses of care, accompanied by full disclosure of the participants, methods, evidence, and criteria used to arrive at these statements; and
- review and critique of all these elements by methodologists, clinicians, and other relevant parties not involved in the original process."

Challenging as the development of guidelines is, their implementation is an even more formidable task. Just as the effectiveness of a dental treatment cannot be assumed, neither can the effectiveness of practice guidelines. Research to evaluate their impact on behavior and patient outcomes is essential, and faculties in dental schools should have an important role to play in initiating and undertaking such research. In addition to research

---

[4]The 1992 IOM report included an instrument to assess the soundness of a set of guidelines. The instrument, which underwent preliminary testing during its development, is being used by other groups to assist their assessments of guidelines.

undertaken in dental school facilities, other opportunities for outcomes research should be pursued with suitable dental public health programs, health maintenance organizations, dental service units of the Department of Veterans Affairs medical centers, and similar organizations or groups. Chapter 5 reiterates this proposal.

COMMITTEE FINDINGS AND RECOMMENDATIONS

This committee did not attempt to assess independently the specific health status goals established by Oral Health 2000 or other groups; neither did it attempt to revise the quantitative targets over a longer time period. Rather, the committee focused on four broad health objectives, namely,

1. *reducing disparities in oral health status and services* experienced by disadvantaged economic, racial, or other groups;
2. *improving our knowledge of what works and what does not work* to prevent, diagnose, or treat oral health problems;
3. *encouraging prevention* at both the *individual level* (e.g., feeding practices that prevent baby bottle tooth decay; reduced use of tobacco) and the *community level* (e.g., fluoridation of community water supplies and school-based prevention programs); and
4. *promoting attention to oral health* (including the oral manifestations of other health problems) not just among dental practitioners but also *among other primary care providers, geriatricians, educators, and public officials.*

These emphases are consistent with the focus in dental education, and in public policy more broadly, on the general practitioner and on primary care.[5] They essentially assume the continued technical competence of dental practitioners in using both established and new technologies (e.g., in placing sealants or dental implants). In their focus on disadvantaged groups and on prevention, these emphases are also generally consistent with the rec-

---

[5]Primary care is defined by the kind of care provided *not* by the professional category of the provider (IOM, 1978, 1984, 1994c). Primary care providers are, ideally, the initial and continuing source of care for a broad array of common health problems. They help to integrate specialist and community health and health-related services so that patient care is coordinated and not fragmented. By most definitions, primary care also considers and serves community health needs (WHO, 1978; Isman, 1993). These aspects of primary care are reflected in the guiding principles for this report as stated in Chapter 1.

ommendations of the 1980 IOM study of dental health options. Some committee members were concerned, however, that the Department of Health and Human Services lacked a real organizational focus for setting priorities, coordinating activities, and generally making the best use of limited resources for oral health.

Although the charge to this committee did not include formulating proposals for reforming dental care financing and delivery, some general policy implications flow from the principles that oral health is an integral part of total health and that a focus on health outcomes is essential. Rather than be categorically excluded by public or private programs, coverage for dental care ought to be weighed in terms of its benefits and costs relative to other services being considered for coverage. Following this rationale, the coverage priorities in the 1980 IOM report started with coverage for preventive services and then restorative services for children followed by preventive and then restorative services for adults. This committee believes these priorities remain essentially valid today. Whether or not health care reform legislation is enacted, the goal of improving oral health status through individual and community programs for currently disadvantaged groups—both children and adults—should be a high priority.

For dental education, what are the implications of this discussion? Dental educators have a central role to play in encouraging and promoting basic science and clinical and health services research to distinguish effective and ineffective oral health services; to clarify oral disease patterns or trends and the factors affecting them; and to identify cost-effective strategies likely to help those with the poorest health status and those with limited access to oral health services. Such strategies include both individual and community services and methods for organizing as well as delivering care to those most in need. *Implementation of these strategies requires public support for community service and outreach programs undertaken by dental schools, public health agencies, dental societies, and other groups.*

In addition, health services researchers in dental schools can play an important role in monitoring and analyzing changes in oral health and in the health care system generally. Important changes in health care financing and delivery may emerge slowly or relatively quickly, and they may be long lasting or temporary. The dental community must be cognizant of these possibilities and be prepared to monitor, analyze, and respond to such changes by communicating with policymakers about how the changes proposed might affect the availability, affordability, and effectiveness of dental services and the oral health of the public. As noted in Chapter 6, these changes could significantly affect the patient care mission of the dental school. Although differences among educators and practitioners may sometimes preclude consistent responses, health services researchers can make a contribution to the policy debates with analyses and projections that are objective insofar as possible but that acknowledge the role of value judgments.

As observed throughout this chapter, one limitation facing dental community efforts to improve oral health is a scarcity of consistent, regular information on the oral health status of the population. Another is the modest level of research on the outcomes of alternative interventions.

To support effective and efficient oral health services that improve individual and community health, the committee recommends that dental educators work with public and private organizations to

• maintain a standardized process in the U.S. Department of Health and Human Services to regularly assess the oral health status of the population and identify changing disease patterns at the community and national levels;
• develop and implement a systematic research agenda to evaluate the outcomes of alternative methods of preventing, diagnosing, and treating oral health problems; and
• make use of scientific evidence, outcomes research, and formal consensus processes in devising practice guidelines.

These steps will help prepare dental educators, practitioners, and policymakers to understand and respond to various possible futures. They build on the mission of the dental school to create and disseminate new scientific knowledge and technological innovations.

Armed with better knowledge of oral health trends and effective interventions, the dental community also will be positioned to encourage physicians, nursing home personnel, public officials, and others to be alert to oral health problems among those whom they serve, to provide them with information about good oral health habits, to refer their patients to dental practitioners as appropriate, and to seek advice when they are not certain about what course to take. As part of significant changes now occurring in health care delivery and financing, nurse practitioners are poised to assume more responsibilities for primary and preventive care, and they, like physicians, will need to be alert to patients' oral problems or risks. Dental educators should work with their colleagues in various health professions schools to communicate these themes to medical, nursing, public health, and other students and to experiment with new strategies in didactic and clinical education that reinforce these points.

As discussed further in Chapter 4, realizing the potential for successful medical management of more oral health problems will require continued adaptations in education and practice and, generally, a closer alignment between dentistry and medicine. The growth in numbers of the elderly and the decrease in edentulism in this group also point to the need for curriculum changes, some of which will focus specifically on the geriatric population and some of which will reinforce the medical orientation recommended above.

SUMMARY

Scientific, public health, and other advances have greatly improved the oral health of the American people in recent decades. Nonetheless, significant oral health problems remain common and are concentrated in populations with limited access to dental services. In coming decades, oral health will be affected by further scientific and technological progress, although the timing of specific breakthroughs and their rate of diffusion into practice are hard to predict. Likewise, the degree to which access to oral health services will improve for high-risk or underserved populations is difficult to predict in the midst of a fractious debate over health care reform.

Dental educators have an important role to play in building the scientific, epidemiological, and organizational knowledge base for improved oral health and oral health services. Measuring and evaluating progress in oral health, however, requires more consistent and regular information on oral health status and more research on the outcomes of established and new oral health interventions. Making full use of growing knowledge will, in turn, require dental educators to revise how and what the students are taught and to adjust the ways in which patient care is provided within the dental school. The next three chapters pursue these points.

APPENDIX 3.A OBJECTIVES FOR ORAL HEALTH FROM HEALTHY PEOPLE 2000

13.1 **Reduce dental caries (cavities) so that the proportion of children with one or more caries (in permanent or primary teeth) is no more than 35 percent among children aged 6 through 8 and no more than 60 percent among adolescents aged 15. (Baseline: 53 percent of children aged 6 through 8 in 1986-1987; 78 percent of adolescents aged 15 in 1986-1987).**

	Special Population Targets	
Caries Prevalence	1986-1987 Baseline	2000 Target Dental Percent Decrease
13.1a Children aged 6-8 whose parents have less than high school education	70%	45%
13.1b American Indian/Alaska Native children aged 6-8	92%[a] 52%[b]	45%
13.1c Black children aged 6-8	61%	40%
13.1d American Indian/Alaska Native adolescents aged 15	93%[b]	70%

13.2 **Reduce untreated dental caries so that the proportion of children with untreated caries (in permanent or primary teeth) is no more than 20 percent among children aged 6 through 8 and no more than 15 percent among adolescents aged 15. (Baseline: 27 percent of children aged 6 through 8 in 1986; 23 percent of adolescents aged 15 in 1986-1987)**

	Special Population Targets	
Dental Caries	1986-1987 Baseline	2000 Target Untreated Percent Decrease
Among Children		
13.2a Children aged 6-8 whose parents have less than high school education	43%	30%
13.2b American Indian/Alaska Native children aged 6-8	64%[c]	35%
13.2c Black children aged 6-8	38%	25%
13.2d Hispanic children aged 6-8	36%[d]	25%
Among Adolescents		
13.2a Adolescents aged 15 whose parents have less than high school education	41%	25%
13.2b American Indian/Alaska Native adolescents aged 15	84%[c]	40%
13.2c Black adolescents aged 15	38%	20%
13.2d Hispanic adolescents aged 15	31%-47%[d]	25%

13.3   Increase to at least 45 percent the proportion of people aged 35 through 44 who have never lost a permanent tooth due to dental caries or periodontal disease. (Baseline: 31 percent of employed adults had never lost a permanent tooth for any reason in 1985-1986)

13.4   Reduce to no more than 20 percent the proportion of people aged 65 and older who have lost all of their natural teeth. (Baseline: 36 percent in 1986)

Complete Tooth Loss Prevalence	Special Population Target	
	1986 Baseline	2000 Target Percent Decrease
13.4a Low-income people (annual family income <$15,000)	46%	25%

13.5   Reduce the prevalence of gingivitis among people aged 35 through 44 to no more than 30 percent. (Baseline: 42 percent in 1985-1986)

Gingivitis Prevalence	Special Population Targets	
	1985 Baseline	2000 Target Gingivitis Percent Decrease
13.5a Low-income people (annual family income <$12,500)	50%	35%
13.5b American Indian/Alaska Native	95%[e]	50%
13.5c Hispanics		50%
Mexican Americans	74%[f]	
Cubans	79%	
Puerto Ricans	82%	

13.6   Reduce destructive periodontal diseases to a prevalence of no more than 15 percent among people aged 35 through 44. (Baseline: 24 percent in 1985-1986)

13.7   Reduce deaths due to cancer of the oral cavity and pharynx to no more than 10.5 per 100,000 men aged 45 through 74 and 4.1 per 100,000 women aged 45 through 74. (Baseline: 12.1 per 100,000 men and 4.1 per 100,000 women in 1987)

13.8   Increase to at least 50 percent the proportion of children who have received protective sealants on the occlusal (chewing) surfaces of permanent molar teeth. (Baseline: 11 percent of children aged 8 and 8 percent of adolescents aged 14 in 1986-1987)

13.9   Increase to at least 75 percent the proportion of people served by community water systems providing optimal levels of fluoride. (Baseline: 62 percent in 1989)

13.10   Increase use of professionally or self-administered topical or systemic (dietary) fluorides to at least 85 percent of people not receiving optimally fluoridated public water. (Baseline: An estimated 50 percent in 1989)

13.11   Increase to at least 75 percent the proportion of parents and caregivers who use feeding practices that prevent baby bottle tooth decay. (Baseline data available in 1991)

Special Population Targets

Appropriate Feeding Practices	Baseline	2000 Target
13.11a Parents and caregivers with less than high school education	—	65%
13.11b American Indian/Alaska Native parents and caregivers	—	65%

13.12 Increase to at least 90 percent the proportion of all children entering school programs for the first time who have received an oral health screening, referral, and followup for necessary diagnostic, preventive, and treatment services. (Baseline: 66 percent of children aged 5 visited a dentist during the previous year in 1986)

13.13 Extend to all long-term institutional facilities the requirement that oral examinations and services be provided no later than 90 days after entry into these facilities. (Baseline: Nursing facilities receiving Medicaid or Medicare reimbursement will be required to provide for oral examinations within 90 days of patient entry beginning in 1990; baseline data unavailable for other institutions)

13.14 Increase to at least 70 percent the proportion of people aged 35 and older using the oral health care system during each year. (Baseline: 54 percent in 1986)

Special Population Targets

Proportion Using Oral Health Care During Each Year	1986 Baseline	2000 Target System Percent Decrease
13.14a Edentulous people	11%	50%
13.14b People aged 65 and older	42%	60%

13.15 Increase to at least 40 the number of States that have an effective system for recording and referring infants with cleft lips and/or palates to craniofacial anomaly teams. (Baseline: In 1988, approximately 25 States had a central recording mechanism for cleft lip and/or palate and approximately 25 States had an organized referral system to craniofacial anomaly teams)

13.16 Extend requirement of the use of effective head, face, eye, and mouth protection to all organizations, agencies, and institutions sponsoring sporting and recreation events that pose risks of injury. (Baseline: Only National Collegiate Athletic Association football, hockey, and lacrosse; high school football; amateur boxing; and amateur ice hockey in 1988)

[a]In primary teeth in 1983-1984.
[b]In permanent teeth in 1983-1984.
[c]1983-1984 baseline.
[d]1982-1984 baseline.
[e]1983-84 baseline.
[f]1982-84 baseline.

SOURCE: U.S. Department of Health and Human Services. *Healthy People 2000: National Health Promotion and Disease Prevention Objectives.* DHHS Publication No. (PHS) 91-5021. Washington, D.C.: U.S. Government Printing Office, 1990, pp. 352-361.

APPENDIX 3.B EXCERPT FROM U.S. PREVENTIVE SERVICES TASK FORCE GUIDELINES FOR COUNSELING TO PREVENT DENTAL DISEASE

CLINICAL INTERVENTIONS

All patients should be encouraged to visit the dentist on a regular basis. The optimal frequency of visits should be determined by the patient's dentist; for most healthy patients, a dental checkup once every one to two years is sufficient. All patients should also be encouraged to brush their teeth daily with a fluoride-containing toothpaste. Adolescents and adults should be advised to clean thoroughly between the teeth with dental floss each day. Those persons with a history of frequent caries may benefit from reduced intake of foods containing refined sugars and by avoiding sugary between-meal snacks. Pregnant women, parents, and caregivers of young children should be counseled to put children to bed without a bottle and to substitute a cup for the bottle when the child reaches 1 year of age. If the child must have a bottle, it should be filled with water.

In accordance with existing guidelines, children living in an area with inadequate water fluoridation (less than 0.7 parts per million [ppm]) should be prescribed daily fluoride drops or tablets. Fluoride tablets should be prescribed for children over age 3; the recommended dose is 1 mg/day if the community water fluoride concentration is less than 0.3 ppm, and 0.50 mg/day if the concentration is 0.3-0.7 ppm. For children 2 to 3 years of age the corresponding doses are 0.50 mg/day and 0.25 mg/day, respectively, and either drops or tablets are appropriate. Children under age 2 should be treated with fluoride drops if the water concentration is less than 0.3 ppm; the recommended dose is 0.25 mg/day.

When examining the mouth, clinicians should be alert for obvious signs of untreated tooth decay, inflamed or cyanotic gingiva, loose teeth, and severe halitosis. Screening for oral cancer should be performed for high risk groups (see Chapter 15), and all patients should be counseled regarding the use of tobacco products (Chapter 48). Children should also be examined for evidence of baby bottle tooth decay, mismatching of upper and lower dental arches, crowding or malalignment of the teeth, premature loss of primary posterior teeth (baby molars), and obvious mouth breathing. Patients with these or other suspected abnormalities should be referred to their dentists for further evaluation.

SOURCE: U.S. Preventive Services Task Force. *Guide to Clinical Preventive Services: An Assessment of the Effectiveness of 169 Interventions.* Baltimore, MD: Williams & Wilkins, 1989, p. 354.

APPENDIX 3.C EXCERPT FROM 1980 IOM REPORT ON PRIORITIES FOR DENTAL COVERAGE UNDER NATIONAL HEALTH INSURANCE

1. Prevention for children and adolescents
   a. Integration of dental health education and plaque control into general education program
   b. Screening examination, prophylaxis (aged 12-17 years only), an appropriate type of fluoride application, and sealants where applicable

2. Comprehensive services (other than prevention) for children and adolescents
   a. Examination
   b. Radiographs
   c. Space maintainers
   d. Extractions
   e. Restorations
   f. Crowns
   g. Endodontic treatment
   h. Treatment of handicapping malocclusion

3. Prevention for adults (18 years and over)
   a. Screening examination and prophylaxis
   b. Prophylaxis

4. Comprehensive services for adults
   a. Examination
   b. Radiographs
   c. Extractions
   d. Periodontal treatment
   e. Restorations
   f. Crowns
   g. Endodontic treatment
   h. Replacement services
      1. Bridges
      2. Full and partial dentures

SOURCE: Institute of Medicine (IOM). *Public Policy Options for Better Dental Health.* Washington, D.C.: National Academy Press, 1980.

APPENDIX 3.D DESIRABLE ATTRIBUTES OF CLINICAL PRACTICE GUIDELINES (IOM)

Attribute	Explanation
VALIDITY	Practice guidelines are valid if, when followed, they lead to the health and cost outcomes projected for them. A prospective assessment of validity will consider the substance and quality of the evidence cited, the means used to evaluate the evidence, and the relationship between the evidence and recommendations.
Strength of Evidence	Practice guidelines should be accompanied by descriptions of the strength of the evidence and the expert judgment behind them.
Estimated Outcomes	Practice guidelines should be accompanied by estimates of the health and cost outcomes expected from the interventions in question, compared with alternative practices. Assessments of relevant health outcomes will consider patient perceptions and preferences.

RELIABILITY/ REPRODUCIBILITY	Practice guidelines are reproducible and reliable (1) if—given the same evidence and methods for guidelines development—another set of experts produces essentially the same statements and (2) if—given the same clinical circumstances—the guidelines are interpreted and applied consistently by practitioners (or other appropriate parties).
CLINICAL APPLICABILITY	Practice guidelines should be as inclusive of appropriately defined patient populations as evidence and expert judgment permit, and they should explicitly state the population(s) to which statements apply.
CLINICAL FLEXIBILITY	Practice guidelines should identify the specifically known or generally expected exceptions to their recommendations and discuss how patient preferences are to be identified and considered.
CLARITY	Practice guidelines must use unambiguous language, define terms precisely, and use logical, easy-to-follow modes of presentation.
MULTIDISCIPLINARY PROCESS	Practice guidelines must be developed by a process that includes participation by representatives of key affected groups. Participation may include serving on panels that develop guidelines, providing evidence and viewpoints to the panels, and reviewing draft guidelines.
SCHEDULED REVIEW	Practice guidelines must include statements about when they should be reviewed to determine whether revisions are warranted, given new clinical evidence or professional consensus (or the lack of it).
DOCUMENTATION	The procedures followed in developing guidelines, the participants involved, the evidence used, the assumptions and rationales accepted, and the analytic methods employed must be meticulously documented and described.

SOURCE: Institute of Medicine. *Guidelines for Clinical Practice: From Development to Use.* M.J. Field and K.N. Lohr, eds. Washington, D.C.: National Academy Press, 1992.

4

The Mission of Education

The most visible mission of dental education is to develop future practitioners. Broadly stated, its basic goals are to *(1) educate students to serve their patients and communities well* and *(2) prepare students to continue to grow in skill and knowledge over their lifetime in practice.* This report throughout refers to "education" rather than "training" to emphasize that dentistry as a profession demands both intellectual and technical skills that depend on clinically relevant education in the basic sciences and scientifically informed education in clinical care.

This chapter starts by putting current curriculum critiques in historical context. It then discusses several major curriculum concerns within the framework of principles established in Chapter 1. Then, because a sound curriculum means little without capable faculty and students, two major sections consider the people who constitute the heart of a dental school and whose careful recruitment and continued development are essential to the educational changes proposed in this chapter. Although the emphasis is on predoctoral education, this chapter also examines the critical relationship between predoctoral and advanced education in general dentistry. Continuing education, sometimes viewed as part of a university's service mission, is here considered to be one more stage of a lifelong learning process that professionals must pursue and dental schools must support. Research and patient care, which are examined in Chapters 5 and 6, are critical in their own right but are also crucial contributors to the kind of educational enterprise recommended in this chapter.

The discussion below tends to focus on dental schools as discrete entities. The committee did not, however, intend to understate the role of organizations such as the American Association of Dental Schools (AADS) or limited-purpose consortia of several dental schools as promoters of change. These groups serve many valuable purposes, for example, by stimulating discussion, facilitating communication about innovative programs, devising model approaches to common problems, providing technical support, collecting and analyzing information, and promoting good relationships with organized dentistry and others. Collective as well as individual effort is essential if the changes recommended are to be achieved.

CURRICULUM IN CONTEXT

A curriculum embodies the values and vision of an institution and a discipline. As expressed in the principles stated in Chapter 1, dental education should be scientifically based, clinically relevant, medically informed, and socially responsible. It should emphasize outcomes as well as services, efficiency as well as effectiveness, and community as well as individual needs. It should prepare students to critically assess both new and old technologies and practices throughout their careers.

Traditionally, faculty have largely controlled school and department decisions about what is taught, by whom, and in what fashion. As discussed in a later section of this chapter, among the most important and difficult factors affecting the direction and pace of curriculum change are those involving the composition, power, and disciplinary organization of faculty.

SEVENTY YEARS OF CURRICULUM CRITIQUES

In the course of this study, the committee heard a lively debate about the strengths and weaknesses of current curricula and the values and vision that curriculum reform should reflect. As the background paper by Tedesco underscores, most critiques of the dental curriculum are long-standing. The core concepts behind changes that are still being advocated date back several decades.

Moreover, if the word "medical" were changed to "dental," the basic points of several persistent critiques of undergraduate medical education could easily apply to dentistry (Enarson and Burg, 1992). The links between the Flexner report (1910) on medical education and the Gies report (1926) on dental education have already been cited in Chapter 2. In the 1960s, the report *Planning for Medical Progress Through Education* (Coggeshall, 1965) foreshadowed the 1993 recommendations of the Pew Health Professions Commission. For example, it envisioned medical education as a "continuum" that begins with preprofessional years (secondary and collegiate), is marked by the M.D. degree as a "midpoint," and extends with continuous education and reeducation "until the professional life of the practitioner is finished" (pp. 39-40). The Coggeshall report also stressed (as does this report) the importance of health professions schools as integral parts of the university. More recently, the 1992 report *Medical Education in Transition* (sponsored by the Robert Wood Johnson Foundation) argued that "there is [an] . . . urgent need for students to appreciate the relevance—and, indeed, the excitement—of applying today's scientific advances to the practice of medicine" (Marston and Jones, 1992, p. vi). That theme likewise runs throughout this report.

One lesson of past reports is that the dental curriculum is not alone as a target for criticism. A more sobering lesson is that it is much easier to analyze and recommend than to act.[1] The practical, political, and procedural demands of major shifts in course offerings and content test the stamina of those attempting change (AAMC, 1992; Hendrickson et al., 1993). As one educator put it, "Most deans would rather take a daily physical beating than try to make significant changes in the traditional [curriculum]" (Garrison, 1993, p. 344).

Recognizing the difficulties of change, various organizations have tried to assist planning processes, demonstration projects, and other activities in dental schools. The Pew National Dental Education Program offers a model of this kind of private support. It funded strategic planning processes in 21 schools and implementation

---

[1]Apropos of this, Renee Fox has observed this about a series of reports on medical education. They have appeared "at periodic, closely spaced intervals [and] . . . contained virtually the same rediscovered principles, . . . [they have included] the same concern over the degree to which these conceptions are being honored more in the breach than in practice, the same explanatory diagnoses [about] what accounts for these deficiencies, along with renewed dedication to remedying them through essentially the same exhortations and reforms" (Fox, 1990, cited in Howell, 1992, p. 717).

activities in 6 (University of California, San Francisco; Columbia University; University of Florida; University of Maryland; Oregon Health Sciences University; and University of Southern California). These projects are summarized in the background paper by Tedesco, and an initial evaluation of the programs is reported in Feldman et al. (1991).

This committee's findings and recommendations are intended to provide additional guidance and leverage for those with the desire and the will to seek further and more widespread reform of dental school curricula. They are also intended to reflect the interconnections of the education, research, and patient care missions of the dental school and to place curriculum objectives in the context of changing concerns about faculty, students, financing, regulatory practices, and work force planning.

BACKGROUND DATA

The major source of quantitative data on the dental school curriculum is a series of annual education surveys conducted and published by the American Dental Association (ADA). The background paper by Tedesco presents additional historical data from many sources. Information from the survey of deans by the Institute of Medicine (IOM) and the American Association of Dental Schools is also included here.

Through its site visits, survey of deans, public hearing, and other activities, the committee sought to supplement quantitative and written information with a more qualitative sense of the curriculum as experienced by students, faculty, and to a limited degree, patients. In some respects, this qualitative sense is another label for realism, an understanding of the practical and political challenges of change.

Variations in Program Length and Density

The dominant model of dental education is a four-year predoctoral program. One school (the last of a group of 16 that tried a three-year schedule during the 1970s) offers a three-calendar-year predoctoral program, and another has offered a five-calendar-year program that it is planning to reduce to four years. The predoctoral program is generally preceded by a baccalaureate degree with appropriate preprofessional coursework in the sciences. For the majority of dental graduates, it is followed by advanced education in general dentistry or a specialty.

Beyond that common base lies substantial variability in program length and density. The length of the predoctoral program ranges from 120 to 187 weeks, with a mean length of 158 weeks.[2] The number of weeks of instruction for the fourth year of dental school averages 38, with a range from 28 to 49 weeks (a 75 percent difference). Summers have increasingly been filled with academic requirements.

For the four-year programs, total clock hours[3] range from 3,450 to 6,635—an almost twofold difference. Clock hours per week range from 20 to 41; the median number of clock hours per week is 30.

Many schools offer optional programs that allow qualifying students to combine baccalaureate and predoctoral coursework in a structured six- or seven-year program. Some schools cooperate with other university programs to offer joint degrees, for example, a D.D.S. and a master's degree in public health, business, or public policy.

VARIATIONS IN INSTRUCTIONAL ALLOCATIONS

The variability in length of the total dental curriculum extends to individual components. Table 4.1 summarizes the two- to sevenfold differences among schools in hours devoted to basic, clinical, and behavioral sciences. The background paper by Tedesco reveals similar variation among schools in the hours allocated for 12 basic science, 24 clinical science, and 5 behavioral science categories.

The background paper also summarizes historical data on clock hours and their distributions over the past 30 years. These data suggest a gradual increase in curriculum requirements. This committee did not chart statistical changes in clock hours by individual school, but the survey of deans, the site visits, and other information once again suggest considerable variation across schools.

In the deans' survey, a near majority of dental school deans (25 of 54) estimated that overall clock hours of instruction had remained about the same for the past 10 years. Only five suggested that

---

[2]Medical school curricula are similarly variable in length, ranging from 119 to 192 weeks, and the mean is 153 weeks (Jonas et al., 1993).

[3]Clock hours may include lecture, laboratory, or clinic hours or some mix of these. They do not convert into credit hours at a fixed rate. For example, according to the 1993-1995 catalog of the University of Illinois at Chicago (University of Illinois, 1993), the first year includes 200 clock hours of gross anatomy for 8 credit hours and 20 clock hours of dental radiology for 1 credit hour. In the third year, 10 clock hours of introduction to research receives 1 credit hour.

TABLE 4.1   Variability in Curriculum Requirements—
Basic Sciences, Clinical Sciences, and Behavioral Sciences

Curriculum	Total Clock Hours			Percentage of Total Hours		
	Low	Median	High	Low	Mean	High
Basic Sciences						
Didactic	447	574	1,770			
Laboratory	52	206	584			
Total	563	787	2,103	12	17	34
Clinical Sciences						
Didactic	678	1,001	1,535			
Laboratory	398	726	1,208			
Patient care intramural	415	1,938	2,740			
Patient care extramural	8	119	1,798			
Total	2,567	3,844	5,400	64	80	87
Behavioral Sciences						
Didactic	57	115	373			
Laboratory	2	12	120			
Total	57	123	373	1	3	5

SOURCE: Excerpted from American Dental Association, 1994c.

hours had increased rather than decreased. A majority of deans reported some or substantial increases in clock hours in clinical sciences, practice management, research methods, and behavioral science instruction. For the next 15 years, a majority expected further increases in these areas, in clinical training at nontraditional sites, and in working with allied personnel. Twelve deans reported decreases in basic science hours, compared to 10 reporting increases. Decreases in preclinical instruction were reported by 14 deans, but 5 reported increases. A majority of deans (30) predicted that preclinical hours of instruction would drop further. The committee could not determine whether decreases in basic science hours represented a desirable pruning of marginally relevant material or a deemphasis of the scientific foundation of dentistry at a time when that base is becoming more important.

ACCREDITATION STANDARDS AND CURRICULUM GUIDELINES

Curriculum content is influenced by the standards of the Commission on Dental Accreditation and the curriculum guidelines developed independently by the AADS. Curriculum guidelines, which are not enforceable in the same way as accreditation standards, are intended to provide useful models for dental schools that neither stifle innovation nor mire schools in detailed regulatory requirements. As described in more depth in the background by Tedesco, the AADS is redrafting the guidelines to focus on competencies that comprise a mix of skills, practices, and attitudes (or understanding) needed by dental practitioners.

The accreditation standards (and the accompanying discussion) emphasize preparation for lifelong learning (5.1.1), education in scientific reasoning and problem solving (5.1.2), and application of basic science principles to clinical care (5.2.1). Patient assessment and coordinated treatment planning are also stressed (5.3). The charge that accreditation standards stifle innovation focuses, in part, on the detailed specifications in clinical areas and on the standard that "early specialization must not be permitted until the student has achieved a standard of minimal clinical competency in all areas necessary to the practice of general dentistry" (5.1.3) (CDA, 1993a, p. 489).

The committee heard the accreditation standards commended for promoting many of the directions discussed below. It also heard complaints that the standards discouraged innovation. As discussed in Chapter 8, the committee's sense is that both arguments have merit.

ISSUES AND CONTROVERSIES

As noted earlier, 70 years of surveys and reports have identified curriculum problems that persist to a considerable extent today. Most criticisms can be grouped into at least five broad concerns. First, basic science concepts and methods are weakly linked to students' clinical education and experience. Second, the curriculum is insufficiently attuned to current and emerging dental science and practice. Third, many problems remain in implementing comprehensive patient care as a model for clinical education. Fourth, linkages between dentistry and medicine are weak. Fifth, the overcrowded dental curriculum gives students too little time to consolidate concepts and develop critical thinking skills that prepare them for lifelong learning.

INTEGRATING THE BASIC AND CLINICAL SCIENCES

Curriculum Structure

As described in Chapter 2 and in the background paper by Tedesco, the 1910 Flexner report and the 1926 report by William Gies called for curricula that embodied the scientific basis of medicine, including dentistry. Intervening years have broadened the case for basic science education to prepare students to become practitioners who can critically appraise new strategies for patient care and apply them when appropriate and who can understand the relevant biological bases of oral health and disease. Education in the basic sciences should also provide the vocabulary and basic concepts for researchers and clinicians to communicate with each other (Ten Cate, 1986).

Figure 4.1 (derived from Formicola, 1991) depicts graphically the traditional Flexner-Gies organizational scheme.[4] It also presents two alternative models that illustrate curriculum innovations adopted after World War II by medical schools at Cornell, Colorado, and what is now Case Western Reserve (Marston and Jones., 1992). These new models also contain other innovative concepts including comprehensive patient care.

The Flexner-Gies model concentrated basic science education in the early part of the medical and dental school curriculum. Over time, as dental schools settled into a four-year schedule, the first two years of the curriculum also incorporated preclinical instruction (e.g., tooth preparation for restorations).

The traditional curriculum, although a great advance over the nonscientific curriculum that preceded it, has been criticized severely for divorcing basic science from clinical practice to such an extent that many students view basic science as a largely irrelevant hurdle that has to be passed before their "real" training begins (Neidle, 1986a; Prockop, 1992). "Pre-clinical curricula are stuffed with too many courses, too many lectures, and too many faculty hobby horses that leave students at the end of two years exhausted [and] disgruntled" (Petersdorf, 1987, p. 19).

More specific criticisms include the following (see Vevier, 1987; Marston and Jones, 1992; Prockop, 1992; Pew Health Professions Commission, 1993). First, expectations that students can master the core basic science disciplines in the equivalent of four semesters are unsustainable and counterproductive given the explosion of scientific knowledge. Second, the emphasis on mastering facts

---

[4]This model is also called the horizontal model because it has often been graphed with years on the vertical axis so that the last two years of clinical science are stacked horizontally above the first two years of basic science. Figure 4.1A shows a vertical rather than horizontal division because school years are consistently placed on the horizontal axis for each model.

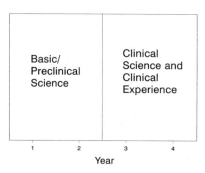

A. Traditional Curriculum: Structure of Basic Science and Clinical Education

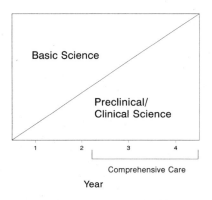

B. Diagonal Curriculum: Structure of Basic Science and Clinical Education

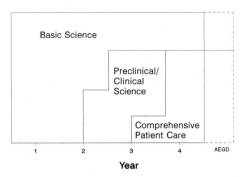

C. Integrated Curriculum: Structure of Basic Science and Clinical Education

FIGURE 4.1 Alternative configurations of basic and clinical science education. NOTE: AEGD = advanced education in general dentistry. SOURCE: Derived from Formicola, 1991.

still prevails over mastering principles and methods. Third, Ph.D.-trained basic scientists are not, in isolation, well prepared to focus their courses on the concepts and knowledge that are most clinically relevant. Fourth, the preparation and focus of National Board examinations, despite revisions, reinforce these problems. Fifth, some of the more esoteric areas of the basic sciences are not really relevant to clinicians and should be identified and dropped.

Although these criticisms have been directed at both medical and dental education, dental students face additional burdens under a traditional curriculum. Besides the basic science courses, they must fit a considerable volume of preclinical laboratory work into their first two years.

More generally, it was suggested to the committee that locating basic science faculty in the medical school can contribute to a lack of accountability to the dental school and thereby to curriculum immobility and low research productivity. For the majority of dental schools (29 in 1992), the basic science faculty are shared with the medical school, and instruction for dental and other health professions students is negotiated (ADA, 1993f). Although these dental schools may contribute 10 to 20 percent of their budgets to medical schools for basic science faculty positions, they do not have direct control over the faculty, and this may make it difficult for them to influence course content, for example, the inclusion of clinically relevant topics and examples. Some interviews suggested that schools may receive little in return beyond instructional hours (e.g., no participation in research related to oral health issues). If more shared faculty can be interested in oral health issues, then the larger and more diverse pool of basic scientists available on such a basis may be an asset. Such a pool is also created when academic health centers organize all basic science faculty in a separate unit.

Alternatives to the traditional curriculum propose a more gradual shift in emphasis from basic science to clinical education. The objectives, which this committee endorses, are to reduce the disjuncture between instruction in the basic and clinical sciences and to encourage more "correlation" between the two throughout the predoctoral program. As depicted simply in Figure 4.1B, the goal is a gradual shift in educational emphasis rather than an abrupt chronological divide. In actuality, because coursework is generally blocked into discrete units (e.g., hours), the shift is better depicted as a stepwise rather than a continuous progression (Figure 4.1C). The revised figure still oversimplifies by omitting coursework in areas such as the behavioral sciences.

Curriculum reorganization can do only so much, however. The link between science and practice must be demonstrated by faculty in both the classroom and the clinic. Thus, the modes as well as the content of education are important.

Modes of Education

Another shift from the traditional curriculum involves the introduction of instructional methods that attempt to reduce student alienation and disinterest by melding basic science principles and information with realistic analyses of clinical dental problems. Problem-based learning is perhaps the most notable example of such new approaches. Rather than view dental students as "repositories of facts with psychomotor skills" (Tedesco et al., 1992), advocates of problem-based learning see students as acquiring an intellectual framework for practice and an understanding of the scientific method. In a sense, education is "what you have left after you've forgotten the facts" (Smith, 1985, cited by DePaola, 1986).

At the risk of some oversimplification, traditional instruction and problem-based learning can be contrasted as follows.

Traditional Instruction	Problem-Based Learning
Fact-oriented science	Concept- and problem-oriented science
Discipline-focused courses	Interdisciplinary education
Abstract knowledge	Clinically related problems
Larger classes	Smaller classes
Lectures	Guided discussions
Multiple-choice examinations	Analytic examinations

A number of dental schools have introduced problem-based learning in recent years, but little research documents its educational outcomes to date. Some medical schools, however, have up to 20 years experience with the approach. Two recent reviews of research on outcomes of problem-based versus traditional instructional methods indicate that the former was associated with greater student satisfaction; higher faculty evaluations; better clinical functioning; better performance on Part III of the medical board examinations (the problem-solving segment); and poorer performance on the Part I (fact-based) examination (Albanese and Mitchell, 1993; Vernon and Blake, 1993; see also Norman and Schmidt, 1992, and the background paper by Tedesco). One of these reviews (Albanese and Mitchell) recommended caution in curriculum-wide conversion to the strategy until more evidence is available on costs and effectiveness of different methods of problem-based learning, in particular, more and less directive approaches.

If problem-based learning is successful in encouraging critical thinking, it should prompt students and faculty to question variations in approaches to different clinical problems and to become more focused on the outcomes of alternative patterns of care. The committee learned that some schools, in an effort to standardize some aspects of clinical instruction and reduce inconsistent assessments of student performance, have begun to identify variations among faculty in clinical preferences and practices; to secure agreement on preferred practices by using scientific evidence and formal consensus processes; and to develop the case for acceptable variations. Such processes are politically sensitive and time consuming. Furthermore, the paucity of outcomes research and systematically developed practice guidelines is a problem. Chapter 3 has already discussed this deficiency and recommended increased support for both outcomes research and practice guidelines. The background paper by Bader and Shugars explores these topics in depth. It notes research indicating that dental faculty are as variable in their clinical preferences and practices as other dentists.

Computer-based and other self-paced instructional materials and the use of standardized patients can also help in encouraging critical thinking and relating basic science principles to clinical examples.[5] They generally involve conscious, multidisciplinary efforts to construct learning opportunities that are less dependent than traditional instruction on the talents and biases of individual faculty.

The committee recognizes that costs are a barrier to the introduction of new instructional methods that may require additional spending for faculty to develop and teach smaller classes, acquisition of computer hardware and software, physical space reconfiguration, and faculty training in new teaching methods. In some cases, however, computer-based instruction might replace some faculty instruction, and reductions in total curriculum hours, as recom-

---

[5]Standardized patients are not real patients but individuals who are specially trained to present consistent behavior and descriptions of symptoms. They are used primarily in the teaching or evaluation of diagnostic and treatment planning skills. In addition to sparing real patients the experience of serving as "teaching material," these individuals are more easily scheduled for the convenience of students and faculty.

mended below, should free some resources for new uses. Further, special appeals to alumni and industry may attract funds for capital investments in up-to-date computer capacity that would not be forthcoming for other purposes.

CURRENT CONCEPTS AND PRACTICE

The committee heard arguments that dental school curricula—and faculty—are too often oriented to past oral health problems and practices. Specifically, curricula have not kept pace with changes in oral health problems (e.g, the increasing proportion of patients with complex medical conditions); scientific knowledge and technologies (e.g., in areas such as pharmacology and implants); information management tools and techniques; and society's expectations for health professionals (e.g., attention to informing patients about their choices).

In addition, the committee was impressed with arguments that students spend too much time on preclinical and laboratory activities (e.g., fabrication of crowns and prostheses) that today are most often performed by technicians and other personnel. More generally, financial and other constraints mean that many students receive an inadequate education in effective and efficient team practice with dental hygienists, assistants, and technicians.

An annual AADS survey of dental school seniors (Solomon and Whiton, 1991; AADS, 1992) asks for their views on curriculum components that were under- and overstressed. As presented in Figure 4.2, the 1992 survey found that a quarter or more students rated curriculum attention to orthodontics, practice administration, geriatric dentistry, emergency treatment, and community dentistry as inadequate. Attention to dental materials, basic medical science, and periodontics was rated as excessive by more than 10 percent of the respondents.

In the committee's view, several factors contribute to resistance to curriculum change. They include faculty conservatism, slow change in licensure examinations, and economic limits on changes that require capital expenditures or recruitment of additional personnel.

Faculty conservatism can be attributed to at least three factors beyond personal attachment to familiar arrangements and anxiety about the possible negative consequences of change. First, despite the recent growth of advanced education programs in general dentistry, many generalist faculty lack such training and are also not involved with advanced students who should be better prepared than predoctoral students to question traditional prac-

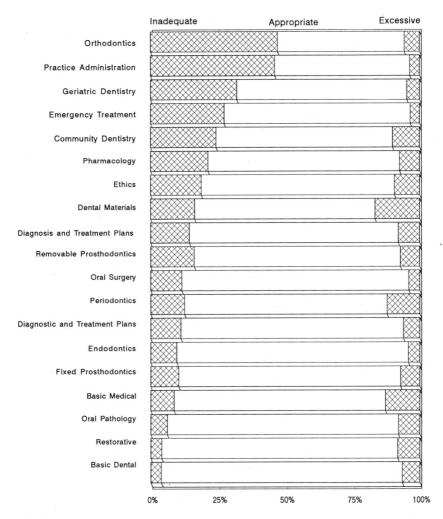

FIGURE 4.2 Survey of dental school seniors: Ratings of curriculum emphasis.
SOURCE: American Association of Dental Schools, 1992.

tices. Second, some clinical faculty are unable or unwilling to participate in faculty practice plans or interact clinically with those in private, community-based practice, which may limit their exposure to current practice and expectations. Third, clinical faculty who are not involved in research may be less familiar with scientific and technological advances. On occasion, the committee heard that some full-time faculty are viewed as not conversant with newer materials, techniques, and debates. By default, students may look to part-time faculty as models for up-to-date practice. Whether these perceptions have a basis in fact or are just one more sign of tensions between educators and practitioners, they were disquieting to the committee and warrant attention from educators, for example, through continuing education or alumni and community relations programs.

As noted earlier, one problem with oral health services (indeed, health services generally) is limited evidence about the effectiveness of many preventive, diagnostic, and therapeutic interventions. As the evidence base related to both new and established dental procedures and technologies expands and as more science-based practice guidelines are developed, dental educators will be better positioned to assess and shape current practice. Well-designed and presented outcomes studies and practice guidelines should, in the future, prove to be useful educational tools (IOM, 1992).

COMPREHENSIVE PATIENT CARE

Traditionally, dental schools organize clinical experience for students through rotations in discipline-based clinics. That is, students spend fixed amounts of time in up to nine specialty clinics (e.g., fixed prosthodontics, periodontics) supervised by specialty faculty.

In contrast, the premise of the comprehensive care model of clinical education is that students should learn to provide patient care in a manner and setting similar to those found in an efficient dental practice (Vining, 1984; see, generally, *Journal of Dental Education,* June 1984 supplement). The continuum of care learned by predoctoral students should be that provided by the general dentist including (1) patient examination and evaluation; (2) diagnosis and treatment planning; (3) direct treatment for a range of common dental problems; (4) use of allied dental personnel; and (5) referral to dental specialists, physicians, or others as appropriate.

Again at the risk of oversimplifying, the traditional and comprehensive care approaches to clinical education can be contrasted as follows:

Traditional Care	Comprehensive Care
Specialist role model	Generalist role model
Student-centered instruction	Patient-centered education
Segmented patient care	Continuity of patient care
Procedure focus	Evaluation and management focus
Numerical requirements	Competency criteria

Chapter 6 argues that these tenets of comprehensive care are supportive of the patient care mission of the dental school and better prepare students to be sensitive to patient needs and less narrowly focused on technique. It argues further that unless academic programs offer patient-centered education, they will fare poorly in the restructured health care system of the future.

Although many schools have adopted some elements of comprehensive care, most have considerable progress to make in providing patient-centered, continuous care and in evaluating students based on competency rather than numerical requirements. A 1993 survey estimated that 40 dental schools had comprehensive care programs, up from 25 schools identified in 1989 (Baughan et al., 1993; Dodge et al., 1993). The structure of these programs varied substantially with respect to the features listed above. For example, some drew faculty from specialty departments, whereas others relied on faculty from departments of general practice; numerical criteria for evaluating student performance remain commonplace. One innovative variant of the comprehensive care model, the "Pennsylvania experiment," took a subset of students out of the large school-based clinic and linked them to faculty-based private practices (Cohen et al., 1985, 1991). In general, differences in the way schools implement comprehensive care involve both practical realities and pedagogical concerns.

The practical challenges of implementing comprehensive care in dental schools are taxing. They involve (1) finding and financing appropriate physical space; (2) recruiting patients and matching patient needs with individual student needs to gain competency in specific procedures; (3) increasing faculty work loads and accountability; (4) locating and integrating qualified part-time faculty; and (5) managing disciplinary tensions. Many of these challenges are discussed further in Chapter 6, which considers the patient care activities of the dental school from a patient's rather than a student's perspective. In general, "some features of practice, such as the total management of each patient, the care of large and diverse groups of patients, and the operation of a dental office are not easily simulated in a dental school" (AADS and Kellogg Foundation, 1980, p. 20).

Most of the schools visited by the committee acknowledged that their implementation of comprehensive care involved less-than-ideal compromises—political, logistical, and financial. For example, the University of Pennsylvania dental school, despite concluding that its experimental practice was educationally desirable and financially feasible on a small scale, has not found it feasible to expand the model to cover all students (Cohen et al., 1991).

Columbia University concluded both that introduction to comprehensive care in the third dental year was premature and that a single (fourth) year of comprehensive care was insufficient preparation for entry-level practice (Formicola, 1991). Accordingly, Columbia concluded, as did Pennsylvania, that a postgraduate year was an essential supplement to its predoctoral comprehensive care program (Cohen, 1985; Formicola, 1991). A later section of this chapter discusses the need for a postgraduate year of education in general dentistry.

A pedagogic debate in comprehensive care focuses on the use of general faculty to instruct students in basic specialty procedures that are frequently performed by general dentists (Hasler, 1984). Some dental educators argue that few generalist faculty have advanced training in the procedures they supervise. Others are concerned that "calibrating" assessments of student competency will be difficult if comprehensive care faculty come from different disciplines. This is a particular issue in comprehensive care clinics because of their greater attention to the nonprocedural elements of care (e.g., evaluation and treatment planning) (Baughan et al., 1993).

EDUCATIONAL INEFFICIENCIES

Although dental schools vary considerably and detailed comparative data are generally unavailable, the committee became concerned that many if not most dental students learn in settings that are neither clinically nor educationally efficient. Students stand in line for supplies, collect patient payments, lack assistance from allied personnel, wait for faculty review of their work, and undertake clerical functions neither essential to their education nor routine in practice. The emphasis on procedures rather than on patient care means that students may be assigned to complete procedures from start to finish even when they are so inexperienced that hours of extra time are required. In some schools, outdated arrangements of facilities produce some gross wastes of student time (for example, in one school, students must run up and down the escalators from the clinic floor to the cashier floor to handle patient payments).

These inefficiencies add to the student's overcrowded week, squander patient time, and provide an inappropriate model of patient care. Dental educators recognized the minimal educational value of having students collect patient payments, but clinic managers told the committee that they could not afford to hire clerks to handle this responsibility and that patient payment before receipt of service was essential to financial survival. Similarly, educators often acknowledged that student clinics are generally understaffed with allied dental professionals but argued that they would further increase the clinic deficit by hiring more such personnel. Several of the schools visited by the committee were acutely aware of physical plant problems and had substantial renovations of their patient care space planned, under way, or recently completed.

Chapter 6, which looks at these circumstances from a patient's perspective, argues that dental schools must change their approach to patient care for ethical and practical reasons. In a health care environment marked by significant restructuring and serious challenges to the economic position of academic health centers, dental school clinics are poorly positioned to attract the growing numbers of insured patients (with or without health care reform) and to help the academic health center compete for health plan contracts.

In the broader context of the university and academic health center, efficiency considerations may argue for studies to determine whether consolidation of some aspects of the dental curriculum with other educational programs could generate administrative and personnel savings with no harm to (and, possibly, enhancement of) educational objectives. Although not a matter of efficiency per se, opening some dental school courses to students from other programs such as physical anthropology would make a modest contribution to reducing the isolation of dental schools, as discussed further in Chapter 7.

REBALANCING AN OVERCROWDED CURRICULUM

The combination of scientific and technological advances, academic traditions, and commitment to a four-year program has generated a curriculum widely regarded as overcrowded. With the conventional 40-hour work week used for comparison, the average dental student spends 30 hours in scheduled lectures, laboratory, or clinic work and has just 10 (theoretically) unscheduled daytime hours. Little of the formal curriculum is organized around the active learning strategies described earlier, and little time is left for critical reflection, consolidation of concepts and information, supplementary reading, or consultation with faculty.

The year as well as the week is packed with requirements. Only a handful of schools leave summers free for students to refresh themselves physically and mentally or to enlarge their education through discretionary research projects or off-campus clinical experience. Free summers would also allow students to earn money for tuition and might alleviate the need for outside employment during the school year.

Virtually every dean who met with committee members spoke of efforts to reevaluate and redesign the curriculum so as to reduce inappropriate duplication or overlap among courses; to set priorities for identifying content that has greater relevance for today's students and tomorrow's practitioners; and to find more time-efficient ways of teaching. Severe financial pressure can stimulate "downsizing," but the political realities of academia may lead to cuts based more on the relative power of different disciplines and individuals than on expectations about the educational needs of future practitioners. In its site visits, the committee found instances in which the curriculum had been pruned, but efforts to prevent regrowth were not always successful. That is, if a curriculum committee was successful in cutting back in certain areas, the pressure to add elsewhere was difficult to resist.

One challenge in curriculum change involves the cost—or even the feasibility—of obtaining data, for example, that (1) identify the specific courses in a given school that have overlapping material; (2) correlate the emphases in clinical instruction with the actual and desirable content of current dental practice; and (3) document the effectiveness (related to cost) of alternative instructional methods. As described in the background paper by Bader and Shugars and in Chapter 8, the third task is complicated by questions about the validity and reliability of measures of professional competency. Other obstacles relate to shortages of faculty trained to employ new teaching methods and limited availability of instructional software and related hardware tailored to the particular requirements of dental education (which constitutes a relatively small market).

These difficulties notwithstanding, the committee concluded that curriculum restructuring should be a high priority. Among the emphases should be the balance between facts and concepts in basic science courses, and the reexamination of heavy work loads in preclinical technique.

DENTISTRY AND MEDICINE

The environmental changes alluded to above are among the factors contributing to new interest in the relationship between dentistry and medicine. Debates about this relationship are centuries old. In Europe, dentistry was often a specialty of medicine, and all dentists had medical degrees, but the recent trend has been toward separate programs and degrees as found in the United States.

Since the first U.S. dental school was founded a century and a half ago, medical and dental schools have been separate. Integration of classes and other experiences exists in some institutions. For example, the University of Connecticut has completely integrated education in the basic sciences, and Columbia University has integrated most of the lecture portion of basic science education but still groups dental students together for smaller seminars and work groups. Several dental schools provide elective medical clerkships directed by internists. At the graduate level, hospital-based residency programs typically require residents to take medical rotations, and many oral and maxillofacial surgery programs award a medical degree after five years of training.

The scientific, clinical, and epidemiological literature and the committee's interviews with deans, faculty, students, and leaders of dental professional organizations—all point to changes in oral health care that will make the acquisition of additional knowledge of systemic disease and medical interventions more important in the future. Among these changes are the following:

• The technology used to prevent and treat oral diseases will increasingly involve diagnostic, pharmacological, and other interventions that demand medical knowledge. As described in Chapter 3 and in the background papers, advances in the biomedical and clinical sciences will almost certainly accelerate this trend.

• Medically complicated or compromised patients, particularly the elderly, are becoming a larger segment of dental practice. Treatment for these patients must take their systemic health problems and their typical use of multiple prescription drugs and nonprescription drugs into account.

• A growing number of dentists will be employed or practicing in large multispecialty practices, staff and group model health maintenance organizations (HMOs), and similar settings. Appropriate clinical experience in medicine may help them function more comfortably in these environments, particularly if the stress is on a broad scope of generalist care.

Meeting the challenges of changing technology, patient mix, and work setting will require changes in the relationship between dentistry and medicine. The options range from marginal change in dental education to complete integration. The committee discussed this relationship at length. It concluded that marginal change is insufficient but beyond this found considerable disagreement on directions. Although the discussion below focuses on the relationship between medicine and dentistry, the committee notes the important relationships between dentistry and other health professions, a point emphasized in Chapter 3. That chapter recommends that dental educators work with colleagues in the other health professions to emphasize these relationships and to experiment with new strategies in didactic and clinical instruction.

Closer Integration as an Alternative. In the view of most committee members, closer integration of dentistry and medicine is a reasonable and desirable objective, one that might take a number of specific forms and one that a few schools have already adopted in some form. The committee's emphasis was not on institutional arrangements or degrees but on educational and clinical substance.

Although many variants on the details are possible, closer integration would generally involve the following elements. First, dental students would take basic science courses that would be the same as or similar to those taken by medical students and that would generally be taught by the same faculty. The content of courses, whether taught on a separate or an integrated basis, would reflect the principles of clinical relevance and critical thinking discussed earlier in this chapter. Second, basic science courses for dental and medical students, whether or not taught jointly, would include conditions or problems relevant to oral disease and would not, in any case, be divorced from clinical care. Early exposure to patients would, whenever possible, be joint with medical students and thus include a wide range of patients. Third, dental students would have required clerkships in relevant areas of medicine (e.g., physical evaluation of hospitalized and ambulatory patients, urgent care and emergency medicine, pediatrics, and geriatrics), with options for additional training. Fourth, dental faculty would have sufficient experience in clinical medicine so that they—and not just physicians—could impart medical knowledge to dental students and serve as role models for them. Fifth, dental licensure examinations would be redesigned to increase the emphasis on critical thinking and clinically relevant knowledge of systemic disease and physiology. This change is desirable in any case.

Whatever the form, closer integration of dentistry with medicine would still entail fundamental changes for students, faculty, and institutions. These changes would be demanding to plan and implement and could not be expected to occur quickly or painlessly. During site visits, university and dental school officials sympathetic to the concept of closer integration explained to committee members why they were not moving more quickly or fully to integrate medical and dental education. From a purely practical perspective, the lack of large enough classrooms and the complexities of class scheduling are important barriers to joint education. Likewise, building medical knowledge within the dental faculty takes time and money and would likely require a combination of faculty development and recruitment of new faculty.

Another concern involves the preparation of entering students. Entering medical students have higher grade point averages—3.45 compared with 3.09 for dental students (on a 4-point scale) (Jonas et al., 1993). Eighty-six percent of medical students have a baccalaureate degree as their highest degree compared to 65 percent of dental students. Such differences may put dental students at a disadvantage in shared courses. In addition, if dental students still were differentiated by a heavy load of preclinical courses, then they would be at a further disadvantage compared with medical students. The committee has already argued that the necessity of this work load needs to be reexamined.

Student qualifications aside, even educators who favored joint predoctoral education argued that some differentiation in curriculum was essential. Oral biology and other topics of special relevance to dental practitioners require special emphasis.

Although more of the burden of change might fall on dental schools, medical schools would also have to make curriculum adjustments and widen their perspectives so that future generalist and specialty physicians would regard oral health as a part of their concern with total health. With or without further integration and as already argued, it is this committee's sense that basic science faculty affiliated with medical schools need to be more accountable for the education of dental students and any other nonmedical students they teach. The research implications of current organizational structures are discussed in Chapter 5, and the financial aspects of various kinds of consolidation are discussed in Chapter 7.

Even without such additional challenges, change in medical schools is not easy. Early on, this chapter noted that medical education as currently organized has been seriously criticized for inadequacies in predoctoral basic science education and overspecialization in graduate medical education. Moreover, many medical schools are likely to be preoccupied in coming years with the pressures created by health care restructuring (as discussed more generally in Chapter 6). Many of these changes should, however, bring the schools closer to the prevention and primary care orientation of dentistry.

Despite its recognition of the difficulties of more closely integrating dental and medical education, the majority of the committee believed that such integration is necessary to prepare dental practitioners for a future characterized by more medical management of oral health problems and more patients with complex medical problems. Within the general framework suggested above, dental and medical educators have a variety of options they can test and revise.

Dentistry as a Medical Specialty? The most far-reaching option is for dentistry to become a medical specialty fully integrated with medicine in the way that otolaryngology and ophthalmology are. Although some committee members believed this was a desirable long-term direction, the majority of the committee disagreed or was unconvinced. Despite this disagreement, however, the committee felt that steps by individual universities and states to test this or similar approaches would be desirable and instructive if undertaken with foundation or government support for a formal, integrated evaluation of the effort.

The case for this option rests, in large part, on the scientific, demographic, and organizational trends noted above. Combining courses and faculty also could help counter what some see as unsustainable increases in the cost of medical and dental education. In addition, as dentistry moves closer to medicine and as medicine moves toward generalist practice, practitioners will become better prepared to work as part of a health care team in a more integrated health care system.

Against complete integration are arguments that clinical, organizational, legal, economic, and cultural considerations make the objective sufficiently unrealistic that it would distract attention from more achievable but still major changes. These considerations include the need for significant, politically difficult revisions of state practice acts; the requirement that major university components be restructured; the realignment of responsibilities across existing and possibly new professional categories; and the uncertain impact of such realignments on the quality of care. A further argument against converting dentistry to a medical specialty that requires additional years of specialty training (following the pattern of ophthalmology or otolaryngology) is that the cost of education for general dental practice could increase substantially, which, in turn, could lead to higher fees for dentists' services.

To reduce the length of the total pre- and postdoctoral program for those who sought careers in dentistry and thereby trim educational costs, an alternative to the traditional medical model might be devised that would create an early specialization track for dentistry at the predoctoral level. Medicine and dentistry have, generally, rejected predoctoral specialization, so this would be a considerable innovation. In any case, it is not clear whether a special track for dentistry within medical schools would qualify as "complete integration" rather than "closer integration" of medicine and dentistry.

A more conventional (but still controversial) approach to cost concerns would be to delegate more care to allied dental personnel working under the supervision of dentist physicians who provide more complex medical and surgical services. Proponents of this view cite evidence that existing or new categories of allied dental practitioners can be trained to perform safely and effectively some of the more common tasks now performed by dentists (Burt and Eklund, 1992; Freed and Perry, 1992; see also the background paper by Tedesco). A more complex and difficult alternative would be the creation of a new category of advanced allied dental professionals whose education and scope of practice include many restorative services and whose education might involve a five-year baccalaureate program similar to that for pharmacists.

Although some redefinition of professional roles appears crucial to the feasibility of converting dentistry into a medical specialty, this committee did not have the resources to estimate the net effects on costs and quality of care of the options suggested above. It encourages the appropriate government agencies to pursue these questions and to support further testing of these and other strategies for the use of allied dental personnel. The committee was also unanimous in encouraging dental and medical schools to continue and expand experiments with combined medicine-dentistry programs for interested students and residents. This combination of experiments with new steps and extensions of previously tested strategies should help prepare future policymakers and educators to make more informed judgments about the oral health work force in the face of continued scientific, technological, economic, and other changes.

ADVANCED EDUCATION

Today, dental school graduates have two broad options in pursuing advanced clinical training—one that focuses on general dentistry and the other, on education in one of the dental specialties.

The first option was the subject of the most controversy and attention during the committee's work.

Currently, first-year postdoctoral positions are available for approximately 60 percent of graduating dentists. These positions are split about evenly between eight specialist and two general dentistry categories (Table 4.2). Virtually all of the growth in the number of positions has been accounted for by the growth in general dentistry positions. The total number of specialty positions has stayed essentially steady. However, because the number of dental graduates has decreased since the 1970s, the proportion of all dentists who are specialists has been increasing.

ADVANCED EDUCATION IN GENERAL DENTISTRY

In contrast to medicine, substantial numbers of dental students do not pursue residency training after graduation. Yet, the emphasis in most dental schools on preparing students to be competent, entry-level general practitioners upon graduation puts a considerable burden on both schools and students. As discussed earlier, some have concluded that students need a postgraduate year of broad but supervised experience in general dentistry to make the transition from dental graduate to competent entry-level practitioner.

History and Development

Hospital-based general practice residency (GPR) programs have been formally evaluated and accredited since the late 1940s, although such residencies date back at least to the 1920s (Santangelo, 1987; AADS, 1994a). Other postgraduate programs in specialty areas were not explicitly approved until the 1960s. In 1977, the AADS urged that programs of advanced education in general dentistry (AEGD) be approved for nonhospital sites, consistent with dentistry's focus on comprehensive care and care outside the inpatient setting. In 1979, the ADA authorized this step.

The concept of advanced education in general dentistry was given a strong boost in 1980 by an AADS task force funded by the W.H. Kellogg Foundation. That group recommended that "the number of positions in general practice residencies and other advanced dental education programs . . . be increased to accommodate approximately one-half of the dental school graduates by the mid-1980s" (AADS and W.K. Kellogg Foundation, 1980, p. 6).

The postgraduate year in general dentistry (PGY1) has sometimes been referred to as a fifth year, but this terminology implies

TABLE 4.2 First-Year Enrollment in Advanced General and Specialty Education Programs

Program	1971	1975	1977	1979	1981	1983	1985	1987	1989	1991	1992
Postdoctoral General Dentistry											
GPR	516	694	753	923	942	917	943	903	877	903	863
AEGD	NA	NA	NA	NA	27	98	120	243	297	366	398
Total	516	694	753	923	969	1,015	1,063	1,146	1,174	1,269	1,261
Specialty Programs											
Dental public health	26	35	11	23	28	20	21	25	22	20	24
Endodontics	113	134	140	141	143	139	131	130	143	156	157
Oral pathology	24	25	26	23	22	19	20	11	14	16	14
Oral surgery	242	223	221	226	206	216	211	212	208	215	214
Orthodontics	320	304	296	283	288	297	294	302	295	285	279
Pediatric dentistry	163	176	166	181	175	149	157	165	168	177	161
Periodontics	171	178	190	190	195	183	179	195	208	195	207
Prosthodontics	144	152	164	170	159	178	195	179	191	192	194
Combined programs	NA	NA	NA	3	3	1	1	1	2	3	2
Total	1,203	1,227	1,214	1,240	1,219	1,202	1,209	1,230	1,251	1,259	1,252
Advanced Education											
All first-year positions	1,719	1,921	1,967	2,163	2,188	2,217	2,272	2,376	2,425	2,528	2,513

NOTE: AEGD = advanced education in general dentistry; GPR = general practice residency; NA = not available.

SOURCE: American Association of Dental Schools, 1993b.

to many a fifth predoctoral year (Gray, 1987). As recommended by this committee, neither the AEGD nor the GPR should be regarded as an extension or revision of the predoctoral curriculum; rather, each should provide a period of greater independence and responsibility for complex patient care.

Although GPR positions outnumber AEGD positions, the number of GPR slots has been declining, and changes in Medicare payments for graduate medical education may lead to further declines. Since 1978, the federal government has invested nearly $40 million in support of postgraduate general dentistry (Handelman et al., 1993). For FY 1993, the appropriation for this area was $3,730,000.

It does not appear that advanced education in general dentistry serves as a prelude to specialization. One recent study indicates that nearly 90 percent of graduates with such training remained in general practice (Handelman et al., 1993).

Britain now requires dental graduates to participate in what is termed a "vocational" year of office-based training before they begin general practice, and other European nations appear to be moving in this direction (AADS, 1994a). Many advocate a similar requirement for this country under the AEGD or PGY1 label.

Issues and Controversies

As described in an earlier section, the existing predoctoral curriculum is so burdened with coursework and acquisition of technical skills that students have little time to integrate their skills and knowledge as envisioned in the concept of comprehensive patient care. This deficiency is a particular problem for general dentists, whose responsibilities for primary care require comprehensive management of all patient care, whether it is provided directly or referred to specialists as appropriate. The problem is analogous to that in medicine before graduate medical education was universally accepted. A year of postgraduate or advanced education in general dentistry would allow students to gain speed and confidence in procedures, broaden their patient management skills to cover more complex problems, and mature in the nontechnical aspects of patient care.

Curriculum reform that emphasizes comprehensive patient care and other restructuring and pruning of the dental curriculum should improve student readiness to enter practice. The postgraduate year should *not* be seen as a way of avoiding such reform. Conversely, predoctoral curriculum change is not a substitute for a postgraduate year. This committee believes that all graduates of U.S. dental schools should have the opportunity to round out and refine their predoctoral work through a supervised and accredited postgraduate experience. This is not possible now.

One estimate is that demand for AEGD or GPR positions exceeds supply by about 400 positions (AADS, 1994a). During site visits, liaison panel meetings, and other activities, the committee often heard that those most in need of the advanced year were the least successful in competing for available positions (see also Little St. Simons Conference, 1993). The demand for AEGD and general practice residencies is cited by some as evidence that students do not feel adequately prepared for practice (Garrison, 1993).

An exception to this supply-demand imbalance was reported by the U.S. Department of Defense (DOD) in its testimony to the committee (Martin, 1993). In contrast to the past, the department now cannot fill all its one-year GPR positions. The testimony cited the increased number of residencies in the civilian sector (often in more appealing locations) as well as DOD's relatively low salaries and limited provisions for scholarships or loan forgiveness. Dental educators and DOD officials have a mutual interest in identifying how unfilled residencies might be made more attractive, for example, through changes in federal or other policies regarding loan forgiveness or payback arrangements.

The expectation of postgraduate experience would increase the flexibility of dental schools to modify their predoctoral curricula to encompass advances in dental practice and research. More than three-quarters of the deans agreed that building or sustaining a strong postdoctoral *general* dentistry program was a priority, although a slightly higher percentage agreed that a strong postdoctoral *specialty* program was a priority. Slightly more than 60 percent of deans surveyed for this report agreed that a year of postgraduate training should be *required* by 2005.

The qualifications to the endorsement of a required postgraduate year are primarily practical not philosophical. The major obstacles to such a requirement and indeed to the more modest recommendation of this committee are fiscal. Financial pressures on hospitals have resulted in a modest decline in the number of hospital-based general dentistry programs, and uncertainties over future funding for graduate medical education may have some spillover effects on dentistry.[6] Startup funding from the U.S. Pub-

---

[6]However, a 1985 AADS survey indicated that many hospitals were not claiming Medicare reimbursement for GPR programs (AADS, 1994b). Although Medicare beneficiaries generally are not covered for dental services, GPR programs and some AEGD positions may be eligible for funds under Medicare's provisions for direct and indirect support of graduate medical education.

lic Health Service is often available for AEGD programs, but continued funding generally requires creative efforts to supplement routine patient care revenues with additional funding sources including federal and state programs for disadvantaged groups. To the extent that faculty practice plans expand their patient base and revenues, they may also offer opportunities for postgraduate training. Creating appropriately structured, stipend-paying residency positions demands a substantial investment of administrative and faculty time—and favorable local conditions.

In addition, to make postgraduate education a requirement for licensure, each state would have to revise its statutes, a daunting prospect. Another consideration is student resistance; some students say they do not need additional training and balk at the economic opportunity cost of delaying their entrance into private practice. In light of these concerns, the committee chose to recommend increased opportunities rather than requirements for residencies. As these opportunities are expanded and their relative benefits and costs are studied further, the case for or against a requirement should become clearer.

Other concerns involve the availability of general practice faculty to teach advanced students and a shortage of patients with treatment needs consistent with students' educational program. The latter is already a problem for some predoctoral student clinics. Although expanded coverage of dental care under health care reform might not make predoctoral clinics more attractive, AEGD clinics might very well be able to attract patients newly able to afford dental care. Two models proposed to expand the availability of postgraduate positions would place students in university-affiliated private offices and in community clinics such as those funded by the federal government to provide care in underserved areas. In some instances, the development of additional sites for advanced education may lay the foundation for schools to use the same sites for extramural predoctoral education.

ADVANCED SPECIALTY EDUCATION

As described in Chapter 2, the first specialty programs were established a century ago, but they were slow to proliferate. Specialty standards were first developed in the 1940s but an accreditation program did not begin until the 1960s. Today, eight recognized dental specialties have 421 accredited programs in dental schools and other institutions. Table 4.2 lists the specialties and their first-year enrollments. Chapter 8 and the background paper consider regulatory issues related to dental specialties.

Many of the issues raised in the discussion of predoctoral education apply broadly to all aspects of dental education and practice. These issues can be rephrased so that they speak to the importance of advanced specialty education that

1. emphasizes the scientific basis of the specialty;
2. promotes critical thinking about the effectiveness of alternative treatments including the options of generalist care or continued observation;
3. focuses on the patient not the procedure; and
4. prepares practitioners to treat medically complicated patients and work with medical specialists and generalists as appropriate.

As presented to this committee, the primary concerns about the distinctive content and quality of specialist education dealt with how they prepared individuals for research or teaching rather than clinical careers. Although most specialist curricula include exposure to the scientific method and literature, the primary focus is clinical proficiency, not the generation or evaluation of new knowledge. Some schools provide more scientific training in programs leading to a master's degree than in programs leading to a specialty certificate, but this is not universal. Such programs may help prepare clinical faculty to teach with a greater appreciation of dentistry's science base and to participate as partners in clinical research under the direction of full-fledged researchers. Notwithstanding these benefits, such program do not and should not be expected to prepare students for a research career.

Accordingly, those involved in faculty recruitment and development should not mistake acquisition of a master's degree with academic preparation for a research career. Likewise, educators interested in developing a serious research training component within a dental school should focus on programs leading to a doctorate not a master's degree. This argument is reinforced in Chapter 5.

In presentations to the committee, some groups were worried that insufficient numbers were being trained in particular specialties, for instance, pediatric and public health dentistry (AAPD, 1993; AAPHD, 1993; ABDPH, 1993; ASTDD, 1993).[7] In site vis-

---

[7]Dental public health differs from the other recognized specialties in that its primary emphasis is the oral health status of communities (including groups

its, schools expressed concern about the availability of oral pathologists. More common was a concern that the proportion of specialists was increasing in dentistry because the number of specialists being trained had remained fairly steady while the number of dental graduates had dropped. These concerns do not relate, for the most part, to specialty curricula but to work force issues. In Chapter 9, the committee cautions against a decrease in dental schools' focus on generalist education, but it found few data or analyses on which to base conclusions about requirements for individual specialties. Unlike medicine, restrictions on dental specialty training have not figured in the debates about health care reform.

A quite different set of concerns about advanced specialty education related to its reinforcing of faculty organization by specialty category. The committee heard arguments that curriculum reform is impeded by this organizational structure and by faculty interests and attachments to particular specialties. Further, legitimate questions can be asked about whether disproportionate resources are devoted to graduate specialty education. The committee found few data on the allocation of resources between predoctoral and advanced dental education. One dean reported that 30 percent of faculty effort at his school is directed to advanced education, which accounts for 10 percent of enrollment—but 45 percent of clinic revenues (Hunt, 1993). An expert in financial administration reported that the cost of educating a graduate specialty student is 70 percent higher than the cost of educating a predoctoral student (Consani, 1993). Whether these figures are typical or, in any case, whether they represent disproportionate emphasis, the committee could not determine.

CONTINUING EDUCATION

One of the guiding principles for this study was that *learning is a lifelong enterprise for dental practitioners. It cannot stop with the awarding of a degree or the completion of a residency pro-*

---

with less than average health status) not clinical services for individuals. Because their work constitutes a public good and because the income expectations for public health dentist are comparatively low, subsidized education programs in this specialty were cited as especially important. Congress reauthorized dental public health training in 1992 but adequate funding is in doubt. Oral pathology is another specialty that does not emphasize individual patient care.

gram. Continuing dental education is part of the continuum of education, and dental schools are obvious sources of continuing education that covers advances in relevant scientific fields, provides critical appraisals of new technologies, and incorporates an evaluation component that draws on faculty research skills to assess the impact of different approaches to continuing education. Interest in the effectiveness of continuing education is likely to grow as more public attention focuses on methods of documenting and continuously improving the performance of established practitioners (Nash et al., 1993; Horn and Hopkins, 1994). Although evidence of the positive—or negative—effects of traditional programs is limited (Bader, 1987; Davis et al., 1992), the issue for educators and policymakers is not whether continuing education is necessary but what methods or formats are most effective in reaching particular educational objectives.

In the deans' survey, continuing education was rated as highly or very highly important for 41 of the 54 schools. Only one dean reported it low in importance, and 12 responded that it was moderately important. Thirty-two deans (59 percent) responded that continuing education would be either more or much more important in the future. None of the deans reported that providing continuing education would be less important in the future. Questions remain, however, about whether dental and medical schools are prepared to invest resources in lifelong learning programs for dental professionals that are based on practitioners' concerns, patients' needs, and practice realities (Chambers, 1992b; Davis and Parboosingh, 1993).

OPTIONS FOR CONTINUING EDUCATION

The committee found a range of continuing education offerings, representing wide differences in intensity and scope. The offerings are not easily ranked in quality and depth. Some obviously provide more complete education and evaluation than others, and some might actually be harmful if they provide inadequate instruction but give participants a false sense of competency. Some programs include clinical experience; others are purely didactic. Not all qualify for continuing education credits.

The array of course media includes audio and video cassettes, computer modules, cable TV programs, and personal instruction. Instruction may occur in quite disparate settings. Some involve weekend or day courses at hotels or resorts or sessions at professional conferences. Informal study clubs may meet in participants' homes or offices. Dental schools offer a variety of programs both on-site and in outlying locations arranged by the schools. Every major general dentistry and specialty organization, many producers of dental equipment and other products, and a variety of other organizations sponsor continuing education courses.

In its site visits, the committee found varying levels of dental school involvement in continuing education. School location, traditions, faculty interest, and available market influence school decisions. One school visited by the committee was increasing its continuing education programs to improve relations between alumni and practitioner. Continuing education programs may, like faculty practice plans, provide a way to supplement faculty salaries. Some schools, however, reported that the costs of providing continuing education exceeded the revenues generated from course fees, making it a financial drain on the school when it was expected to generate a surplus.

In principle, dental schools have the advantage of facilities specifically designed for clinical education and ready access to a diverse faculty including educators, researchers, and practitioners. In actuality, they may not successfully mobilize or build upon these advantages to serve and attract practitioners (Chambers, 1992b). In the future, educational and other support might come in unconventional formats such as computer-based information or interactive consulting services. Improved communication links between schools and practitioners also may offer a base for extending research opportunities as discussed in Chapter 5.

Active state support for the area health education centers (AHEC) program facilitates dental school involvement in continuing education. At the University of North Carolina (UNC) at Chapel Hill, for example, the AHEC program supports continuing health professions education by deploying the university's faculty throughout the state. The state has designated specific funds for a portion of faculty time, facilities, transportation, and similar costs. Because the AHEC program is academic health center wide, it also links the dental school to other health professions schools at the UNC. In Washington State, which also has a strong AHEC program, the University of Washington dental school is extensively involved in continuing dental education.

ACCREDITATION AND EVALUATION

Following the path of other health professions, the AADS section on continuing education has endorsed a set of accreditation standards for sponsors and providers (AADS, 1992).[8] In 1989, the ADA Board of Trustees adopted a resolution to consider an evaluation and approval mechanism for continuing education that would address concerns about quality and the need for certification of programs and instructors (ADA, 1992c). After considerable work on an initial proposal by the Council on Dental Education, the ADA board appointed a committee to work with representatives from each of the specialties, the American Association of Dental Examiners (AADE), the AADS, and the Academy of General Dentistry (AGD) to develop a continuing dental education Provider Recognition Program (PRP). That committee recommended adoption of a PRP that would certify providers or programs, not individual courses, to ensure quality and reputability. The committee also recommended establishment of a PRP steering committee and a review committee on continuing dental education. In early 1993, the Continuing Education Recognition Program was established under the auspices of the ADA in cooperation with 11 other national dental organizations (ADA, CERP, 1993a).

As noted above, little is known about the effectiveness of alternative methods of continuing education or about the specific methods best suited for topics as diverse as patient education and implant materials and techniques. Moreover, the availability of a sound continuing education course does not guarantee that those who enroll will actually participate, learn, and then practice what they learn. Skepticism about the value of participation in continuing education courses as a proxy for competency in practice is common, even among its supporters. This skepticism echoes more general reservations about the impact of education and information as vehicles for influencing practitioner behavior (Eisenberg, 1986; Lomas, 1991; Kibbe et al., 1994). It reinforces the call for a *stronger emphasis on evaluation of the effectiveness of different methods and formats*; such evaluation should, in turn, provide dental faculty with additional research opportunities.

---

[8]The Accreditation Council for Continuing Medical Education accredits most providers of continuing medical education to ensure some degree of consistency. These providers and sponsors include medical schools, specialty societies (national, state, and local), teaching hospitals, community hospitals, pharmaceutical and medical device firms, educational companies, and voluntary health organizations (USDHHS, OIG, 1994, B-1).

REQUIREMENTS FOR CONTINUING EDUCATION

Prior to 1980, only 9 of the 52 states and territories (including the District of Columbia and Puerto Rico) required continued education for dentists (ADA, Department of State Government Affairs, 1994). By January 1994, 40 of 52 dental boards required—as a condition for relicensure—some sort of continuing education credit hours for dentists over a one- to five-year period; 43 required such credits of dental hygienists. Continuing education requirements are relatively uncontroversial among practitioners compared to other measures such as periodic written or clinical examinations or review of patient records.

Although the committee viewed continuing education as part of the process of continued professional development, it also believed that state boards should move beyond continuing education requirements as a measure of continued competency. Boards should work with others in the dental community to develop pilot projects to identify practical methods of measuring professional performance for established practitioners. A recent draft report from the AADE describes several alternatives including in-office audits, simulated case evaluations, the AGD's fellowship examination, and the diplomate examinations administered by specialty societies (AADE, 1993a). Chapter 8 examines this issue in the context of state licensure requirements.

FACULTY

The day-to-day fulfillment of the educational mission of dental schools depends on the quality and commitment of their faculty. Whether students enter practice with appropriate clinical skills and with critical thinking skills to guide them throughout their careers and whether they leave with positive attitudes about dental education depend largely on faculty. In addition, faculty contribute significantly to the development of new knowledge in oral health and to the care of patients.

It is the sense of this committee that several of the problems described in this report arise, in part, because dental faculty are too little involved with educational, clinical, and scientific contacts outside their clinical or basic science departments. They are thus isolated

- from the rest of the university and academic health center;
- from researchers in government, industry, and other universities;
- from the challenges and demands of active patient care; and
- from dentist colleagues in the community.

The task of reducing isolation is addressed throughout this report. This section focuses on initiatives by dental schools to achieve new relationships among faculty and between faculty and university administration. Among the dental schools visited by the committee, such initiatives had included the consolidation of traditional departments into larger units, the establishment of active curriculum committees, the formal study of the content and interrelationships of courses, the introduction or expansion of faculty development programs, and even the adoption of early retirement programs.

Such structural and procedural changes have the potential positive effects of focusing governance arguments on the relative contribution of parts to the whole rather than on the merits of the parts in isolation. If carefully implemented, they may reduce the administrative costs associated with small departments, make it easier to gather empirical information about what is actually happening in the school, and disturb practices justified mainly by their long existence.

Even if undertaken in a spirit of sensitivity and cooperation, however, these initiatives have potential negative effects as well. For example, they may create new organizational layers, interests, and paperwork. Some steps, such as early retirement programs, may divert resources away from other, perhaps better, uses and may create jealousy. Departmental consolidation may hamper recruitment of talented individuals who see traditional units as providing greater autonomy and control over resources. Restructuring may have the added purpose of saving money, but such savings may prove elusive. If the changes do not work as promised, they may reinforce the not inconsiderable cynicism that already exists inside and outside the university about proposals for educational restructuring and reform.

Provisions for tenure and legal prohibitions against mandatory retirement make it difficult to restructure the faculty, particularly during periods of relative stasis or decline in resources. Universities like most organizations have considerable reluctance to disrupt current personnel and constituencies in favor of personnel and constituencies whose influence—indeed existence—lies largely in the future.

The discussion below starts with a statistical profile of the dental faculty and continues with an overview of several central issues including faculty isolation, scholarship, tenure, and faculty development.

STATISTICAL PROFILE

In 1968, before the surge in dental school enrollments, the 52 existing dental schools had about 2,800 full-time basic science and clinical faculty, not quite 4,400 part-time faculty, and 15,400 students. Eighty-five percent of the part-time faculty—about 925 full-time equivalent positions—were clinical (AADS, 1993b).

In 1992, after the number of schools had grown to 60 and then fallen back to 55, dental schools had more than 3,300 full-time faculty in the basic and clinical sciences, more than 6,700 part-time faculty, and slightly less than 16,000 students. About 93 percent of the part-time faculty (or 1,275 full-time equivalents [FTEs]) were on the clinical side. As a percentage of full-time faculty, those in basic science dropped from 42 to 25 percent of the total during the same period.

Figure 4.3 show trends in the numbers of full-time and part-time faculty in the sciences. As a percentage of FTE clinical positions, part-time faculty dropped from 36 percent of the total in 1968 to 28 percent in 1992. ADA figures for 1992-1993 show that

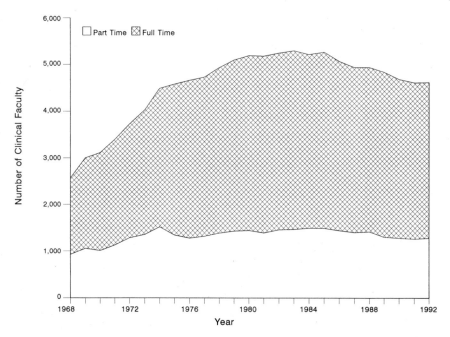

FIGURE 4.3 Trends in numbers of full-time and part-time clinical faculty. SOURCE: American Association of Dental Schools, 1993b.

part-time clinical faculty range from lows of 0 and 17 percent of the total clinical faculty at the University of North Carolina and the University of Florida (both public schools) to highs of 93 and 94 percent at Tufts University and the University of Southern California (both private schools).

According to AADS figures, in 1992, 19 percent of dental school faculty were women, and the percentages varied little between full-time and part-time faculty. About 4 percent of faculty were African-Americans; other minorities comprised about 8 percent.

ISSUES

Dental school faculty are clearly a diverse group with quite varied training, responsibilities, and concerns. Basic science and clinical faculty tend to have quite different responsibilities, work loads, and interactions with students. In general, clinical faculty spend more hours teaching or supervising clinic work and, thus, spend more time with students. The combination of these hours and any hours spent in a faculty practice plan will tend to leave clinical faculty with less time for research compared with basic science faculty.

Among clinical faculty, some have dental degrees, others have Ph.D.s, and some have both. Some have postgraduate specialty training; others have none. Some teach full-time; others, part-time. Some full-time faculty participate in faculty practice plans; others have no patients for whom they are directly responsible. Some are active researchers, but many clinical faculty have little or no involvement in research. Some have close ties to organized dentistry and local practitioners; others find such involvement uncomfortable. Faculty diversity enriches education, research, and patient care, but managing this diversity to achieve a balanced, high-quality faculty is a demanding task.

Faculty Development

One commentary recently observed that most schools spend a lot of time on recruitment, what they called the "fish-and-catch" phase of managing faculty resources (Bland and Ridky, 1993). The support and continual development of faculty once they are hired (i.e., caught) have been relatively neglected, with the major postrecruitment effort focused on tenure decisions. The reasons for this neglect of faculty development include lack of interest, and even resistance, from faculty themselves; management inattention; funding problems; and methodological questions that are both typical of educational efforts generally and specific to those aimed at faculty (Blackburn, 1991). Evaluations of faculty development strategies are limited.

The development or even retraining of faculty at all stages of their careers is, however, becoming a practical if not a philosophical concern of the university and the dental school as they have had to cope with resource limitations, increased public scrutiny, deteriorating faculty morale, and faculty composition influenced by tenure as well as educational needs (Schuster and Wheeler, 1990; Parker, 1991). Because many current faculty are products of the very educational approaches critiqued in this chapter, implementation of new strategies may require that faculty be educated both to understand the rationales for change and to learn new skills. The same argument holds for the new expectations with respect to research and patient care outlined in Chapters 5 and 6.

The importance of faculty development is increasingly being recognized in dental schools. In 1990, the AADS identified faculty development as an action priority (see, generally, the *Journal of Dental Education*, October 1991). The standards of the Commission on Dental Accreditation state that "there must be a professional development program available for full-time faculty of dental schools" (CDA, 1993a, p. 4). In the committee's survey one question asked deans to rate priorities for faculty development over the next 15 years. Table 4.3 presents their responses. In an added

TABLE 4.3   Survey of Deans' Priorities for Dental School Faculty Development over the Next 15 Years

Weighted Rank	Area
In the next 15 years, what priority would you place on faculty development in these areas?	
1	a Increasing sensitivity to student needs and concerns
8	b. Developing administrative and management skills
7	c. Developing facility with problem-based learning or similar strategies
4	d. Developing competency-based evaluations of student clinical skills
6	e. Using computer-based instructional tools
3	f. Improving instructional tools
5	g. Improving research skills
2	h. Increasing emphasis on patient outcomes assessment

SOURCE: Institute of Medicine and American Association of Dental Schools, 1994.

comment, one dean noted that faculty development demanded a very heavy commitment of resources. Not only does it require resources to plan, develop, staff, and evaluate internal activities or to send faculty to outside programs, the more intensive efforts—for example, research training—may require that faculty be freed from other obligations. This, in turn, may require schools to bring in clinicians from the community to fill in for absent clinical faculty (Dirksen, 1992). Finding the appropriate person may be difficult, particularly in smaller communities. These difficulties notwithstanding, the committee believes that faculty development programs are an important part of dental school efforts to adapt to a changing and resource-constrained environment.

As was evident in the committee's site visits and other activities, faculty development can take many forms and focus on a variety of objectives. The forms include seminars, workshops, written materials, editorial or technical assistance, peer assessment and guidance, and mentoring (Wheeler, 1991; Stritter, 1993). The broad objectives may be to develop teaching abilities, writing skills, research capabilities, or leadership talents. Less tangible than any of these objectives and methods is a much broader and more complex aim—building and sustaining talented and energetic faculty that are committed to the multiple missions of the dental school and the larger university and are intent on communicating their knowledge, enthusiasm, and dedication to students.

Faculty as Role Models

A related philosophical issue involves the ways in which faculty should serve as role models for students. To the extent that clinical faculty are not themselves engaged in patient care beyond the student clinic, they are often criticized as poor role models for their students, the great majority of whom will become full-time practitioners. Faculty who practice what they teach should find it easier to keep abreast of changing technologies and patient expectations. Being teachers as well as dentists, however, clinical faculty are particularly obligated to serve as role models of critical thinking in practice.

Faculty practice plans were recommended to the committee as a dual-purpose strategy to strengthen dental school faculties. On the one hand, they permit faculty salaries to be supplemented and made more competitive with private practice. On the other hand, they enhance faculty stature and experience by keeping them in touch with the realities of practice and the challenges of critical thinking in that environment.

Two other dimensions of faculty as role models involve research, which is covered in the next chapter, and responsibility for student education in comprehensive patient care. As noted earlier, the committee heard competing views about the latter issue. One argument is that generalist faculty should take the lead in educating students in comprehensive patient care because they can best exemplify the general practice model and philosophy that is the foundation of most predoctoral programs. The competing view is that instruction in the kinds of periodontic, endodontic, and other conditions seen by general dentists—and either treated by them or referred—requires faculty with advanced training. It is likely that both models can work if designed, implemented, and evaluated carefully.

In any case, the committee urges that one objective of faculty recruitment and development efforts be the establishing of faculty who are regarded as master clinicians in general practice, that is, qualified beyond the average general dentist. This objective, unfortunately, may conflict with the conventions of academic employment, in particular, compensation levels and tenure. More generally, because dental students tend to emerge from predoctoral and advanced education programs with very high levels of debt, graduates interested in academic careers may find that an entry-level academic appointment will make debt repayment difficult. Once they are established in private practice, these individuals may be reluctant to relinquish its pecuniary rewards even after they have reduced or eliminated their education debt. A number of the schools visited by the committee noted the irony of not being able to afford to hire their own top—but highly indebted—graduates.

Compensation

In common with other professional schools, dental schools can face difficulties in attracting qualified clinicians as educators and researchers because such individuals generally earn substantially higher incomes in private practice. Salary levels are typically higher in professional schools than elsewhere in universities, which may create jealousies elsewhere on campus.

Although the nonpecuniary benefits of teaching the next generation and of generating and disseminating new knowledge must be valued by faculty and nurtured by university and public officials, competitive salaries and benefits are essential. Unfortunately, in combination with the physical plant and equipment requirements of dental education, such compensation helps make dental schools expensive parts of their parent universities and academic health centers.

In medical schools, a major strategy for augmenting salaries for clinical faculties has been the faculty practice plan. This strategy, already mentioned in the discussion of role models, is examined further in the discussion of financing dental education in Chapter 7. That discussion notes that most revenues generated by practice plans are consumed either in patient care expenses or in supplements to faculty salaries, with little left for other educational purposes. Faculty practice also has nonfinancial benefits, particularly, as noted above, the increased involvement of faculty in actual patient care, not just in the supervision of patient care.

Tenure

In 1992, the percentage of full-time clinical faculty in dental schools who were tenured ranged from a low of 7 percent at Loma Linda University to a high of 96 percent at the State University of New York at Stony Brook. On average, about half of all such faculty are tenured. The percentage of full-time clinical faculty not eligible for tenure ranged from less than 5 percent at five schools to at least 50 percent at five other schools. Both the low end and the high end of the tenure continuum raised concerns for the committee. Earlier sections of this chapter have noted that tenure limits the flexibility of dental school in adapting to change and in restructuring the curriculum to remedy long-standing problems, and tenure may also act as a constraint on recruitment of a faculty that is more representative of the country's population. Very low levels of tenure combined with high ratios of part-time faculty may, however, deprive a school of a core of faculty committed primarily to the missions of the dental school rather than to the exigencies of private practice.

In principle, tenure rewards academic quality and protects intellectual freedom. The guiding statement on tenure, issued in 1940 by the American Association of University Professors, entitled "Statement of Principles on Academic Freedom and Tenure," refers to careful consideration of "accomplishments in teaching, scholarship, and college or university service" (AAUP, 1990). For health professions schools, the concept of service includes service to individual patients, and for higher education in general, the concept now more generally includes service to the community and nation.

Most educators acknowledge that very few faculty can be "triple threats," excelling in research, teaching, and service, and those who excel primarily in the latter areas often have not fared well in tenure decisions. For that reason, many schools have altered tenure practices. One approach has been to revise the criteria for tenure to grant more recognition to teaching and service. If the principle of scholarly excellence is to be maintained and if "teaching [is] to be equal to research," then it must be "vigorously assessed," a step that requires better methods for measuring performance (Boyer, 1990, p. 37; Stritter, 1993). Likewise, service must be assessed on the basis of academic as well as social relevance. In some cases, it is not clear what academic standards are being applied. The result may be a perception that teaching and patient care are relegated to second-class status (Scheetz and Mendel, 1993). The concern about how to assess performance in teaching for tenure-related purposes reinforces questions about measuring educational outcomes that are troublesome in many contexts including curriculum reform, licensure policies, and accreditation standards.

Rather than revise the terms of tenure, a second strategy has been to devise alternatives to tenure that may, to varying degrees, coexist with it and with institutional standards of excellence. These alternatives are highly varied, ranging from renewable contracts to increased reliance on part-time faculty to more generous sabbatical policies and other benefits for those who forgo tenure (Honan, 1994a).

Concerns about tenure have been intensified by the 1986 Age Discrimination in Employment Act, which prohibits mandatory retirement for most workers. Until 1994, colleges and universities were allowed to maintain mandatory retirement at age 70. A congressionally mandated study by the National Academy of Sciences concluded that most faculty would retire before age 70 at most institutions but that some research universities might have a high proportion of faculty working beyond that age (NRC, 1991). The study concluded that age itself did not affect institutional quality but that reduced faculty turnover and limited hiring flexibility did. They also affect efforts to create a faculty more representative of the broader population. Another 1991 study suggested that up to 10 percent of faculty at both private and public institutions of higher education would be over age 70 by the year 2000 (Honan, 1994b).

In this study's survey of deans, slightly more than 60 percent reported that their institutions had modified tenure criteria or adopted alternatives, and another 10 percent reported that they were being considered. Nearly 80 percent of the deans favored alternative tracks.

STUDENTS

A historic and not always fair charge against colleges, universities, and academic health science centers is that students are often viewed as a peripheral burden by administrators and faculty, who are preoccupied with organizational charts, salaries and benefits, research, private practice or consulting activities, and academic politics. The committee was not surprised to hear this charge sometimes directed at dental schools, often by faculty and administrators as well as practitioners. Indeed, research on medical and dental student perceptions suggests that an unpleasant atmosphere created by clinical faculty is among the most stressful aspects of school life (Wolff et al., 1992; Westerman et al., 1993).

That dental educators have been reexamining their attitudes, practices, and objectives about students is suggested by responses to the committee's survey of deans cited above in Table 4.3. The most uniformly cited priority for faculty development was programs to increase faculty sensitivity to student needs and concerns: of 54 deans, 43 rated such programs a high priority, and 8 a moderate priority.

Regardless of the merits of charges about past behavior, several factors have made careful regard for students a priority for universities generally and dental schools in particular. Demographics—notably, the so-called baby bust and its accompanying "shortage" in the pool of young adults—has prompted educators to work harder to attract and retain students. The 1980s saw a substantial decrease in applications for admission to dental school combined with a decline in the "quality" of applicants as measured by grades and test scores, which are admittedly limited—although widely used—measures of qualifications. Schools risked closure if they could not attract a sufficient number and quality of students to satisfy university academic standards and maintain tuition revenues. Without the influx of women students described below, the situation would be much worse.

Statistical Profile

In 1993, 54 dental schools enrolled nearly 16,000 predoctoral dental students and graduated more than 3,800 (AADS, 1993b). An array of postdoctoral programs in both university and nonuniversity (e.g., hospital) settings enrolls nearly 4,600 students. In Table 4.2, first-year enrollments in advanced programs are listed. In

addition, university, community college, and other programs enroll about 10,000 dental hygienists, 6,000 dental assistants, and
1,000 dental laboratory technicians (AADS, 1993b).

In 1992, total predoctoral enrollment of dental students ranged
from lows of 109 and 111 at Harvard and the State University of
New York at Stony Brook, respectively (excluding Loyola, which
closed in 1993), to highs of 520 and 1,145 at the University of
Southern California and New York University, respectively.[9] Figure 4.4 graphs dental schools grouped according to enrollment.

Among the 54 schools currently in operation, predoctoral enrollment has decreased since 1983 for 45 schools and increased for
9; all but 2 of the latter are private or private state-related schools.
Between 1982 and 1992, total enrollment dropped 30 percent—
from 22,235 to 15,980. The decreases are negligible for several
schools, but others have cut enrollment by a quarter or even a
half. Of the six public schools with more than 500 predoctoral
students in 1983, none has as many as 400 students now. Of the
seven private or private state-related schools with more than 500
students in 1983, two have closed, one has remained roughly steady
in size, three have downsized by more than 20 percent, and one
has increased its total enrollment by 80 percent.

Student enrollment statistics show great variability in state residence, gender, race, ethnicity, and graduation from foreign dental
schools (ADA, 1993a, b, c). Nonresident enrollments range from 0
to 60 percent among public schools and from 7 to 94 percent among
private and private state-related schools. The proportion of female
students ranges from less than 15 percent at one school to slightly
more than 50 percent at two schools. Two schools have majority
African-American enrollments, but no other schools appear to have
African-American enrollments equal to the group's representation
in the general population. A few schools have near-majority enrollments of students of Asian origin, and Hispanic students constitute
more than 20 percent of enrollment at a few schools. In Chapter 9,
which considers a dental work force for the future, strategies to
increase participation by underrepresented minorities are discussed.

Enrollment of foreign dental graduates ranges from a low of 0
in 20 schools (and only one or two students at 11 more schools) to

---

[9]By way of comparison, there are about 66,000 medical predoctoral students
in 126 schools (Jonas et al., 1993). In size, medical schools (excluding Duluth,
which offers only the first two years) range from 157 students at Morehouse
University to 1,284 at Wayne State University.

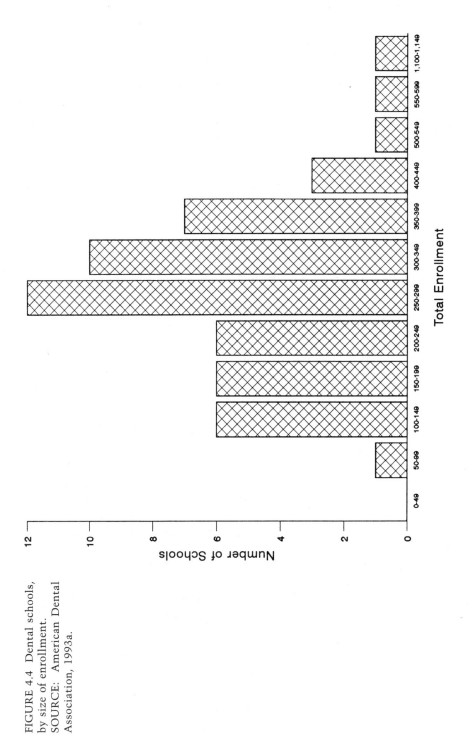

FIGURE 4.4 Dental schools, by size of enrollment. SOURCE: American Dental Association, 1993a.

highs of 17 percent in two schools and 41 percent at one school (ADA, 1993e). The last school alone accounted for nearly half of all enrolled foreign dental graduates, and two-thirds of such graduates were enrolled in just four private institutions. As noted in the background paper by Capilouto et al., the number of foreign dental graduates admitted with advanced standing to U.S. dental schools has grown sharply, nearly doubling from 1990 to 1992.

QUALITY OF APPLICANTS AND GRADUATES

Improving the quality of applicants and admitted students was clearly a priority (either self-chosen or externally dictated) at several of the schools visited by the committee. These schools pointed to recent improvements in student credentials but acknowledged that they could not say whether these improvements reflected their recruiting efforts or other factors such as the decreasing attractiveness of M.B.A. programs.

In the 1970s, increases in the number of dental school applicants and the ratio of applicants to enrollees were accompanied by increases in grade point averages and dental admission test scores (AADS, 1993b). The 1980s saw decreases in each area. Recent trends indicate improvements in applicant ratios and grade point averages. In addition, the attrition rate has dropped. In their survey responses, three-quarters of dental school deans agreed that dental school applicants were "better" today than five years ago. Although grade point averages were often mentioned during site visits and other meetings, the committee concluded that dental educators' views on shifts in student quality were not limited to this indicator but were also based on their first-hand experience with students over the course of many years.

The earlier apparent drop-off in student qualifications may now be reverberating in initially higher failure rates on board and licensure examinations. For example, the percentage of U.S. graduates failing Part I of the National Board examinations increased fairly steadily from 9.6 in 1982 to 16.0 in 1992; for Part II, the failure rate went from 8.0 to 13.2 percent during the same period (ADA, 1993d).[10] These trends may be another factor prompting schools

---

[10]The Part II examination and scoring system was changed in 1992, but ADA tests of the new examination suggest the change did not affect failure rates (David Demarais, ADA staff, personal communication, August 23, 1994). In the three years preceding 1992, the failure rates were 13.4, 15.3, and 15.2.

to pay more attention to how they recruit and educate their students. The relationships among the entering qualifications of dental students, their achievements in dental school, their success on licensure examinations, their subsequent performance in dental practice, and school evaluations during the accreditation process are discussed further in Chapter 8.

In considering the quality of dental students and graduates, the committee developed some particular questions about graduates of foreign dental schools. ADA data indicate that these students are more likely to fail the National Board Dental Examinations (ADA, 1993c). For example, 48 and 39 percent failed the 1992 Part I and II examinations, compared to 16 and 13 percent of U.S. students, respectively.[11] The committee found no data on the proportions of foreign dental graduates who never passed the examination and no follow-up data on those who eventually did pass. Information on clinical examination performance is not available.

The committee recognizes that foreign dental graduates who do become licensed in the United States may provide needed services, and it opposes discrimination on the basis of nationality. Nonetheless, as discussed further in Chapter 8, the committee is troubled by shortcomings in the processes for assessing student performance and graduate competency, and it is concerned that these shortcomings may be even more serious for foreign dental graduates who enter with advanced standing. The committee urges dental educators, accrediting organizations, and related groups to assess current policies for the admission, education, graduation, and licensure of graduates of foreign dental schools and to eliminate admissions policies or other practices that may exploit these students or threaten the quality of patient care.

TUITION AND DEBT LOAD

In its visits to dental schools, the committee heard countervailing worries about tuition. On the one hand, tuition cannot continue to go up at the same rate as in the past; on the other hand, tuition is a major source of revenue for many schools.

---

[11]This information is consistent with limited data on examination results for foreign medical graduates (Page, 1994). The medical examination data also indicate that American graduates of foreign medical schools have even higher failure rates.

High student tuition is one of the most acute quality-of-life problems for many dental students and a major worry for dental educators. Figure 4.5 shows the change in tuition (in constant dollars) charged by public and private dental schools from 1970 to 1991. In 1970, tuition ranged from $67 dollars for in-state students at the least expensive school to $2,750 for all students at the most expensive. In 1991, the range was from $3,126 to $33,195. Other fees and living expenses add to total costs. For example, instrument purchase or rental can add thousands of dollars to students' costs. Not surprisingly, many dental students leave school with considerable debt, as illustrated in Figure 4.6. The high cost of dental education contributes to concerns that students from low- and middle-income families will lose access and that only those from wealthy families and those poor enough to qualify for substantial income-based financial aid will be able to afford dental school.

In addition to considering the implications of the tuition and debt situations for both students and schools, the committee was

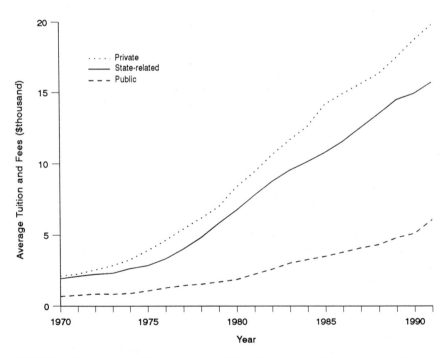

FIGURE 4.5 Average resident tuition and fees in constant dollars by school type. SOURCE: American Association of Dental Schools, 1992.

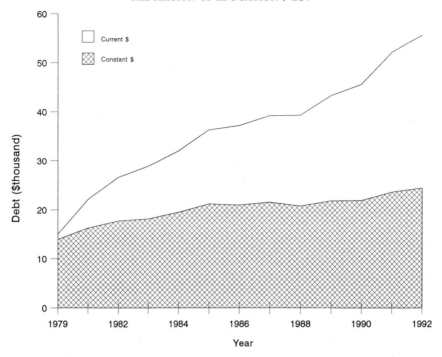

FIGURE 4.6 Student debt in constant dollars. SOURCE: American Association of Dental Schools, 1993b.

concerned about the implications for practitioners and patients. During almost every site visit, the committee heard students admit that debt limited their options after graduation. Among the options discouraged are rural practice, short-term or career military service, practice in low-income areas, and academic or research careers. Several of these options involve settings with a shortage of practitioners. For example, the Department of Defense (1993, p. 1) testified to the committee that "the high level of indebtedness . . . [means that] many . . . who would consider serving in the armed services . . . cannot afford such a career. . . . All three services are well short of their recruiting needs."

Some students who would prefer to go into practice say they opt for advanced education in part to put off debt repayment. For some but not all loan categories, interest charges are suspended during the training period. An additional incentive is the prospect of higher income with which to repay debt. Conversely, other students feel that they must start earning immediately after graduation, even if they would prefer a general practice residency or postgraduate specialty training. The fact that several categories of postgraduate training in dentistry neither pay a stipend nor waive tuition only adds to the difficulty. (Stipends are the norm in hospital-based programs, primarily for oral and maxillofacial surgery and general practice residencies; they are common if not universal in pediatrics and advanced general dentistry.)

Efforts to control tuition and educational costs generally are discussed in Chapter 7 and in the background paper by Douglass and Fein. In addition to trying to control tuition costs, policymakers may ameliorate the debt problem to some degree by adopting or expanding programs of national service that link debt forgiveness to a period of practice in underserved areas.[12]

In simple numerical terms, existing programs fall short as either debt relief or access improvement. Between FY 1991 and FY 1993, the National Health Service Corps (NHSC) increased the number of loan repayment positions from 11 to 55 (J. Rosetti, personal communication to M. Allukian, April 4, 1994). For 1994, 75 loan repayment positions were approved, but approximately 350 dentists were on a waiting list. Between FY 1991 and FY 1993, the number of scholarships decreased from 22 to 5, and none are projected in the future. In fact, the brochure describing the NHSC scholarship program does not even mention dentistry (AADS, 1994b).

---

[12]The 1992 reauthorization of the Higher Education Act (HEA) changed the terms and conditions of many borrowing programs, particularly in the areas of deferment, interest capitalization, and repayment schedules. For example, the HEA created a direct loan demonstration program for institutions, in which participating schools will be designing programs that would allow income-sensitive repayment schedules. In the case of the most commonly used federal loan program, the Stafford, there is an increased focus on borrowers' needs in the allocation of interest subsidies. Instead of offering the same interest rate to all borrowers, an unsubsidized Stafford loan program has been created for those who do not show a need for interest subsidies.

Most students are subject to interest capitalization during their undergraduate education unless the borrower makes interest payments while in school or qualifies for the need-based interest subsidy. Students pursuing postdoctoral educational opportunities are eligible for loan deferment with interest capitalization (except those awarded need-based interest subsidies). In addition, a loan consolidation program is available, that allows consolidation of certain loans with the option of graduated and income-sensitive repayment schedules and extended payback (up to 30 years, depending on the level of indebtedness).

In FY 1993, the Health Resource Services Administration listed more than 1,000 dental shortage areas in need of over 2,000 dentists. The limitations of the NHSC program as a vehicle for improving access to care in underserved areas are discussed further in Chapter 9. Without greater public funding of this program, it will meet neither the primary goal of improved access nor the important secondary goal of helping students who are not wealthy retain access to dental education.

QUALITY OF STUDENT LIFE

During site visits, several specific initiatives to improve student instruction and quality of life were cited. Most of these initiatives were also expected to improve the quality of education. Specifically,

1. upgraded admission standards would avoid the distress created for and by students who are not academically qualified (given available resources and reasonable expectations for special remediation programs) to tackle predoctoral coursework;

2. revisions in instructional methods would discourage authoritarian and rote teaching, thereby reducing the stress associated with numerical requirements and factual recall;

3. attempts to rebalance the curriculum would provide more stimulating education and more time to reflect on it; and

4. efforts to create a sense of community among health professions students and to expand student exposure to the broader offerings of university life would improve the quality of life for dental students.

The second and third of these directions—instructional and curriculum changes—have already been discussed. The fourth area reflects an acknowledgment that although the insularity of most professional schools—and dental schools in particular—has its comforts, isolation can be stifling. The committee was impressed by what it heard of efforts to create a sense of community among health professions students. These efforts are designed, in part, to increase the quality of services and support available to students by pooling library, housing, and other resources or activities and, in part, to enrich student life. Joint teaching of dental and other health professions students is intended to broaden the educational experience and promote the concept of health care as an enterprise involving teamwork and consultation. Enrichment of the dental school experience stretches beyond the health professions in the form of joint degrees and coursework involving a range of other schools and programs such as engineering, business, and health administration.

A self-interested reason for dental educators to improve the quality of student life is that unhappy student memories may mean meager alumni contributions. Although such contributions are a relatively small part of school budgets they can relieve some of the pressure caused by cutbacks in public funding and greater competition for research funds. More generally, if practitioners retain negative feelings after they graduate, this may contribute to the tensions between the education and the practice communities noted elsewhere in this report.

FINDINGS AND RECOMMENDATIONS

Because education is the most visible mission of dental schools, the committee commissioned a background paper on curriculum by Tedesco and focused many of its information collection activities on issues related to curriculum, faculty, and students. The committee examined extensive analyses of dental education. It also consulted numerous analyses of medical education to identify parallels and contrasts. The persistence of several common themes is striking and underscores the challenge of achieving change.

The committee feels confident that most of those involved in dental education would agree that the following problems persist. Basic and clinical science teaching do not stress the basic sciences as a relevant foundation for clinical practice. Individual courses and the overall curriculum often reflect past rather than current practice and knowledge. Comprehensive care is more an ideal than a reality in clinical education, and instruction still focuses too heavily on procedures. Linkages between medicine and dentistry are insufficient to prepare students to comprehend and apply the growing medical core of dental practice. The curriculum is crowded with redundant or marginally useful material and gives students too little time to consolidate concepts or to develop critical thinking skills. Lack of flexible tenure and promotion policies and of adequate resources for faculty development limits efforts to match the faculty to educational needs. Despite progress, insensitivity to student needs is still a concern. All of these weaknesses undermine efforts to prepare students for lifelong learning.

Many other reports have argued for movement away from these traditions and problems and have suggested specific alternatives including curriculum reform, education using active learning strategies such as problem-based learning, closer relationships between dentistry and medicine, new approaches to comprehensive care, and revised accreditation standards. The problem is not so much agreement on directions for change but difficulty in overcoming the obstacles to change. These include lack of specific information on course content, limited evaluation of educational impact, university policy restrictions, faculty conservatism, and regulatory and financial constraints. Suggestions and recommendations here or in other chapters address most of these obstacles, but each institution will have to tailor strategies to its specific circumstances. More generally, the kind of leadership and commitment emphasized in Chapter 7 is not something that can be transmitted through a report, although this report may—as stated early in this chapter—provide guidance and some leverage.

The following recommendations emphasize curriculum reform, closer relationships with medicine, clinical experience in efficient practice settings, and student debt. They offer a mix of aspirations and instrumental actions to move toward desired goals. They need to be considered in conjunction with Chapter 6's recommendations about the patient care mission of dental schools, Chapter 8's consideration of licensure and accreditation policies, and Chapter 9's discussion of work force policies.

To stimulate progress toward curriculum goals long endorsed in dental education, the committee recommends that dental schools set explicit targets, procedures, and timetables for modernizing courses, eliminating marginally useful and redundant course content, and reducing excessive course loads. The process should include steps to

• design an integrated basic and clinical science curriculum that provides clinically relevant education in the basic sciences and scientifically based education in clinical care;

• incorporate in all educational activities a focus on outcomes and an emphasis on the relevance of scientific knowledge and thinking to clinical choices;

• shift more curriculum hours from lectures to guided seminars and other active learning strategies that develop critical thinking and problem-solving skills;

• identify and decrease the hours spent in low priority preclinical technique, clinical laboratory work, and lectures; and

• complement clinic hours with scheduled time for discussion of specific diagnosis, planning, and treatment-completion issues that arise in clinic sessions.

To prepare future practitioners for more medically based modes of oral health care and more medically complicated patients, dental educators should work with their colleagues in medical schools and academic health centers to

• move toward integrated basic science education for dental and medical students;
• require and provide for dental students at least one rotation, clerkship, or equivalent experience in relevant areas of medicine, and offer opportunities for additional elective experience in hospitals, nursing homes, ambulatory care clinics, and other settings;
• continue and expand experiments with combined M.D.-D.D.S. programs and similar programs for interested students and residents; and
• increase the experience of dental faculty in clinical medicine so that they—and not just physicians—can impart medical knowledge to dental students and serve as role models for them.

To prepare students and faculty for an environment that will demand increasing efficiency, accountability, and evidence of effectiveness, the committee recommends that dental students and faculty participate in efficiently managed clinics and faculty practices in which

• patient-centered, comprehensive care is the norm;
• patients' preferences and their social, economic, and emotional circumstances are sensitively considered;
• teamwork and cost-effective use of well-trained allied dental personnel are stressed;
• evaluations of practice patterns and of the outcomes of care guide actions to improve both the quality and the efficiency of such care;
• general dentists serve as role models in the appropriate treatment and referral of patients needing advanced therapies; and
• larger numbers of patients, including those with more diverse characteristics and clinical problems, are served.

The committee recommends that postdoctoral education in a general dentistry or specialty program be available for every dental graduate, that the goal be to achieve this within five to ten years, and that the emphasis be on creating new positions in advanced general dentistry and discouraging additional specialty residencies unless warranted by shortages of services that cannot be provided effectively by other personnel.

To permit faculty hiring and promotion practices that better reflect educational objectives and changing needs, the committee recommends that dental schools and their universities supplement tenure-track positions with other full-time nontenured clinical or research positions that provide greater flexibility in achieving teaching, research, and patient care objectives.

To improve the availability of dental care in underserved areas and to limit the negative effects of high student debt, Congress and the states should act to increase the number of dentists serving in the National Health Service Corps and other federal or state programs that link financial assistance to work in underserved areas.

SUMMARY

The education of future practitioners is the central mission of dental schools. The content and method of dental education have been the subject of many criticisms over the years related to the weak links between basic science and clinical education or experience, the overcrowded dental curriculum, and the isolation of faculty both individually and collectively from the world beyond departmental boundaries. Linkages between dentistry and medicine are weaker than the nature of oral health problems and the growth of medically oriented interventions warrant. Problems remain in implementing comprehensive patient-centered care. The persistence of these problems testifies to the difficulty of change. Although the next two chapters of this report catalog yet more problems in the areas of research and patient care, their recommendations focus on steps that would address not only those problems but also some identified in this chapter. For example, greater research involvement by clinical faculty would almost certainly reinforce the links between basic science and clinic education, and revitalization of the patient care mission would likewise help make clinically current and patient-centered education a reality.

5

The Mission of Research

Oral health researchers in U.S. dental schools and universities, together with researchers in government, postgraduate institutes, and industry, have built a base of scientific and clinical knowledge that has been widely communicated and used to improve oral health. Their ongoing research initiatives combined with broad advances in the biomedical sciences will add to these achievements in the future. Discoveries in genetics, molecular and cell biology, immunology, and pharmacology, as well as in materials and computer sciences, will reshape the character and focus of dental practice and dental education itself. Vaccines against caries and periodontal disease, new anti-infectious agents, sophisticated simulation models, even genetic therapies are all likely to materialize in the future. The main questions are not whether but *when* they will arrive and in what specific form.

Many of the basic science discoveries that will be most influential in shaping future oral health and oral health practice will occur outside dental schools—in university science departments, in medical schools, and in government, industrial, and other research laboratories. This means that dental school research programs must be linked to basic research programs outside the school. Involvement with medical school and other university research activities will be increasingly important.

Some dental schools are vital centers for the creation of new knowledge about oral diseases and their prevention or treatment.

Nonetheless, many dental schools and dental faculty still have little or no involvement with research or, more broadly, scholarship. Twenty percent of the dental schools received two-thirds of the research and training funds distributed by the National Institute of Dental Research (NIDR) in 1991. As described in Chapter 2, NIDR was created in 1948 to bolster the very limited research and research training capacity of dental schools as well as to conduct its own research program. It remains the major source of support for oral health research and for training of oral health researchers.

This chapter begins with a discussion of broad goals for dental schools. It then reviews basic data on funding sources, amounts, and targets of oral health research. Later sections discuss major issues and concerns, in particular, funding constraints and shortages of well-trained oral health researchers. The background papers by Greenspan and by Jeffcoat and Clark provide a selective overview of the current state of, and future prospects for, oral health science and technology and of the role of dental schools in technology transfer. The paper by Bader and Shugars focuses on outcomes and health services research.

BROAD GOALS FOR RESEARCH IN THE DENTAL SCHOOL

As stated in Chapter 1, the committee strongly believes that dental education should be scientifically based and undertaken in an environment in which the creation and acquisition of new scientific and clinical knowledge are valued and vigorously pursued. The research standards for dental schools published by the Commission on Dental Accreditation support this goal (Table 5.1).

In addition to creating new knowledge, the research mission includes disseminating such knowledge, educating clinicians to critically assess scientific and technological innovations, and educating future researchers. Conceptualized somewhat differently, these dimensions include a mix of scholarly activities: *discovery, integration, application, and teaching* (Boyer, 1990; Bepko, 1991). However categorized, these elements of research and scholarship are linked by the broad common goal of improved oral health and should influence all elements of the dental school curriculum. Their scope is sufficiently broad that they offer opportunities for faculty contributions beyond the laboratory or clinical trial—important as those traditional venues of research are.

The *creation or discovery of new knowledge* is the heart of the university's research mission. Within the diverse components of

TABLE 5.1 Research Standards for Accreditation

1. *Research, the process of scientific inquiry involved in the development and dissemination of new or improved knowledge, must be an integral component of the mission of each dental educational institution.*

As the advancement of the profession, and ultimately the health of the public, depends upon the development and dissemination of new or improved knowledge, dental education institutions must accept the obligation to do research. Research, whether basic, clinical, behavioral or that leading to improved oral health care delivery, must be in evidence.

Although it is recognized that institutional priorities will vary in relation to research, education and service, research efforts must be of such quantity and quality as to support the stated mission of the institution. In addition, there should be an appropriate balance among these three activities to ensure that institutional objectives are being fully realized.

2. *A formal research development plan must be evident to ensure the continual support of the research mission of the institution.*

The administrative responsibilities for the development, monitoring and continuance of research activities should be clearly outlined.

3. *The amount of time and resources available for faculty research should be sufficient to support the objectives of the institution.*

There should be clearly evident a mechanism whereby interested faculty and students at all levels might become meaningfully involved in research endeavors. Institutional resources should be available to provide interim support for faculty in the event that funds for sponsored research lapse.

SOURCE: CDA, 1993a.

the modern university, discovery can take varied forms. Past Institute of Medicine (IOM) studies of health research have identified a "continuum" of relevant research fields, including: "the *biomedical sciences*, which inquire into the basic nature of life through deeper understanding of life process; the *clinical sciences*, which translate fundamental research into medical practice; *population-based sciences*, such as epidemiology and biostatistics; the *behavioral and social sciences; biophysics, bioengineering*, and clinically oriented *medical engineering and physics*; the *hybrid sciences*, such as nutritional and environmental sciences; *health services research*, which studies the health care system; and *technology transfer*" (IOM, 1979, 1990d, p. 30, emphasis added).

The creation of new knowledge often involves studies that cross disciplines. For dental faculty, interdisciplinary research—particularly when it involves clinical faculty—has the additional benefit of reducing the isolation for which dental schools have sometimes been criticized (Hogness, 1982; McCallum, 1983; Ranney,

1989; Littleton, 1992). The focus of such integrating research is highly varied and includes basic biological processes at the cellular and molecular levels, pharmacological methods for preventing or treating oral disease, biomaterials development, "hard tissue engineering" (involving bone and tooth structures), and oral health epidemiology and behavior. The background paper by Greenspan, for example, discusses how approaches combining molecular biology, molecular immunology, and epidemiology are advancing basic scientific knowledge of periodontal diseases.

In addition to basic and clinical research, both behavioral research and health services research are essential for the improvement of oral health in individuals and populations. Basic scientific discoveries and clinical advances do not automatically benefit individuals or communities. Access to these advances may be limited by organizational, behavioral, financial, or other barriers, and clinical advances may not directly address the problems of particular population subgroups. A major goal of behavioral, epidemiological, and health services research is to identify the factors that encourage or thwart the various steps required to move from scientific knowledge to improved health. Basic, clinical, and health services research, taken together, can reinforce and support the emphasis on health outcomes that is demanded in today's health care system.

In addition to creating knowledge, dental schools are also important vehicles for *disseminating and integrating knowledge* through their predoctoral, graduate, and continuing education programs. They play a role in the process of *technology transfer*, which involves the movement of new applications of knowledge from academic, governmental, and commercial research centers to the practice setting.

At their best, dental school faculty and curricula act as critical filters that help students and practitioners to separate well-founded from ill-founded claims for the effectiveness of specific new—and old—interventions. At their worst, as this committee heard on occasion, faculty are neither immersed in advances in science and technology nor prepared to scrutinize rigorously claims for the effectiveness of new (to say nothing of established) clinical practices.[1] The committee's site visits produced repeated references

---

[1]The somewhat tenuous standing of oral research in the broader research community is suggested by the periodic reports on needs and training for biomedical and behavioral sciences developed by the Office of Scientific and Engineering

to the archetype of the nonscholarly faculty member—the "checker" who inspects student work but makes no contribution through critical thinking or research.[2]

In disseminating knowledge and participating in technology transfer, the objectives for dental education are not merely to promote the appropriate adoption of new techniques, drugs, or materials but more generally to *promote informed and intelligent practice.* This requires the curricular framework described in Chapter 4, one that provides a practice-relevant foundation in the basic sciences and that incorporates research findings and evaluation in classroom and chairside clinical instruction. Coursework in research methods and participation in research projects are other components of a curriculum designed to promote professional inquisitiveness, intellectual confidence, and critical appraisal skills that students will take with them into practice. Further, faculty who are actively involved in the conduct and evaluation of research can exemplify the critical cast of mind that all health professionals should possess.

Continuing education programs offer a potentially important opportunity for dental schools to help clinicians learn about scientific and clinical advances and to evaluate their effectiveness critically. In the committee's site visits, faculty and practitioners argued that dental schools can go beyond the narrow technique and product focus of many commercial programs to present practitioners with an evidence- and outcomes-oriented assessment of new technologies. Such assessments are particularly important for practitioners whose formal education did not provide the evaluative skills and perspectives advocated in this report and who, thus, may be more vulnerable to enthusiastically promoted but inadequately tested new technologies.

Finally, with the active support of NIDR, dental schools have a major responsibility for *educating future dental researchers.* Small

---

Personnel (OSEP) of the National Academy of Sciences. In 1985, training for oral health research was covered solely under the topic of clinical sciences; the 1989 report did not even consider it (NAs, 1985, 1989). Putting oral health research on the agenda for the 1994 OSEP report required a special effort from the dental research community. The results of that effort are reflected in the proceedings of a workshop held in July 1993 and in the sections of the 1994 report discussed later in this chapter.

[2]Apropos of this is Meskin's tongue-in-check dictionary definition of research: "1. a state to be avoided at all costs 2. less common, an unnatural act required of dental faculty in order to achieve the state of tenure 3. much less common, an arduous task fraught with pain but achievable 4. much, much less common . . . an enjoyable pursuit to achieve academic excellence" (Meskin, 1983).

but important support for research training also comes from private foundations (e.g., the Robert Wood Johnson clinical scholars program) and industry. Oral health research does and should draw on researchers trained in medical schools and graduate schools, but a stronger dental school role in research education is an important means to strengthen the link between the basic and clinical sciences in dental schools, solidify the position of dental schools in research-intensive universities and academic health centers, and direct research to oral health problems. Expanding and strengthening the pool of capable basic science and, especially, clinical researchers are, at the same time, preconditions for expanding and strengthening the research productivity of dental schools.

RESEARCH REVENUES, EXPENDITURES, AND PUBLICATIONS

Measuring the *output* of research activities in dental schools is difficult. Therefore, this summary focuses on *inputs*, in particular, research funding. It also includes some information on research productivity as measured by publications.

Data on research revenues and expenditures for dental schools come from two primary sources, the American Dental Association (ADA) and the National Institute of Dental Research. ADA data do not include institutions that offer only postgraduate dental education programs such as the Eastman Dental Center and the Mayo Graduate School of Medicine. To the extent that dental faculty are involved in multidisciplinary research projects that are administered by other units (e.g., medical schools), dental school involvement in research may be understated. In addition, the research activity of dental school faculty may not be reflected in the financial figures for other reasons, for example, if foundations refuse to pay full overhead costs for research contracts, schools may categorize the funds they do provide as gift income not research revenues.

The ADA reports dental school *expenditures* for research in four categories: basic science, clinical science, behavioral science, and training grants (Table 5.2). As measured by expenditures, the major focus of research is clinical, followed by basic science, training, and—a very distance fourth—behavioral science research. ADA data for 1993 show that 46 of 55 schools reported expenditures for clinical research, 38 for basic science, 34 for training, and 11 for behavioral research.

For the reporting year ending June 30, 1993, *revenues* from sponsored education, research, and research training accounted for more than

$125 million out of total dental school revenues of more than $1 billion.[3]   The contribution of sponsored education, research, and training to total revenues varies enormously across schools.   It ranges from less than 2 percent at nine schools to 56 percent at one school.   For the next highest school, the figure drops to just under 28 percent (ADA, 1994a).   The mean for all schools is about 10 percent.   By way of comparison, federal research grants and contracts alone account for 12 percent of medical school revenues, and all sources of research and training grants and contracts contribute about 20 percent of their revenues (Krakower et al., 1993).

In 1993, more than 70 percent of dental school research revenues came from the federal government, while 22 percent came from nongovernmental sources and 7 percent from state and local governments (Table 5.3).   The great majority of federal support comes from NIDR, with other agencies—including other divisions of the National Institutes of Health—contributing the remainder. The committee found no comprehensive data on these other sources.[4]

NIDR spending for its external or extramural research program falls into several categories as depicted in Figure 5.1.   The entire extramural program receives not quite 75 percent of the total NIDR budget, about 90 percent of which goes for specific research projects, support for research centers, and other research.   About one-third of NIDR extramural research funds are provided to institutions other than dental schools (e.g., advanced education institutions and medical schools).

A commonly used measure of research productivity relies on individual or institutional publications (Harrington, 1987; McGuire et al., 1988).   The rationale is that the number of scientific publications and the type of these publication are useful indicators of "an institution's contribution to knowledge" (Lipton, 1990).   One analysis found 50 dental institutions worldwide (including advanced education institutions) with 40 or more articles published in 1987 and 1988 in journals included in the Science Citation Index.   Thirteen of these 50 institutions had 90 or more articles.   (Of the 4,300

---

[3]About 10 percent of these revenues involve sponsored educational programs.
[4]Examples can, however, illustrate the range of organizations that might reasonably fund research in dental schools: the National Cancer Institute for work on oral cancer; the National Institute for Arthritis and Musculoskeletal and Skin Diseases for research on connective tissue biochemistry and bone mineralization; the National Institute on Aging for studies of oral health problems in geriatric populations; and the National Institute of Allergy and Infectious Disease for AIDS research.

TABLE 5.2 Dental School Expenditures (dollars) for Research, 1993

Sponsored Research and Training	Public		Private		All	
Basic science	42,321,201	(46%)	11,440,330	(54%)	53,761,532	(47%)
Clinical science	43,639,741	(47%)	6,499,781	(31%)	50,139,523	(44%)
Behavioral science	955,682	(1%)	145,949	(1%)	1,141,631	(1%)
Training grants	5,677,073	(6%)	3,044,359	(14%)	8,721,432	(8%)
Total	92,633,697	(100%)	21,130,419	(100%)	113,764,118	(100%)

SOURCE: Data compiled from American Dental Association, 1994a.

TABLE 5.3 Dental School Revenues (dollars) from Research, 1993

Sponsored Research and Training	Public		Private		All	
Nongovernment	22,017,372	(23%)	5,492,424	(20%)	27,509,796	(22%)
State or local government	5,864,445	(6%)	2,849,836	(10%)	8,714,281	(7%)
Federal government	69,243,174	(71%)	19,554,257	(70%)	88,797,431	(71%)
Total	97,144,991	(100%)	27,896,517	(100%)	125,021,508	(100%)

SOURCE: Data compiled from American Dental Association, 1994a.

journals indexed, 29 focused on dentistry.) Twenty-two of the first group of 50 institutions and seven of the second group of 13 most productive schools were located in the United States; three of the six foreign institutions were in Scandinavian countries (Lipton, 1990).

FOCUS OF RESEARCH AND RESEARCH TRAINING

As indicated by the ADA expenditure data reported above, clinical research accounts for the major part of dental school research, with basic research a relatively close second. Although ADA reports do not further identify the substantive focus of research, NIDR data are helpful here.

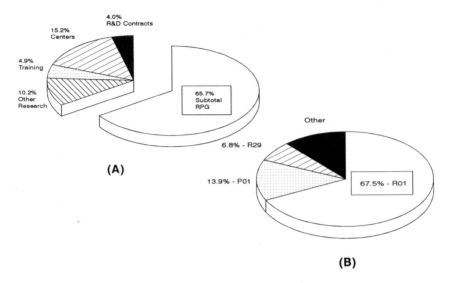

FIGURE 5.1 Percentage distribution of National Institute of Dental Research (NIDR) extramural obligations, FY 1993 (total extramural program = $118,363,000; research projects = $77,805,000). A: All programs; B: Research project grants (RPGs). NOTE: R01 = traditional project grants; R29 = first independent research support and transition (FIRST) award; and P01 = research program projects. Center grants: P20, P30, and P50. SOURCE: NIDR, 1993a.

The focus of NIDR funding has shifted considerably over the institute's history. As reported by Harris (1989), 37 percent of research grants in the NIDR's first three award years were devoted to caries, fluoride, and restorative materials; 10 percent to periodontal disease; 10 percent to nutrition; and 8 percent to craniofacial abnormalities. By 1985, caries and restorative materials accounted for 28 percent of funding; periodontal and soft tissue disease for 34 percent; and craniofacial development, pain, and behavioral science research for 27 percent. Figure 5.2 shows the distribution of NIDR extramural funds across 19 research areas in 1993.

NIDR data do not distinguish between basic and clinical research projects. Data reported by Harris (1989) indicate that the majority of articles published by extramural researchers supported by NIDR concerned "bioscientific" topics not confined to oral conditions.

In addition to individual research projects, NIDR supports 29 research centers, most of them affiliated with dental schools. The varied foci of these centers are revealed in Table 5.4. In FY 1993,

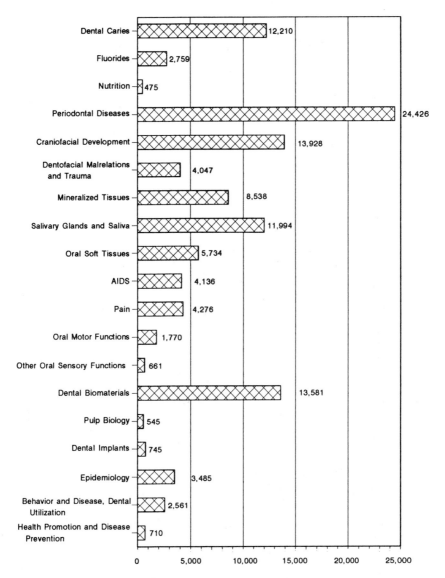

FIGURE 5.2 Distribution of total FY 1993 National Institute of Dental Research (NIDR) extramural funds by research areas ($thousands). SOURCE: NIDR, 1993a.

TABLE 5.4 NIDR Research Centers Support: Number of Projects and Number of Subprojects by Type of Center and Institution, FY 1993

Type of Center and Institution	Department	No. of Projects	No. of Subprojects	Awarded Amounts
Research Centers in Oral Biology		5	27	$ 4,720,173
State University of New York at Buffalo	Oral Biology			
University of Alabama at Birmingham	Oral Biology			
University of California at San Francisco	Stomatology			
University of Pennsylvania	Research Center in Oral Biology			
University of Washington	Oral Biology			
Research Centers on Oral Health in Aging		2	8	1,252,581
University of Iowa	Dows Institute for Dental Research			
University of Texas Health Science Center at San Antonio	Dental Diagnostic Science			
Caries Research Centers		2	11	1,570,588
Forsyth Dental Center	Clinical Trials/Experimentation			
University of Rochester	Dental Research			
Craniofacial Anomalies Research Centers		3	12	2,074,512
University of Iowa	Biology			
University of Pennsylvania	Human Genetics			
University of Southern California	Basic Sciences			
Materials Science Research Centers		3	12	2,070,843
American Dental Association Health Foundation	Paffenbarger Research Center			
University of Florida	Dental Biomaterials			
University of Michigan at Ann Arbor	Biologic and Materials Sciences			

	Department			
Orofacial Pain Research Centers		1	4	626,018
University of California at San Francisco	Oral and Maxillofacial Surgery			
Periodontal Diseases Research Centers		3	11	1,797,353
Forsyth Dental Center	Microbiology			
State University of New York at Buffalo	Oral Biology			
Virginia Commonwealth University	None			
Clinical Core Centers		3	14	1,706,443
University of Iowa	Dows Institute for Dental Research			
University of Minnesota, Twin Cities	Polymer Science and Engineering			
University of Washington	Center for Research in Oral Biology			
Developmental Centers		6	30	2,109,414
Meharry Medical College	None			
New York University	Dental Materials Science			
University of California at Los Angeles	Public Health and Preventive Dentistry			
University of Maryland, Baltimore Professional School	Pathology			
University of Medicine and Dentistry of New Jersey	Pediatric Dentistry			
University of Texas Health Science Center at San Antonio	Pediatric Dentistry			
HIV Center (cofunding support)		1	1	46,650
New York State Psychiatric Institute	Psychiatry			
Total		29	130	$17,974,575

SOURCE: National Institute of Dental Research, 1993a.

about 15 percent of the extramural budget was directed to research centers (NIDR, 1993a).

Not surprisingly, nongovernmental research sponsored by pharmaceutical and other commercial companies appears to be product oriented. One major segment focuses on products such as bonding agents, amalgams, and other restorative materials. Another segment emphasizes pharmaceuticals including antibacterials, remineralization agents, saliva substitutes, and anti-inflammatory drugs.

Slightly less than 5 percent of NIDR extramural funds were allocated for training in FY 1993 (NIDR, 1993a). Of the $5,860,000 for training, 11 percent went directly to individuals, with the remainder channeled through institutional training programs. The total training allocation in 1993 was *less* than it was in 1970, even before adjustment for inflation. The National Research Service Award (NRSA) program, established in 1974, supports short-term training (e.g., in designing clinical trials) and longer-term training including post-D.D.S./D.M.D. training leading to a Ph.D. In 1993, NIDR supported 177 trainees and 23 fellows. The Physician Scientist Award for Dentists, created in 1984, and the Dentist Scientist Award (DSA) program, created in 1985, supported 118 trainees in 1993. The NRSA and DSA programs together, according to one recent estimate (NAS, 1994), produce "on average, fewer than one clinical scholar or potential clinical scholar per dental school per year."

THE RESEARCH WORK FORCE

Data on the oral health research work force come largely from surveys of dental faculty conducted by the American Association of Dental Schools (AADS). A recent analysis of these data (Solomon, 1993) conservatively defined oral health research workers as full-time faculty at dental schools or advanced dental education institutions who had a primary appointment in the dental institution and who either had a Ph.D. or held a primary research appointment (i.e., spent at least 80 percent of their time on research and other noninstructional activities). The AADS analysis identified 910 oral health research workers in 1992-1993, scarcely changed from the 906 such workers in 1986-1987 and 925 in 1989-1990. Given the 14 percent decrease in dental school enrollments during the period, the author of the analysis suggested that these steady numbers probably reflect an increased emphasis on research.

The *exclusion* of faculty with joint medical-dental school appointments and of non-Ph.D. researchers that spend less than 80 percent of their time on research undoubtedly makes the above figures a considerable *underestimate* of those actively involved in oral health research, especially clinical research. The American Association for Dental Research has about 5,000 members, although not all are actively and significantly involved in research. The actual dental research work force that may be mobilized by a dental school, of course, also includes technical personnel, postdoctoral students or fellows, and to a much lesser extent, predoctoral students. Faculty from other professional schools within the university may also support a school's research activities.

Like the health sciences research work force and the population in general (IOM, 1990d), the average age of the oral health research work force is increasing. New members of the work force are somewhat less likely than departing members to hold Ph.D.s, may not "have rigorous academic training in research," and may be "severely handicapped in the highly competitive race for scarce research grants" (Solomon, 1993, p. 825).

EXPANDING RESEARCH CAPACITY AND ACCOMPLISHMENTS

If new knowledge is to continue to advance the oral health of the public, the dental school must support the fundamental commitment of the university to research and scholarship. The research mission, however, poses significant challenges for dental schools. As described in Chapter 2, most dental schools at midcentury lacked the resources and perhaps the will to conduct serious research, despite calls for such initiative from leading practitioners. Research is still a low priority at many schools (AADR, 1993).

In the survey of deans undertaken by the committee with the assistance of the American Association of Dental Schools almost half the deans cited developing new knowledge as of "very high" importance to their schools. It was, however, outranked as a priority by educating general practitioners, providing patient care, contributing to the intellectual and organizational life of the university or academic health science center, promoting a strong dental profession, and educating specialty practitioners. Contributing to new clinical knowledge was ranked more important than contributing to new knowledge in the basic sciences. The majority of the deans believed that developing new knowledge would be "more important" or "much more important" to their schools in the future. Only one expected this objective to become less important (in the area of basic sciences). A recent survey also suggested that deans were weighing faculty scholarship more heavily and that a successful bid for tenure required a considerably higher level of publications than in the past (Scheetz and Mendel, 1993).

Common obstacles to increased dental school involvement in research and research training include limited discretionary funds for research training; heavy time demands on faculty for "intensive, direct, and constant supervision" of students engaged in often irreversible clinical procedures; a technique-oriented culture; and lack of mentors and role models for young investigators (IOM, 1994b). Many established programs also face the perennial financial burden of modernizing or replacing facilities or equipment outdated by time and technological advances. As noted in an earlier IOM report, unsuitable research facilities hamper both research performance and research education (IOM, 1990d). That report argued generally for the development of a coherent federal policy to set priorities for renewing and expanding the health sciences research infrastructure.

For schools that do not now have a significant research program, initiating such a program is a formidable undertaking. It requires concentrated groundwork related to several major questions (McCallum, 1983; Ranney, 1989) including the following: (1) What funds are available to recruit a critical mass of new faculty and establish a sustainable research group? (2) Does any existing discipline or department within the school offer a core research capacity? (3) Can visiting or other short-term appointments help stimulate research activity? (4) Does the organization of the basic science and clinical departments obstruct wider research capacity? (5) What collaborative or other resources can be found elsewhere in the university or academic health center?

Answering these questions and implementing a developmental strategy demand leadership from the level of the department chair through the dean to the senior levels of the university and academic health center. Department chairs, however, may be unwilling or unable to provide leadership unless they have strong research backgrounds. Deans may be willing but not able to lead without outside support. And university officials may be capable of leading but unwilling to commit their attention and resources. If they are willing to lead, university officials can support the dean financially and politically in working through or around obstacles to change.

Given the expense and complexity of pursuing important research topics, Ranney (1989, p. 80) argues that "dental schools in and of themselves will not be able to develop the manpower and facilities to keep abreast of and capture for their programs those advances in knowledge that facilitate advances in oral health care. If we don't participate [in the parent university], someone else will do it without us." Not incidentally, if oral health researchers successfully collaborate, they also demonstrate their value to their parent institution (DePaola, 1989; Ranney, 1989).

The challenges facing the individual dental school are to a considerable degree replicated at the national level. In particular, strengthening aggregate capacity in oral health research faces twin problems of limited overall funding and limited research capacity.

FUNDING

The best organizational predictors of dental school research productivity, according to a 1987 study, were level of NIDR funding, student-to-faculty ratio, and number of dental-related books in the library (Harrington, 1987). The study also concluded that the single best predictor of institutional academic reputation was research productivity (measured by number of publications).

As noted earlier, 20 percent of the dental schools received two-thirds of the research and training funds distributed by NIDR in 1991. Twenty years earlier, 20 percent of dental schools received more than three-quarters of these funds. Thus, research activity has become somewhat less narrowly concentrated than in the past.

At the same time that research activity has become somewhat more *widely distributed*, funding has become more *thinly spread*. Total NIDR appropriations have not kept pace with inflation in the biomedical research and development sector. As Table 5.5 reveals, when calculated in constant dollars with 1970 as a base year, NIDR appropriations were lower in 1993 than in 1973. Although the committee would certainly like to see funding for oral health research grow, it recognizes the budget constraints under which policymakers are operating. Dentistry has to make a strong case for the need for more resources and its capacity to use them effectively.

Paradoxically, some university officials and deans of dental schools view research as an added source of revenue, whereas others fear that it may be a net drain on resources.[5] As one IOM report noted, "there is speculation that many institutions underreport

---

[5]As a potential strategy for acquiring new financial resources, the utility of increasing sponsored research was rated high or very high by about 60 percent of the deans, a somewhat greater percentage than those citing postdoctoral general dentistry programs, alumni contributions, or private practice plans.

TABLE 5.5 Total NIDR Appropriations FY 1970-1973 in
Current and Constant Dollars

Fiscal Year	Current Dollars (thousands)	BRDPI Base (FY 1970)	Constant 1970 Dollars (thousands)
1970	28,754	100.0	28,754
1971	35,440	105.8	33,497
1972	43,388	111.1	39,053
1973	46,991	116.4	40,370
1974	43,959	123.8	35,508
1975	50,033	137.0	36,520
1976	51,291	147.2	34,844
1977	55,573	159.0	34,952
1978	61,728	170.7	36,162
1979	65,213	184.9	35,269
1980	68,303	202.1	33,797
1981	71,114	221.8	32,062
1982	71,983	241.0	29,868
1983	79,292	254.9	31,107
1984	88,674	269.6	32,891
1985	100,688	283.8	35,479
1986	98,841	295.7	33,426
1987	117,945	311.4	37,876
1988	126,297	327.0	38,623
1989	130,752	344.0	38,009
1990	135,451	363.1	37,304
1991	148,916	380.9	39,096
1992	158,917	398.7	39,859
1993	161,142	413.6	38,961

NOTE: BRDPI = Biomedical Research and Development Price Index.

SOURCES: Calculations from National Institute of Dental Research, Financial Management Section, March 1994.

indirect costs to keep the overall costs of research low, thus helping their individual institutions remain competitive nationally" (IOM, 1990d, p. 155). In order to guard against the latter possibility, university officials, deans, and faculty need to reach agreement about the costs to be covered in sponsored research. Definition of indirect costs and support for faculty salaries are major issues.[6] Health professions schools have become increasingly con-

[6]Indirect costs are negotiated between individual institutions and the government according to guidelines on reimbursable expenses. For a given institution, one of the federal agencies sponsoring research at the institution negotiates a rate that

cerned about recovering the indirect costs of research, but it is not clear how successful this effort has been.

Schools have become increasingly aggressive in seeking private support, primarily from industry, but data are not available to track their success. Industry may support student fellowships, provide grants for basic science research, collaborate in faculty-initiated research, and award contracts for research using protocols provided by the sponsor. Of all U.S. spending on health research and development in 1992, an estimated 48.3 percent came from industry compared to slightly more than 47 percent from public sources (NIH, 1993, p. 2). Industry is more likely to conduct research in its own facilities rather than to fund research elsewhere. In contrast, about 24 percent of federally funded health and development research is conducted in government laboratories compared to 52.7 percent in institutions of higher education (NIH, 1993, p. 4).

One industry-based researcher has described what dental schools interested in support from industry should be capable of doing to meet industry expectations (Sakkab, 1983). He cites (1) the ability to recruit patients with appropriate problems or characteristics; (2) the availability of clinical faculty able to measure variables of interest to industry (e.g., stain removal, loss of attachment); (3) the existence of written protocols to protect against bias and conflict of interest; and (4) the stability to maintain multiyear studies.

Although data are scarce on such efforts, a number of schools have drawn on the resources of the larger university to create collaborative research relationships with medical, public health, engineering, and other programs. This strategy has the additional advantage of helping integrate the school with other parts of the university.

---

will apply to all federal agencies that fund research at the institution. Three categories of indirect costs are relatively straightforward: operation and maintenance expenses, use charges for buildings and equipment, and library expenses. For specific research projects, it is more difficult to define indirect costs associated with sponsored projects administration, general administration, student administration and services, and departmental administration. Indirect costs became increasingly important beginning in 1966 when the federal government shifted from a policy of direct support for physical plant maintenance and replacement to support through the indirect cost component for research. The small (2 percent) depreciation component of indirect costs assumes a 50-year life span for buildings, a figure that might be reasonable for classrooms or dormitories but may be too long for many research facilities (IOM, 1990d).

Data on involvement in internally supported and unsponsored research are virtually nonexistent. Involvement in such intramural research or scholarship may be more a sign of commitment to scholarship or to preparation for sponsored research than a significant contribution to the research mission of the dental school (or its financing). Such involvement is, however, important. It may provide ideas for future research, influence students' education in critical thinking, and enliven the intellectual environment.

HUMAN RESOURCES

Although funding limits dental schools efforts to fulfill their research mission, the dearth of capable researchers is perhaps a more fundamental (albeit related) problem. A recent committee of the National Research Council's Office of Scientific and Engineering Personnel (OSEP) cited an "alarming shortage of trained researchers in oral health." It called for "at least 200 graduates per year" to supply dental schools' needs. That is roughly four times the current number. OSEP also recommended that "at least half of a dental school faculty should be clinical scholars . . . The other half . . . should be scholarly clinicians" (NAS, 1994). This committee concurs in the spirit of that recommendation.

At the level of the individual dental school, the options for increasing faculty research capacity are basically two: (1) train or recruit new faculty or (2) retrain or develop existing faculty. Collectively, the recruitment strategy requires training more new researchers. If this does not happen, schools will merely be raiding each other for the same small group.

Creating Dentist Scientists

Although dental schools recruit basic scientists without dental training, they also need to recruit or train research faculty who are dentists to help focus research on oral health problems rather than on problems that other research sites could pursue equally well. Since its birth, NIDR has made the training of dental scientists a high priority. NIDR provides institutional support for research training programs in eight schools (another four programs are being or have been phased out). The agency is now considering the initiation of a D.D.S./Ph.D. program similar to that in medicine, an emphasis recommended in the OSEP report (NAS, 1994). Such an approach has the advantages of targeting people who are—from the start—interested in a research career and of limiting their debt load, a burden that can deter dental graduates from research training. It requires, however, a commitment of dental schools and universities to provide the appropriate educational opportunities.

In an attempt to assess the productivity of its research training programs, NIDR has tracked the number of trainees in different programs who have later submitted applications for its funds and received awards. This short-term analysis is presented in Table 5.6. The data indicate a fairly low yield in applications and awards for some programs, and NIDR is proposing to restructure some of them. The committee noted, however, that short-term training programs to improve student and faculty awareness and appreciation of research and research methods should not be expected to produce research grants and, thus, cannot be appropriately evaluated with conventional measures. This activity accounts for a small proportion of training funds and, in the committee's view, warrants continuation as a small but visible sign that an appreciation and understanding of research is important for nonresearchers.

A number of problems with the dental scientist program were noted in the committee's site visits, liaison panel meetings, and other information collection activities. One is the competitiveness gap and, relatedly, the tenure issue mentioned earlier. A second problem, reported by dental school deans, involves salary disparities. The stipend for those in some NIDR training programs may be higher than starting salaries at dental schools. NIDR is planning to adjust stipends to avoid such disparities.

A recent task force created for an Institute of Medicine study of career paths in clinical research set forth priorities for expanding the research capacity (Appendix B in IOM, 1994b, reprinted in the June 1994 issue of the *Journal of Dental Education*). The group distinguished three categories of research talent: (1) the senior dental clinical scientist who has specialty training,[7] a Ph.D., and postdoctoral training in research methods, who can plan and manage major clinical research projects; (2) the dentist scientist who has specialty training, preferably a basic science Ph.D., and research experience, who can become involved in clinical research in collaboration with research methodologists and other clinical investigators; and (3) dental clinical research associates, who have

---

[7]This category may include those with education in advanced general dentistry beyond the first postgraduate year.

TABLE 5.6 Research Grant Activity (FY 1985-1992) of Physician (K11) and Dentist (K15, K16) Scientists

Mechanism	No. of Appointees	No. of Graduates	No. of Grant Applicants (% of graduates)	No. of Applications	No. of Grantees (% of graduates)	No. of Grants	Grants as Percentage of Applicants
K11	40	23	13 (57%)	38	8 (35%)	13	34
K15	41	24	7 (29%)	23	2 (8%)	4	17
K16	145	59	13 (22%)	23	8 (14%)	8	35
Total	226	106	33 (31%)	84	18 (17%)	25	30

SOURCE: National Institute of Dental Research, 1993a.

little formal research training but are excellent clinicians able to be active participants in research. This committee supports these distinctions and directions but would add that advanced general dentistry be considered as a form of specialty training in this context.

In addition, the committee notes that training need not result in a Ph.D. to increase clinical research capacity. For example, although Chapter 4 argues that a master's degree in a dental specialty is not sufficient training for a research career, it can help prepare clinical faculty to participate as partners in clinical research under the direction of fully trained researchers. In addition, those in specialty fellowship programs could be placed in clinical research centers or laboratories of established investigators inside or outside the dental school to learn the scientific method by participation.

Faculty Development Programs

A major objective of many faculty development programs is to improve research skills. In the responses of the deans surveyed, however, this objective was outranked as a priority for faculty development by four other areas.[8] One of these areas, patient outcomes assessment, however, covers some similar methodological and conceptual ground.

Limits of (existing) faculty development strategies should be noted. To free faculty time for research training requires financial resources. It may also require schools to bring in clinicians from the community to fill in for absent clinical faculty, and finding the appropriate person may be difficult, particularly in smaller communities (Dirksen, 1992). Nonetheless the committee believes all schools should attempt to build faculty capacity even when circumstances are difficult.

OTHER ISSUES

Other problems also complicate dental school efforts to build and maintain a research faculty. These problems involve personnel policies, organizational arrangements, and physical location.

---

[8]The higher-ranking priorities were increasing sensitivity to student needs and concerns, increasing emphasis on patient outcomes assessment, improving instructional skills, and developing competency-based evaluations of student clinical skills.

As noted in Chapter 4, many dental and medical schools have revised unduly restrictive personnel policies by creating nontenure career tracks for clinical faculty and sometimes research faculty (Kennedy, 1984; Kalkwarf, 1986). This special track strategy acknowledges that many valuable faculty may not be "triple threats" in research, teaching, and service. It aims less at the problem of adding research capacity than at obstacles to the sensible use and rewarding of trained researchers.

The organizational structure of universities and academic health centers may also create difficulties for dental schools. On the one hand, when basic science faculty are part of the medical school, they may have little attachment to the research and educational missions of the dental school. On the other hand, when these faculty are located in the dental school, they may lack the critical mass to generate fundable research. Some of these problems might be resolved by a separate basic sciences unit designed and managed to serve the research and teaching missions of all the health professions schools (and, to some degree, other parts of the university). Depending on particular institutional circumstances, a freestanding department could create additional overhead and coordination costs; or it could permit some economies of scale in both stimulating and conducting multidisciplinary research.

Some dental schools are physically and organizationally isolated from their parent university or academic health center. This isolation impairs communication (even with the advent of electronic mail); imposes bureaucratic costs; and limits the sharing of expensive facilities, equipment, and support staff. These are not insignificant problems, although the existence of multiuniversity and even multinational research projects demonstrates that collaborative work among physically separate researchers is possible.

Dental schools may structure their research activities in several different ways. Some are organized along traditional departmental structures. As indicated above, some schools have created research centers with support from NIDR, and others have created centers with different sources of support (e.g., the periodontal research center at the University of Alabama at Birmingham, which receives support from other public and private sources).

EXTENDING RESEARCH OPPORTUNITIES

In addition to building oral health research capacity by training more and better researchers and seeking additional research funds, researchers and policymakers should also explore creative strategies to extend traditional avenues for acquiring clinical knowledge and to make use of untapped faculty resources. Such strategies will also help schools to respond to patient and purchaser pressure for more and quicker information about the effectiveness of different clinical strategies.

Used carefully and critically, quasi-experimental and nonexperimental (e.g., survey and epidemiological) research can help build understanding of what works and what does not work in health care. The focus of such strategies tends to be on clinical and behavioral rather than basic science research. The idea is *not* to replace or undermine the most demanding of traditional research strategies but to supplement them.

The exacting requirements and high expense (and sometimes ethical or practical infeasibility) of randomized controlled clinical trials (RCTs) restrict their use and probably contribute to faults in their practical implementation (Moher et al., 1994; Schulz et al., 1994). A poorly designed or executed RCT may provide less valid and reliable information than another, theoretically less rigorous strategy. In addition, because RCTs aim to ascertain *efficacy* (effects under controlled conditions) rather than *effectiveness* (results under actual conditions of practice), their value to clinicians may be limited.

Alternatives to the classical RCT include "large simple trials" (Zelen, 1993),[9] analyses of large data bases collected for other purposes (e.g., insurance claims) (Tilson, 1993; IOM, 1994d),[10] and

---

[9]Such trials are "simple" only by comparison to RCTs. Zelen proposes, for example, an open protocol system that would allow patients and clinicians anywhere in the United States to participate in a trial under defined conditions of eligibility according to specific treatment protocols. Among the key elements are sophisticated statistical controls, broad eligibility requirements, and streamlined data collection. Implementation would require regional training programs, a national support hotline and electronic mail network, and a roster of participating clinicians who would be paid for data collection and have their records audited periodically. Zelen insists that trials must always be randomized and always include a treatment (i.e., never include "watchful waiting" or a placebo). Such trials would not be inexpensive or easy to organize.

[10]In general, better data exist for inpatient care than for ambulatory care, even though many such data, whether in the form of hospital discharge summaries or insurance claims, suffer from numerous inadequacies. However, in both health care generally and dentistry specifically, improvements in computer-based patient records, electronic transmission of images and other patient data, and refinements in claims forms (similar to those designed for Medicare and private health insurance) are being encouraged and pursued to build a future research data base for ambulatory services. As in any research, the limitations of specific data need to be carefully evaluated (OTA, 1994).

nonrandomized clinical practice studies (Horn and Hopkins, 1994). Clinical practice studies generally focus on areas in which important patient outcomes (e.g., postsurgicial infections) occur and can be measured within a short period rather than over many months or years.[11] They are often relatively easily replicated and thus amenable to confirming tests in additional sites. In discussions of the merits of simpler research strategies, randomization and physical rather than statistical control of patient variability are among the most controversial issues.

At their best, simpler clinical studies would generate outcomes information that is superior to the impressionistic and anecdotal "knowledge" base that must often be relied upon today. They would require (1) careful selection of target clinical processes, patients, and outcomes of interest; (2) definition, application, and monitoring of replicable study protocols; (3) valid and reliable measures of key variables; (4) statistical procedures to control for other factors that might influence outcomes (e.g., age of patient; comorbid conditions); and (5) adequate systems for recording, retrieving, and analyzing information. In principle, research sites could included general and specialty student clinics, faculty practice plans, extramural clinics, and even private practices. In any research that extends across multiple research sites, the strict adherence of investigators to research protocols is an important concern as demonstrated by the controversy over the violations discovered in the National Surgical Adjuvant Breast and Bowel Project (Angell and Kassirer, 1994).

Dental schools, dental societies, and other organizations interested in oral health research (e.g., NIDR, AADS, American Association of Dental Researchers, ADA, American Dental Hygienists' Association) should evaluate the opportunities for expanded use of simple clinical studies in dentistry and consider collaborating on protocols and priorities for such studies. They might, for example, (1) identify important clinical questions to which relatively inexpensive research strategies could make a contribution; (2) develop standardized designs, measures, software and communications networks, and reporting formats that could be used or modified by clinical faculty; (3) test and replicate the approach in selected schools; (4) develop supportive training programs and an ongoing clearinghouse function; and (5) seek funding for these

---

[11]Recent examples of inexpensive, nonrandomized, nonblinded controlled clinical trials are described in East et al., 1992; Horn and Hopkins, 1994; McDonald and Overhage, 1994; and Stiell et al., 1994.

activities from government, industry, foundations, health agencies (e.g., American Cancer Society), and intramural university sources.

Dental schools provide a practical place to conduct clinical studies because they have available large numbers of eligible patients who, in the normal course of events, will receive treatments of interest to researchers. The simplest studies would impose protocols to structure clinical observations and assessments, while more ambitious studies could attempt quasi-experimental designs.[12] As with any such studies, threats to internal and external validity of findings would have to be carefully considered to assess, for example, the possible impact of special characteristics of the patient population or the extent to which patients were lost to follow-up.

In their background paper, Bader and Shugars suggest that "practitioner networks" based on study clubs, continuing education courses, and general practice residencies could be employed to extend the range of research. Dental schools and dental societies could play a role in structuring and facilitating the activities of these groups, for example, by helping establish computer links for the easy exchange of protocols, data, and questions. Such involvement would have the added advantage of increasing communication between the schools and the practice community and guiding inquiry to issues of direct concern to practitioners.

To repeat, the call here is not for casual or uncritical research but for the careful planning and discriminating application of research strategies to extend knowledge and encourage broader faculty participation in research.[13] Given, however, the history of

---

[12]To cite an example of a possible descriptive study topic, when replacement of an amalgam restoration is planned because margins have deteriorated but no caries are evident, clinicians could record what they found when the restoration was removed. A observation protocol would provide for standardized clinical criteria to be used to characterize (1) the extent of margin deterioration; (2) the patient's level of risk for caries; and (3) the presence or absence of caries after the restoration is removed. One pilot study has suggested a minimal association between caries risk and margin deterioration, but no larger study of this common dental practice has been undertaken (Maryniuk and Brunson, 1989). To illustrate a more ambitious project, a study could randomly assign established clinic patients (with their consent) to 6-, 12-, and 24-month recall intervals and then compare their health status and disease experience using appropriate annualized measures of caries incidence, surface replacements, and attachment loss.

[13]Nonetheless, weak studies can have some value as part of a learning process if at least one capable researcher is periodically available for a "post mortem" review of research deficits. For example, a school could phase in procedures for

disputes over the allocation of resources between basic and applied research in many fields of science, decisionmakers should be prepared to manage similar conflicts and protect research integrity if the directions discussed here are pursued. In addition, innovative research strategies need to be scrutinized for potential harms to patients including failure to secure informed consent when appropriate.

RESEARCH AND THE MISSION OF EDUCATION

The ardent pursuit of research funding and reputation can strengthen or weaken the educational mission of the dental school. A research-oriented school also needs to recognize and reward excellence in teaching, incorporate a scientific perspective into all elements of dental education, and invigorate the curriculum with the spirit of faculty research. In addition, interested students should have a direct opportunity to learn research methods, to undertake research projects as part of regular classes, and to participate in faculty and independent research projects. Providing the latter opportunity requires the following: faculty to teach and to guide or mentor students; facilities accessible to students; some funds for materials and supplies; time aside from the crush of required coursework and clinical experience; and a showcase for students to present their research (Clarkson and Kremenak, 1983; Gibson, 1993; Keller et al., 1993; Winston, 1993). These requirements, in turn, dictate that schools designate a faculty member or administrator responsible for seeing that these conditions are met. The results of student research (in process or final) can be presented through "table clinics" and poster sessions at individual schools, professional conferences, and similar settings. In particular, presentations at the annual meeting of the American Association for Dental Research offer exposure to the broader dental research community.

---

enrolling all patients in a clinical protocol for some problem and then tracking them over time. Participants could learn about the "controllable" ways that information is lost or compromised, for example, through poor adherence to protocols and incomplete or imprecise record keeping. By assessing the impact of these and other less controllable problems such as the loss of patients to follow-up, clinicians could ask the critical question: Is some information (what has been collected) better than none, or is the information so flawed as to be seriously misleading? Even if the answer in the initial stages is the latter, a base has been laid for better future performance.

Beyond broadly encouraging scientific habits of mind in students, dental schools should continue to seek, identify, and inspire predoctoral students with the requisite interest and talents to pursue research careers. Creating research opportunities for students and providing faculty mentors are important strategies for doing so (Hein, 1983). Since 1979 the NIDR has provided short-term training grants to support and stimulate student research programs. With its lower research profile, dentistry may be less attractive than medicine to students with the interests, background, and mind-set that would make them candidates for a research career, but it is still important to search for and encourage such students.

FINDINGS AND RECOMMENDATIONS

Too many dental schools and dental faculty are minimally involved in research and scholarship. The low priority placed on research has important negative consequences. First, faculty in such schools contribute little to the knowledge base for improving oral health or increasing the effectiveness and efficiency of oral health services. Second, students in these schools miss the stimulation and critical edge provided by a research-engaged faculty. Third, schools with low research productivity put themselves in jeopardy in most universities and academic health centers, and they may detract from the reputation of dental research and education more generally. Fourth, lack of research and scholarship within a dental school tends to diminish the school's role as a disseminator of critically evaluated practice advice to dental practitioners.

The committee concurs generally in the finding of the National Academy of Sciences' Office of Scientific and Engineering Personnel that a substantial increase in oral health research graduates is needed (NAS, 1994). It also recognizes the problems facing schools that are trying to build or maintain a strong research program. These include, most notably, limited funding and a dearth of capable researchers. The organizational structure of the basic science faculty may contribute as well.

Other problems include the time demands on many clinical faculty and their frequent isolation from possible collaborators elsewhere in the university or academic health center. Institutions without a strong track record in research may lack the administrative and departmental leadership necessary to plan and achieve change. For institutions committed to research, achieving a reasonable balance between research and educational missions may be a challenge.

The committee urges dental schools to work together and to involve national and local professional societies in devising new avenues for clinical knowledge development. In doing so, they can take advantage of the statistical, data base, communications, measurement, and other research techniques and protocols that are emerging from the growing field of outcomes research.

The committee understands that dental schools will differ in how they define the specifics of their research mission. Schools will need to be selective and set priorities for establishing and maintaining research capacity based on a critical mass of faculty talent, physical facilities, funding, and other resources. Some schools can reasonably aspire to be real centers of research excellence; all dental schools should value scholarship and the creation of new knowledge.

To expand oral health knowledge and to affirm the importance of research and scholarship, each dental school should

• **support a research program that includes clinical research, evaluation and dissemination of new scientific and clinical findings, and research on outcomes, health services, and behavior related to oral health;**
• **extend its research program, when feasible, to the basic sciences and to the transformation of new scientific knowledge into clinically useful applications;**
• **meet or exceed the standard for research and scholarship expected by its parent university or academic health center;**
• **expect all faculty to be critically knowledgeable about scientific advances in their fields and to stay current in their teaching and practice; and**
• **encourage all faculty to participate in research and scholarship.**

To build research capacity and resources, as well as foster relationships with other researchers, all dental schools should develop and pursue collaborative research strategies that start with the academic health center or the university and extend to industry, government, dental societies, and other institutions able to support or assist basic science, clinical, or health services research.

To strengthen the research capacity of dental schools and

faculty, the committee recommends that the National Institute of Dental Research

- continue to evaluate and improve its extramural training and development programs;
- focus more resources on those extramural programs with greater demonstrated productivity in strengthening the oral health research capacity of dental schools and faculties; and
- preserve some funding for short-term training programs intended primarily to increase research understanding and appreciation among clinical teaching faculty and future practitioners.

SUMMARY

Research is a fundamental mission of dental education, but one not uniformly honored among schools. Certainly, the situation is vastly improved from the 1940s and 1950s, thanks largely to training programs supported by the National Institute for Dental Research. Nonetheless, the field still suffers from a shortage of well-trained researchers, particularly clinical researchers.

Improving research productivity in dentistry will require leadership from inside and outside—that is, from the university and the academic health center, from the public and private sectors, and from the practice community. The key objectives are to establish research as a priority; to secure new funding and redistribute existing resources; to develop creative strategies to extend the scope of oral health research; to attract qualified new people and develop existing faculty; and to sustain this capacity over time.

6

The Mission of Patient Care

T his chapter focuses on dental schools' health-related service to individuals and communities. It calls for dental educators to affirm or reaffirm that patient care is a distinct mission that is related but not subservient to the missions of education and research. It argues further for major shifts in schools' patient care objectives and activities, shifts that cannot occur without the support of community dentists and dental organizations. The committee believes that such support will be forthcoming because educators and practitioners ultimately will agree that the best education occurs in a setting of exemplary patient care.

The committee found little in the dental education literature that examined patient care in the dental school from a patient's perspective. Even the discussions of comprehensive care cited in Chapter 4 focus primarily on how to educate students to be patient oriented. This chapter, thus, draws heavily on the committee's site visits and other activities, its broad understanding of the forces reshaping health care delivery and financing, and its judgments about the fit between patient care in the dental school and a restructured health care system.

CONTEXT

An examination of patient care activities in the dental school and academic health center must consider the patient as an individual, as a member of a health insurance plan, and as a part of a community. This triple focus complicates the already intricate balancing act that characterizes patient care in the health professions schools. Not only do schools have to consider differences in individual patients' characteristics and manage possible conflicts between individual and community needs, they must also take into account differences in the objectives and policies of the health plans that increasingly manage or arrange for services for employer, governmental, or other sponsors. Sometimes the interests of these health plans closely parallel those of their individual members, but they may at other times conflict (e.g., when plans restrict member's choice of provider or impose bureaucratic hurdles before care can be provided). When they do, the health care provider can be caught in the middle. As discussed in this chapter, the provider's position is even more difficult if it is also an academic institution with educational and research missions.

Further confounding the patient care responsibilities of the dental school are the varied views of these responsibilities by different individuals and groups. To indigent patients, the student dental clinic may be the only source of care. Similarly, to politicians in a state with public or private state-related dental schools, the clinic may be a vehicle for meeting the needs of the underserved. The community dentist may view a faculty practice plan as a good place to refer complicated patients such as those with AIDS, infectious tuberculosis, or severe behavioral problems. The community dentist might also view the plan and the student clinic as competitors. To the administration of a university or academic health center, the outpatient clinics of a dental school may be a mystery—different from any component of the medical school and in chronic need of subsidy. These varied perspectives challenge dental schools to clearly articulate the value and requirements of their patient care mission.

Such an articulation of the contribution of dental schools to the parent institutions and communities is also important because, even if substantially restructured, patient care in dental schools will include some inefficiencies associated with the educational process. Student clinics are unlikely to be able to cover their full costs through patient fees. Moreover, many educators expect that dental schools' economic advantage—low cost or "free" care for patients without access to the private practice system—will diminish as dental insurers organize network health plans and demand price and other changes from community practitioners. Thus, dental educators with the help of others in the dental community must make the case for public support of the educational and community service aspects of patient care in the dental school. Support from national and local philanthropies and other private sources will also be necessary to help fund the demonstration projects and experiments that will assist schools in making the transition to new models of patient care and community service.

WHO PROVIDES PATIENT CARE IN DENTAL SCHOOLS?

In most dental schools, the majority of patient care activities are provided by students. Many schools delegate to predoctoral students responsibility for both managing and providing a patient's care; faculty assume responsibility for supervising a single visit or procedure at a time. Faculty may provide services incidentally as they oversee student care, and allied health personnel may provide care either as students themselves or as employees. In a few schools, the patient is the responsibility of a designated faculty member (usually a general dentist), although most of the care is still provided by the student. If a specialist faculty member is called in for consultation or procedural direction, the student and generalist faculty member retain responsibility for the patient.

Depending on the array of advanced education programs within a school, advanced education students also provide and oversee patient care in both predoctoral and graduate clinics. One dean has noted that although advanced education students accounted for only 10 percent of his school's enrollment, they generated 45 percent of clinic revenues both because they are more productive and because higher fees can be charged for their services (Hunt, 1993). Schools may let patients choose whether to receive care from a predoctoral student, postdoctoral student, or faculty member.

In the majority of schools, faculty also care for patients in separately housed and staffed faculty practice plans. As discussed further in Chapter 7, a major rationale for faculty practice plans is to supplement faculty salaries. Another rationale, described in Chapter 4, is that they help keep faculty clinically up to date and sensitive to the realities of practice. Involvement in these plans by predoctoral students appears to be limited.

WHERE IS CARE PROVIDED?

The location of patient care activities varies from school to school. All schools operate a dental school clinic on site, and the majority have separate facilities for faculty practice plans. Many schools, but not all, provide care in off-site or extramural facilities, including community clinics, public schools, traveling clinic-vans, and temporary clinics for special populations such as migrant workers. Extramural facilities often provide sites for advanced general dentistry, dental public health, and other residencies. Because relatively few health maintenance organizations (HMOs) or other managed care organizations have significant dental care components, they rarely serve as extramural educational sites.

Student participation in on-site clinics is mandatory and fulfills graduation requirements as measured in procedures, hours, patients treated, or some combination of these. Some schools require student participation in extramural clinical activities and include them as rotations in the third and fourth years. Other schools provide only optional off-site activities because they lack convenient sites or the staff and faculty needed to manage the number of extramural clinics that the entire student population would require.

During its site visits, the committee learned that several schools have cut back or eliminated off-site community service activities due to financial pressures and cuts in state funding. Some schools have attempted to quantify the value of their extramural programs as a way to demonstrate their commitment to the community and underscore the value of state funding.

How Is Care Organized?

The site of care strongly shapes the organization of care. When dental students provide care in extramural facilities in which education is a distinctly secondary goal, their activities and supervision generally conform to the individual facility's scheme for patient care. That scheme will vary considerably from hospital to community clinic to private office.

Within the dental school, care provided by students may be organized around specialty clinics or comprehensive care clinics. Chapter 4 describes these alternatives primarily from an educational perspective but notes that a patient-oriented objective of comprehensive care is to put the patient-general practitioner relationship at the center of the clinic and to provide care in a setting as similar as possible to an efficient private practice or community clinic. Ideally, the student follows the patient through all procedures indicated by the diagnosis and treatment plan, perhaps supervised by a general dentist with involvement by specialists as necessary.

Who Pays for Care in Student Clinics?

Payment for services in dental school clinics typically comes from several sources. Some patients pay the fees from their own resources; some are covered by private insurance; and Medicaid reimburses care for others. States and communities may budget funds for care of indigent and other populations, and schools may also obtain funds from private foundations and alumni contributions or from internal university allocations.

In addition, dental students appear to "subsidize" patient care in two ways. First, if schools do not recover clinic operating costs from fees, appropriations for indigent care, or similar mechanisms, then student tuition may be higher than it otherwise would be. Second, if schools believe they cannot increase clinic operating costs by employing adequate numbers of allied dental and administrative personnel, students may subsidize the clinic by diverting time from their own clinical education to perform tasks that would normally be delegated to others. For example, students often serve as dental assistants, undertake housekeeping components of infection control, collect fees, schedule appointments, and perform other similar tasks that have minimal educational value after an early point. Although the contention is debatable, the income generated by student fees for equipment might also be regarded as a student subsidy of patient care rather than a way of financing education.

No clinic can break even on services provided to patients who cannot pay and whose costs are not reimbursed from other public or private sources. It is not, however, straightforward to determine what constitutes an appropriate "fee" or payment for student services provided to individuals outside the normal market for dental care (discounted or otherwise). To the extent that patient care within the dental school is restructured in the directions outlined in the rest of this chapter, patient or health plan "willingness to pay" may become a more commonplace determinant of prices.

Statistical Profile of Patient Care in Dental Schools

Detailed information on dental services is in relatively short supply, and dental schools are no exception. Because they are part of large organizations that routinely collect and report information, however, dental school utilization statistics may be more complete than data for private practices. Nonetheless, data may not be comparable across schools, and demographic, clinical, economic, and other information about patients is virtually nonexistent.

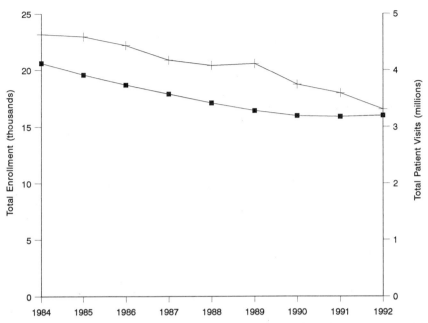

FIGURE 6.1 Trends in dental school enrollments (■) and total patient visits (+), 1984-1992. SOURCE: American Association of Dental Schools, 1993b.

Aggregate Data

From 1984 to 1992, dental school enrollments decreased 22 percent. With fewer students to provide patient care, patient visits in dental schools declined by 29 percent and the number of patients screened decreased by 13 percent (Figure 6.1). Numerically, patient visits fell from 4.63 million in 1984 to 3.31 million in 1992, and total patients screened dropped from a high of 396,000 in 1985 to 343,000 in 1992.

On a *per D.D.S. student equivalent* basis,[1] patient visits de-

---

[1]The D.D.S. equivalent enrollment is the weighted sum of all students (D.D.S./ D.M.D., advanced specialty, advanced nonspecialty, and allied dental) enrolled in the school (AADS, 1993b). How well it summarizes the overall resource demands or other characteristics of a diverse student population (on average or for specific institutions) is unclear, but some adjustment for different levels of students is reasonable.

creased from 216 in 1984 to 207 in 1992; at the same time, patients screened per student increased from 18 in 1984 to 21 in 1992. The *ratio of visits to patients* decreased from 12 per patient screened to 9.6. These changes appear to reflect increased efficiency (e.g., treatment plans completed with fewer visits) and more restrictive standards for accepting screened patients for comprehensive care. In addition, because oral health has improved even in the relatively disadvantaged populations served by most dental schools, dental schools today have to screen more patients to secure an adequate yield of clinical problems (numbers and types) for educational purposes.

From 1985 to 1992, clinic *income* increased from $104.9 million to $171.9 million (AADS, 1993b). In constant dollars, however, total clinic income during this period decreased from $104.9 million to $102.6 million, which is consistent with the decrease in numbers of patients and visits.[2]

As many dental educators and university administrators are all too aware, dental school clinics operate at a loss. In FY 1993, the total revenue of all U.S. dental school clinics was $188,182,280 and the total expense was $230,603,802. The overall net deficit is more than $42,000,000 (on average, more than $785,000 per dental school) (ADA, 1993b). (Unlike teaching hospitals, dental school clinics do not benefit from direct or indirect educational support under Medicare.)

Variations Across Schools

In on-campus clinics, the number of *patient visits* during 1992-1993 varied from lows of 7,500 and 7,732 for two schools to highs of 139,000 and 261,975 for two others (ADA, 1993a). The mean for all schools was 54,890 and the median (which is not influenced by extreme outliers) was 48,169.

The number of *patients screened* varied from a low of 1,050 to a high of 28,930, with a mean of 5,245 (ADA, 1993a). The ratio of patient visits to patients screened was calculated to provide another measure of clinic activity on a per-school basis. This ratio showed wide variances as well. The highest ratios were 38.8 and 34.8, and the lowest was 1.1; the median was 12.9.

---

[2]Constant dollars calculated by using the Consumer Price Index of Medical Care Prices (U.S. Department of Commerce, 1993, p. 114).

Clinic revenue on a per-student basis is also highly variable, ranging from highs of $15,905 and $14,042 per student to lows of $895 and $1,866 per student in 1992; the mean was $5,515 (median of $5,180) (ADA, 1993b). Private schools had a higher mean ($6,255), but also much greater variability as evidenced by a range of revenue ($895 to $15,905).

Similarly, clinic revenue as a *percentage of total revenue* varies from 2.5 to 36.4 percent, with a mean of 12.4 (ADA, 1993b). Again, the mean of 10 percent for public schools is lower than the mean of 16.5 percent for private institutions.[3]

Why do schools vary so much? One answer may be the scheduling practices of the dental school clinic. Differences in the faculty and staff ratios, which would allow more patients to be seen, are likely contributions to variation. Another factor may be the size of the surrounding community or the extent to which the clinic has a "captive" patient population, that is, those for whom private care is not an option. In addition, the ratio of patient visits to patients screened may not capture all of the complexities of dental school clinic operations. For example, a patient may be screened in one academic year but have visits that carry over into the next year. Patients at some schools may be more likely to decline the services recommended in the treatment plan based on the screening visit.

ISSUES AND CHALLENGES

The mixed missions of clinical education and patient care in the dental school make trade-offs almost inevitable regardless of the way that education is structured and overseen. Dental students must gain sufficient clinical experience in a variety of technical procedures to become competent entry-level practitioners, qualified to graduate and become licensed. A procedure-driven learning process does not necessarily translate into efficient, high-quality patient care, particularly when student care is further constrained by low budgets for clinical and administrative support. Thus, patients who can afford care elsewhere typically seek service in other settings, and health plans that contract with a limited set of providers do not look to dental school clinics first.

---

[3]To determine whether these figures were affected by a few schools with a high proportion of revenues from research sources, the percentages were recalculated with research removed from total revenue figures. The variability across schools remained.

This discussion should not imply that schools and students regard patients merely as teaching material. In the committee's survey of dental school deans, only the education of general dentists rated higher than patient care in importance to deans. Schools educate students about the elements of high-quality, ethical patient care and about their responsibilities to provide such care as students not just as licensed practitioners. For a combination of educational, patient care, and economic reasons, educators are exploring simulations or other exercises that increase student proficiency but minimize patient exposure to inept learners.

Whether viewed from an individual patient or a health plan perspective, the patient care challenges for dental schools are significant. They include issues related to efficiency, quality, competitiveness, accountability, and informed consent. From a community perspective, service to disadvantaged or vulnerable populations is an important issue. On all fronts, shifting or addition of resources will compound the stress on educators.

The following discussion first reviews problems and then considers strategies for change. The focus is on-site predoctoral student clinics rather than faculty practice plans, clinics for advanced students, or off-site settings. For the student and the dental school, the changes discussed below reinforce the call in Chapter 4 for a postgraduate year of additional clinical experience. Likewise, they reinforce the emphasis in Chapter 8 on the need for greater agreement by dental educators and examiners on what constitutes competency and how it should be assessed.

EFFICIENCY OF CARE

Compared with services provided by dental graduates, care provided by students may require more time and more visits.[4] Students are generally slower in completing an individual service than are graduates. For example, a cavity preparation that would take an experienced dentist a few minutes will ordinarily take a beginning student much longer. This difference costs patients time and costs clinics money because students are less productive.

---

[4]The impact of experience is reflected in differences in clinic revenues produced by more and less experienced students. Advanced education in general dentistry (AEGD) students produce $44,478 per year in clinic revenues per student (adjusted for regional fee differences) compared with $9,697 per year for predoctoral students (AADS, 1994c).

In addition, variations in educational strategies have time implications. One traditional approach emphasizes student completion of a few cases of a particular procedure from start to finish. The more inexperienced the student, the more likely are the patient, student, and teacher to stay in the clinic much longer than is reasonable, even in a learning context. This is not patient-centered care.

An alternative approach stresses student participation with faculty and postgraduate students in a much larger number of cases. The faculty member serves as a role model, with the student moving from limited to extensive responsibility based on increasing skill and speed. Although the focus of this strategy is broadly on patient care, not narrowly on procedures, and the learning process is structured differently, procedural competency is still an objective. For the patient, this strategy is likely to mean less time in the clinic.

Patients may also be delayed if faculty are not available in a timely fashion to review and approve student work. Moreover, students may not have allied personnel available to assist them and save time by laying out instruments or similar activities. In addition, students often perform nonclinical tasks such as collecting payments from patients and scheduling appointments, which is almost certainly less efficient than using paid office staff. The student's time is, however, typically regarded as "free" because no direct compensation costs are involved.

Student activities aside, efficient use of the patient's time may be a low priority in other respects. Appointments may not be scheduled individually throughout the day but simply set for the beginning of the morning or afternoon clinic, so waiting times may be long. Patients may have to return for multiple visits for procedures that crosscut departments and require separate appointments for each "subclinic" within the clinic. They may have to go elsewhere for specialized care not within the scope of predoctoral training. University personnel regulations may complicate efforts to establish convenient evening and weekend clinics or otherwise make services more patient-friendly. Investments in modern computer-based information and management systems lag.

The social costs of such inefficiency—missed work hours or school days, excess transportation or child care costs—are rarely tallied. The tolerance of inefficiency may also give students a mixed message about the importance of each patient, especially the patient who cannot afford to go elsewhere.

Still, some patients, particularly older ones, may value clinic visits as a social experience more varied and interesting than a private office visit. Evidence that patients value the relationship is provided every holiday season by the food and other gifts they bring to students and staff.

Although lower-income and retired patients now may be willing to trade time for low-cost care in student clinics, changes in the financing and organization of health care could alter this calculus. That is, newly insured patients may seek alternative sources of care, although required deductibles and other cost sharing may still make a low-cost student clinic attractive to some (Tunnicliff, 1994). Groups of patients covered by health plans may increasingly be directed to a restricted network of employed or contracting providers. It is unlikely that a health plan would include a traditional student clinic in this network.

QUALITY OF CARE

Quality of care has been defined by another Institute of Medicine committee as "the degree to which health services for individuals and populations increase the likelihood of desired health outcomes and are consistent with current professional knowledge" (IOM, 1990e, p. 21). Quality problems may arise from (1) overuse of care, which occurs when more services are used or provided than appropriate (e.g., unnecessary replacement of restorations); (2) underuse of care, which happens when clearly beneficial care is forgone (e.g., untreated caries, extraction of a tooth rather than feasible restoration); and (3) poor technical or interpersonal care (e.g., defective restorations, failure to explain treatment options and consequences).

Quality problems occur in all settings, but the dental school has some particular vulnerabilities. First, care provided by learners may be more physically uncomfortable or painful than care provided by the proficient. Also, slow performance may in and of itself produce emotional and physical distress.

Second, the initial technical quality of care may be inadequate. If the problem is apparent, corrective work must be performed by the student or supervising faculty, which involves additional time and perhaps physical discomfort. Other technical deficiencies, such as an imperfectly bonded restoration, may not be observable until some time has passed.

Third, graduation requirements and evaluation procedures are a potential threat to quality of care. At most schools, a student cannot graduate without completing a defined number of various procedures or acquiring a defined number of points calculated as function of number and types of procedures and their difficulty. If a particular patient's (or group of patients') problems do not fit a student's requirements (e.g., for a crown), the student may be tempted to fit the patient to the service rather than vice versa. The result may be either undercare or overcare or both. In principle, faculty oversight—if not student ethics—should preclude such practices, but the oversight process is viewed by many of those interviewed for this study as uneven both within and across schools. Assessment based on competency levels, whether acquired after four or fourteen procedures, would not eliminate the potential for inappropriate treatment, but it would presumably reduce the risk of unnecessary care from those students who are able to demonstrate competency with fewer repetitions of a procedure.

Fourth, dental schools often serve patients who cannot afford to go elsewhere and whose economic status may lead to less than optimal treatment. For example, a poor patient may have a tooth extracted because indigent care programs do not cover root canals or expensive restorations that would save the tooth. Economic realities also mean that dental school clinics may leave some indigent or partially insured patients untreated or only partly treated. Both of these quality of care problems reflect social policies over which dental schools have little control, although dental schools may lobby for improved Medicaid coverage of dental services, for direct public and private support for their own clinic and outreach programs, and for other community-based programs to which they can refer some patients.

The above discussion emphasizes problems, but the dental school clinic also may have characteristics that are linked to higher-quality care including frequent faculty interaction with peers in the same or other disciplines and a systematic process and explicit criteria for evaluating individual treatments. Independently or in conjunction with efforts throughout an academic health center, student clinics can, in principle, draw on the management, research, and analytic capacities of administration and faculty to evaluate practice patterns, examine outcomes, and establish benchmarks for improving the processes and outcomes of care. The positive social benefits that accrue to some patients (as cited above) also may be attributed to a good interpersonal quality of care in a dental school clinic.

Unfortunately, systematic evidence about the quality of care in dental school clinics (and, for that matter, in private practice) is largely unavailable. Quality assurance programs are, for the most part, new and little tested in dental school clinics. As yet, such programs have not provided valid and reliable information on the process and outcomes of care. A 1990 survey of quality assurance programs in dental schools indicated that barely half the responding schools were reviewing the outcomes of care (Butters et al., 1991). Only three-quarters of the schools reported a responsible individual or formal administrative program for quality assurance, and nearly all such programs had been established for less than six years. Less than 90 percent periodically reviewed infection control activities, a universal expectation of quality assurance programs in most settings. Although about two-thirds of the respondents indicated that they assessed patient satisfaction with services, only 19 percent had written criteria for this assessment.

In general, then, dental educators lack both the programs and the data needed to assess the quality of care in an individual school or to compare alternative models of patient care for differences in timeliness and appropriateness. Such assessments and comparisons could prompt changes in processes of care that would serve both the mission of patient care and the mission of education.

To be fair to dental schools, quality assurance mechanisms are generally less advanced in ambulatory care settings than in hospitals (IOM, 1990e). As quality has become an increasingly important issue to policymakers, providers, health plans, and patients, this is changing. More systems and requirements for quality assessment and assurance are developing. Since the early 1980s, accreditation standards for dental schools, for example, have included certain patient protection provisions (CDA, 1993a). These involve emergency services and training, diagnosis and treatment planning, preventive services, recall procedures, and patient rights (Table 6.1).

Whether a single accreditation process is satisfactory for both education and patient care in the dental school is an important question. Reflecting its traditional reliance on the hospital as an educational site, the medical model separates the roles. The Liaison Committee on Medical Education accredits medical schools, and a variety of independent organizations, notably the Joint Commission on the Accreditation of Health Care Organizations, accredit patient care facilities and programs. Although the Joint Commission has moved beyond its original focus on hospital care, the accreditation of ambulatory care settings is in the hands of multiple, often competing organizations that are still struggling with basic criteria and procedures. As the Joint Commission begins to review ambulatory care programs including hospital-associated dental clinics, the content and source of standards for patient care programs are likely to become a more pervasive issue in the academic health center.

TABLE 6.1 Standard 6—Patient Care and Clinic Management

6.1 Patients, students, faculty, and staff must be informed of the school's patient care policies. The school must have mechanisms to review and revise the procedures used in providing care to patients.

    6.1.1 Institutions must have mechanisms to ensure that patients are informed about and have the potential to receive comprehensive dental care.

    6.1.2 Each institution must develop and distribute to all students, faculty, appropriate staff, and to each patient a written statement of patients' rights.

    6.1.3 Each patient must receive an assessment and diagnosis consistent with the level of care being provided.

    6.1.4 An active recall program must be in operation for all active comprehensive care patients. An individualized prevention program should be an integral component of all comprehensive patient care activities.

    6.1.5 Each institution must provide for all registered patients a dental emergency service accessible at all times.

    6.1.6 A written protocol for the prevention and management of medical emergencies must be developed for all clinical programs; all students, faculty and support staff involved in the direct provision of patient care must be recognized (certified) in basic life support procedures, including cardiopulmonary resuscitation, at intervals not to exceed two years, and be able to manage other medical emergencies.

    6.1.7 Institutions must ensure the safe use of ionizing radiation in their clinics.

6.2 Each institution must develop a system of clinic administration and ensure that appropriate authority is granted to those with the responsibility for clinic administration.

    6.2.1 Each institution must ensure that an appropriate level of direct faculty supervision is available at all times when students are providing patient care.

    6.2.2 Dental education institutions must ensure the availability of an adequate patient pool that permits students the opportunity to obtain clinical competency within a reasonable time.

    6.2.3 Each inception must develop mechanisms to ensure that all patients who enter into active treatment do so as soon as possible after first contact with the admissions process. Mechanisms must be in place to track each patient to ensure continuity of care as treatment progresses.

    6.2.4 Each institution must establish and enforce a mechanism to ensure adequate clinical/preclinical/laboratory asepsis, infection and hazard control and disposal of hazardous waste.

    6.2.5 The patient record must be available at each patient appointment and must be an orderly, standardized and legible document in which all necessary information is readily accessible.

    6.2.6 Each school must provide a formal system of quality assurance that includes a formal record review process and a post-operative patient review process.

SOURCE: Commission on Dental Accreditation, 1993a.

ACCOUNTABILITY AND INFORMED CONSENT

Accountability for individual patient care is a potential problem in most dental school clinics as is proper handling of informed consent by patients. In the traditional dental school clinic, no single student or faculty member may be responsible for comprehensive oversight of a patient. Instead, each department may have various faculty members supervising students whose patients arrive in the clinic for specific treatments. If one student or faculty member does not follow a patient from oral diagnosis through treatment, it may not be clear which student is responsible for patient follow-up or future dental work.

In comprehensive care clinics, a student is typically responsible for all basic services for a given patient, and most services are provided in a single general clinic overseen by faculty. Depending on how faculty are scheduled, however, the same combination of student, patient, and service may be overseen by different faculty members. This tends to dilute faculty accountability.

Concerns about informed consent permeate health care. Practitioners, administrators, and consumer advocates are struggling to devise strategies that permit truly informed consent to care from culturally and clinically diverse patients who receive remarkably varied services in different settings and circumstances. Within the dental school, informed consent collected at the screening stage is insufficient because a plan of treatment has yet to be devised to which a patient can consent. In addition, patients may not be properly informed about who will provide care—predoctoral student, resident, fellow, faculty, or some combination.

COMPETITION

As noted earlier, restructuring of health care delivery and financing is challenging academic health centers.[5] HMOs and other kinds of "managed care" plans generally emphasize primary care and compete heavily on price. The emphasis on price tends to

---

[5]This discussion draws on a growing literature discussing the implications of health care restructuring or reform for academic health centers and the health care system more generally. It includes Vanselow, 1986; Williams et al., 1987; Stemmler, 1989; Heyssel, 1990; AAHC, 1992, 1994; Blumenthal and Meyer, 1993; Fox and Wasserman, 1993; Iglehart, 1993; IOM, 1993b; Miles et al., 1993; Pew Commission, 1993; Ridky and Sheldon, 1993; AAMC, 1994; and Weiner, 1994.

put academic health centers at a disadvantage because of their costly characteristics including clinical teaching and research, extensive tertiary services, and care for indigent patients turned away elsewhere. Many centers also have a dearth of primary care practitioners and facilities to serve the day-to-day needs of health plan members. To the extent that it favors mergers and multihospital systems, the competitive environment poses another problem because many academic health centers are constrained in their decisions by their university affiliations and public sponsorship. Proposals to revamp Medicare payments for graduate medical education—a major source of income for health centers—and to institute residency quotas also threaten the financial health and operating arrangements of academic health centers. (Some of these problems are discussed further in Chapter 7.)

The position of the dental school needs, however, to be distinguished from that of the university hospital or the medical school in certain respects. Rather than relying on a separate hospital as medical schools do, each school operates its own outpatient dental "hospital" in the form of a student clinic. These outpatient clinics do not receive the kind of direct and indirect educational payments from Medicare that teaching hospitals receive. Within the dental school, the imbalance between general and specialist care and faculty is substantially less than in the medical school and medical center hospital. In addition, although the spread of dental insurance has allowed more patients to pay for care from private practitioners, the high cost-sharing requirements of many dental plans continue to make the dental school clinic attractive to lower-income patients.

Today, some dental schools have a backlog of patients, and patients may wait weeks for an appointment (Tunnicliff, 1994). At the same time, these schools and others may worry about a shortage of certain types of patients for their student clinics. One consequence of the reduction in caries among children has, for some schools, been an insufficient number of patients with simple caries. Students may thus face complex patients earlier than they would have in the past, another argument for more faculty involvement in patient care.

Where schools face shortages of "teaching" patients, they may try to be more patient oriented to attract those in need of care. This may be difficult. The efficiency, quality, and accountability deficiencies described in this chapter are not easily overcome, especially when the resources constraints make it difficult to upgrade facilities and staffing. In addition, efforts by dental schools to expand the patient base for student clinics—and faculty practice plans—may encounter opposition from community practitioners. For both dental schools and private dentists, the future may bring more significant competitive threats as those health plans that cover dental services extend selective contracting or employment arrangements to dental care (Bradford, 1992; Keefe, 1994).

As noted above, academic health centers face major challenges from health care restructuring, challenges that differ from community to community depending on the specifics of state policies and local health care markets. Individually and collectively, they are still developing strategies to deal with ongoing and anticipated changes in health system organization and financing. Some are likely to fare better than others, either because their environment is less hostile or because their adaptive strategies are superior.

Not surprisingly, the committee's site visits made clear that dental schools face different environments that relate in part to the size, competitiveness, and other characteristics of their community and in part to the directions being set by university or academic health center leaders. Some institutions have indicated that all components of the academic health center, including the dental school, must become more patient oriented and efficient to survive in a more competitive health care system. This may put additional pressure on dental schools to adopt the comprehensive, faculty-based models of clinical education described in Chapter 4. Faculty practice plans that incorporate care by predoctoral students may, however, not be attractive to health plans that include only a limited set of health care providers.

COMMUNITY SERVICE

During the 1970s, many dental schools developed community dentistry departments or programs that provided clinical experiences in community health settings for most dental students. Funding for these programs came from federal government initiatives such as the Model Cities program and Public Health Service grants. The elimination of these federal programs coupled with reductions in other sources of dental school revenues led many schools to discontinue or limit off-site clinical opportunities for students. Another disincentive is that schools forgo fee income when students are off-site rather than providing services in the dental school clinic. Reduced student and faculty involvement in the larger community increases the isolation of the dental school.

If coverage of basic dental services does not become more wide-spread through either private or public initiative, student clinics are likely to remain significant sources of care for low-income people. Even if dental insurance should become near universal, cost-sharing requirements, low reimbursement rates, and other restrictions might still encourage poor or even middle-class patients to seek lower-cost sources of care.

Financial barriers are, however, not the only obstacles to adequate dental care. As noted in Chapter 3, geographic, educational, and other factors also affect access. What this implies for the role of student-provided dental services will probably vary depending on the characteristics of the service area, the school's physical location, and other factors.

RETHINKING THE MISSION OF PATIENT CARE

GENERAL PRECEPTS

More than missions of education and research, the mission of patient care in the dental school is undergoing necessary and fundamental rethinking. This rethinking is necessary because the environment is changing. It is fundamental because it places patient care in a broader social context, one that extends well beyond the dental school and its current patients or patient care activities. The rethinking process will highlight the relationship of the dental school to the academic health center and the relationship of both to a changing health care delivery and financing system.

Because the health care system is a complex mixture of national, state, and community influences and institutions and because each dental school's situation has its own special characteristics, each school's own reassessment and restructuring process will be different. For example, some schools exist within universities that have no academic health center or that have located the center's components across distant campuses or communities. Even when an academic health center exists, it may or may not welcome stronger ties to the dental school. Other centers may see faculty and student dental clinics as assets. To cite another difference, some schools are located in small communities in which prospects for a "managed care revolution" are uncertain. These differences, although they require strategic consideration, should not be used to rationalize inaction.

Starting Points

In the committee's view, *the starting point for dental schools is an affirmation or reaffirmation that patient care is a distinct mission* that is related but not subservient to the educational and research missions. Dental educators and students must be as conscious as the private practitioner of patient needs, preferences, motivations, and limitations.

In preceding sections of this chapter, some specific options for dental schools to improve their patient care mission are proposed or implied. They include

- strategic planning that anticipates continued restructuring of the health care system;
- adoption of a formal, comprehensive quality assurance and improvement program;
- increased faculty accountability for patient care and more reliance on residents (for schools that have relevant graduate programs);
- more efficient administration of nonclinical activities;
- improvement of information systems to support outcomes research, quality improvement, and effective management;
- possible separation of accreditation programs for education and patient care; and
- integration with the patient care activities of the entire academic health center.

Strategic Planning

Strategic planning considers alternative futures and approaches for dealing with both more and less likely contingencies. For most dental schools, the planning process occurs within the broader framework and constraints of strategic planning for the university or academic health center. Chapter 7 recommends that dental schools, as part of their strategic planning process, undertake a very explicit assessment of their position—assets, deficits, opportunities, constraints—within this larger environment and identify objectives and steps to strengthen their position. Patient care will figure significantly in any such effort.

Almost any future for a dental school will involve most of the elements discussed below, including more patient-oriented care, formal quality assurance processes, and improved information systems. Some schools will see integration in a larger system as a feasible and desirable objective, and some may have such integration essentially dictated by their parent institutions. Other schools may determine that their patient care mission will be best served and sustained if they concentrate on market niches such as selected specialty services. Integration may not be a significant option for schools in more rural communities.

Quality Assurance and Improvement

Quality assurance is a very broad subject that, to some degree, encompasses most of the areas discussed later in this section, for example, accreditation and faculty accountability. It also overlaps with topics such as practice guidelines and outcomes research that have been discussed in other chapters. Patient care within dental schools needs, however, an overarching model of quality assurance and improvement as a reference point. One such model, continuous quality improvement (CQI), has gained wide currency elsewhere in the health care system. Its principles emphasize the following (IOM, 1992, p. 103):

• close relationships between so-called customers and suppliers (that is, the partners in any given health care transaction);
• errors being more often the result of defects in systems (e.g., those for reporting test results or scheduling operating rooms) than the consequence of individual deficiencies ("bad apples");
• planning, control, assessment, and improvement activities grounded in statistical and scientific precepts and techniques;
• reliance on internal (self-) monitoring—as opposed to external (regulatory) inspection—with mistakes viewed as "treasures" that should be used for learning and for resolving problems rather than as an occasion for punishment;
• standardization of processes (decreasing their variability) to reduce the opportunity for error and to link specific care processes to health outcomes;
• feedback to practitioners of statistical information on how their practices may differ from those of their peers or depart from evidence-based standards for practice;
• visible commitment to quality by the top leadership of the organization and involvement by all parts of the organization in processes of quality improvement; and
• a striving for *continuous* improvement in contrast to simply achieving preset goals.

Intricate mechanisms for applying these principles have been set forth and, subsequently, questioned for their costs and impact. Experimentation with implementation strategies continues (see, for example, Batalden et al., 1994; Horn and Hopkins, 1994; and Kibbe et al., 1994). This experimentation generally includes steps to improve information systems and analytic capacity at the institutional and systems levels. In the systems category falls research on the outcomes of patient care and the impact of guidelines for care in improving performance. (Chapter 3 discusses outcomes and guidelines.) Generally, institutions have applied CQI first to administrative processes, moving more slowly into clinical applications. The latter are, however, becoming increasingly important.

The precepts of continuous quality improvement appear to be diffusing among dental schools, albeit at an uneven rate. Fortunately, dental schools have the opportunity to learn from the experience of other institutions in implementing these precepts. For dental schools, an additional attraction of patient-oriented quality improvement strategies is that it presents research opportunities for dental school faculty, for example, in assessing patient priorities, measuring satisfaction with care, and evaluating methods for modifying patient behavior and improving compliance with oral hygiene regimens.

Faculty Accountability

Some dental schools are already moving to increase faculty accountability for patient care. The most definitive step is to assign responsibility for each patient to a faculty member who works with students, other generalist and specialty faculty, allied dental personnel, and administrative staff to match patient problems to student needs and capacities and who ensures comprehensive patient care by providing, overseeing, and coordinating services. This definitive step is by no means simple. It demands more of clinical faculty and typically involves administrative, personnel, and or facility adjustments that are neither quickly nor inexpensively implemented. Serving more fully as role models for students should, however, prove stimulating to those faculty who find satisfaction in both patient care and clinical education.

Greater faculty accountability may be accompanied by another change that could improve patient satisfaction and clinic efficiency. As described earlier, the current model in most schools is for students to learn procedures by doing a few of them perfectly from start to finish. An alternative model is for students to participate in the care of a great many patients, undertaking a few elements of a procedure initially and adding steps as they gain proficiency. Under such a model, time demands for many patients should be significantly less.

For the student, the alternative model brings exposure to a wider array of patients with a broader array of clinical problems—some simple, some complex. As a result, students learn more about the acceptable range of practice in areas such as diagnosis, treatment planning, procedural treatments, teamwork with allied dental personnel, and referral to specialists.

Administrative Efficiency and Information

Better patient care means more efficient clinical care, which, in turn, requires more efficient administrative support. The restructuring of the health care system is reinforcing the pressure on practitioners and institutions to upgrade their information systems, patient records, quality assurance and improvement programs, and ability to report their performance to public and private purchasers. Although dentistry and office-based medical care more generally have been slow to experience some of these pressures, this chapter has argued that this relative exemption will not last.

As noted earlier, dental school clinics are, in principle, in a good position to draw on their faculty and on other components of the academic health center for the knowledge and analytic capacities needed to assess and improve their performance. Steps that schools take to improve information and administrative systems should bring diverse benefits, for example, improving feedback of performance information to students and reducing the clerical and other noneducational components of clinic work. They should also reinforce some of the research strategies proposed in the preceding chapter.

Accreditation

The dental community, most notably the Commission on Dental Accreditation and the American Association of Dental Schools, must address the collective processes for overseeing the quality of dental education and the quality of patient care within the dental school. If dental school clinics follow the path of competition and integration outlined elsewhere in this chapter, the development of a separate organization and process for accrediting or certifying clinics in dental schools may be advisable at some point. That process would best be structured as part of a more comprehensive effort to assess and ensure the quality of dental care including community-based and hospital-affiliated services.

The path toward certification for outpatient care programs has not been a smooth one in either medicine or dentistry, and the design and implementation of quality assurance and improvement programs for ambulatory care encounter particular problems. Difficulties include the number and diversity of ambulatory care settings and services, their traditionally fragmented and incomplete data systems, and the relative scarcity of agreed-upon quality indicators, especially outcomes measures (IOM, 1990e). Improvements in data systems and outcome measures should be priorities for dental school clinics regardless of how external review programs are structured.

Integration with the Academic Health Center

To the extent that the health care system of the future is based on organizations that integrate different types and settings of care, most academic health centers will need to develop a more coherent relationship among their constituent patient care units. Where a center can call upon its dental school, it may be able to develop an advantage over competitors without dental programs if the school's patient care activities become more patient oriented and able to attract patients independently or through referrals. Not only could the school offer services, it could be a productive source of referrals for other parts of the academic health center. Thus, academic health centers may indeed welcome participation by dental educators in reorganizing patient care activities to make them more competitive. Where such participation does not exist or is limited, dental school deans and faculty should take the initiative in exploring closer relationships.

Dental schools that are not part of an academic health center could, in principle, seek integration or involvement with other institutions. Whether they would be attractive partners absent some preexisting connection probably would depend on how attractive patient care within the dental school could be made.

FINDINGS AND RECOMMENDATIONS

Dental schools' perceptions of their patient care mission are still evolving, as are their strategies for fulfilling this mission. The typical dental school clinic, put simply, is not patient-friendly. The focus is still very much on procedures rather than on patients, and sufficient emphasis has not been placed on efficiency, quality, and accountability for care from the *patient's* perspective. Problems in these areas are serious in their own right and will become more acute if current trends in health care delivery and financing continue. Academic health centers are having to compete for patients and for participation in managed care plans of various sorts. Whether a dental school clinic adds or subtracts from the overall institution's market position is likely to be an issue in its future. As currently structured, few dental schools—even when they charge lower fees—are attractive to insured patients.

Over the long term, the committee believes that dental schools have no ethical or practical alternative but to make their programs more patient centered and more economically viable. This will involve very significant changes in the way many dental educators and practitioners view the roles and operation of dental schools. Such changes will not be achieved painlessly or immediately or without the support of community dentists and dental organizations. Financing will be a major challenge.

To affirm that patient care is a distinct mission, each dental school should support a strategic planning process to

• develop objectives for patient-centered care in areas such as appointment scheduling, completeness and timeliness of treatment, and definition of faculty and student responsibilities;
• identify current deficiencies in patient care processes and outcomes, along with physical, financial, legal, and other barriers to their correction; and
• design specific actions—including demonstration projects or experiments—to improve the quality, efficiency, and attractiveness of its patient services.

To respond to changes in roles and expectations for providers of outpatient health services including dental school clinics, the Commission on Dental Accreditation and the American Association of Dental Schools should

• reexamine processes for assessing patient care activities in dental schools and ensuring the quality of care, and
• begin to evaluate new options such as eventual participation by dental schools in separate accreditation programs for their ambulatory care facilities.

To increase access to care and improve the oral health

status of underserved populations, dental educators, practitioners, researchers, and public health officials should work together to

• secure more adequate public and private funding for personal dental services, public health and prevention programs, and community outreach activities, including those undertaken by dental school students and faculty; and
• address the special needs of underserved populations through health services research, curriculum content, and patient services, including more productive use of allied dental personnel.

SUMMARY

This chapter has examined the clinical services of dental schools primarily from the patient and health care system perspective rather than from an educational perspective. Such a perspective has not been typical among dental schools, and most schools' views of their patient care mission are still evolving as are their strategies for fulfilling this mission. Changes in the role of health professions schools and academic health centers both in the university and in the larger health care system will put pressure on dental schools to improve the efficiency and quality of their patient services.

Reshaping the provision of patient care in the average dental school will not be easy or quick because it will require change in long-standing attitudes and administrative practices. In addition, it may require that funds be found to upgrade facilities and staffing. These difficulties will be compounded by broad alterations in health care delivery and financing that are proving difficult for academic health centers, private practitioners, patients, and governments alike. Turmoil and uncertainty may be the most stable features of the next decade.

7

Dental Schools and the University

Even in times of prosperity and comfort, universities reexamine their missions and the match between their missions and activities. Such reexaminations may lead to restructuring, consolidation, and elimination of programs. In times of relative financial strain, the incentives for such reexamination and redesign are markedly more intense, as dental educators can attest. Between 1984 and 1994, six private dental schools closed. During site visits and other discussions, the study committee learned that discontinuation of additional schools is a serious—although not necessarily publicly acknowledged—possibility.

This chapter examines the relationship of the dental school to the university, considers factors that put schools at risk, and assesses strategies for strengthening their position—including their financial position. A basic premise is that *dental schools must remain part of the university* rather than once again become independent institutions—essentially trade schools—without the relationships to other professional, scientific, and humanities programs provided by universities. To preserve and strengthen their position within the university, dental schools must ensure that their contributions are genuine and visible to their parent institutions.

As described in Chapter 2, the first university-based dental school was created at Harvard University in 1867, and the University of Michigan created the first postgraduate programs in 1894. A fundamental goal of William Gies's 1926 report on dental education was to improve the stature of these university-based programs and eliminate nonuniversity programs. Likewise, when the National Institute of Dental Research (NIDR) was established in 1948, it rested its research strategy on the proposition that a university base for dentistry was essential to long-term progress in oral health science. This stance reflected a broader, postwar consensus that scientific research was fundamental to the nation's health, well-being, and security and that the country's universities and colleges had to play a central role in advancing knowledge and developing scientific talent (Bush, 1945).

THE UNIVERSITY IN A CHANGING WORLD

America's universities have, since the end of World War II, experienced phenomenal growth and prosperity followed by some degree of retrenchment and instability born of slow economic growth, rising costs for research and development, and increased competition from other calls on society's resources (Williams et al., 1987; President's Council of Advisors on Science and Technology, 1992). Although the situation varies significantly from school to school and from state to state, the pressures on the university and the academic health center have generally intensified in the last decade.

These pressures include federal policies that have added or shifted responsibilities to other units, including states and academic health centers. Resources often have not been shifted or expanded to reflect costly added responsibilities in areas such as occupational health and safety and indigent health care. Indeed, federal and state resources for many longer-standing programs either have not kept pace with inflation or have declined far below the levels that promoted growth in the 1960s and 1970s. At the same time, budgets in many states have been severely strained by a slow and uneven recovery from a prolonged recession, difficult social problems, and public opposition to taxes for almost any purpose.

Educational costs, in common with costs for other service sectors of the economy, have been increasing at rates considerably higher than family incomes and inflation overall (Baumol, 1992). Most of this differential is attributed to rising labor costs that are difficult to offset by increased productivity, for example, through the replacement of people with machines. One result is concern that tuition may be reaching the limit of affordability, particularly at some private institutions.

Physical facilities added during the expansion years of the 1960s and 1970s are wearing out, and keeping up-to-date technologically is expensive, particularly in academic health centers. Some attribute a large part of health care cost increases to technological innovation (Newhouse, 1992). Success during the 1960s and 1970s in attracting new resources multiplied new programs and units, thereby increasing administrative costs and complexities and adding to the number of interested parties (e.g., faculty, students, interest groups) that resist program cutbacks (Detmer and Finney, 1993). University efforts to cut costs by downsizing or reorganizing have also been limited by the tenure system and by the elimination of mandatory retirement Honan, 1994a,b).[1] In addition, demographic changes have created strains as the "baby boom" generation has aged out of its undergraduate years and been replaced by a new mix of students—more women, minorities, and older students—with different characteristics and expectations of the university.

Moreover, universities have been criticized for arrogance and lack of accountability, for neglecting their fundamental educational role, and for overemphasizing the theoretical at the expense of the practical (see, for example, Boyer, 1990; Searle, 1990; Huber, 1992; Bulger, 1993). States, in particular, expect public universities to return visible economic benefits to their economies.

At the national level, the President's Council of Advisers on Science and Technology (1992) has urged universities to be more selective in supporting programs and to reduce support for those that are not "world class." It also urged the government to refrain from encouraging new university programs for which sustained support is unlikely and from increasing the net capacity of the system of research universities.

One problem universities face in developing coherent responses to environmental threats is a generally decentralized organizational structure based in a long tradition of academic autonomy. Within this environment, academic health centers have a unique

---

[1]Universities are, in fact, scaling back programs. In a widely publicized example of retrenchment related to state economic problems, the University of California at Los Angeles has attempted to eliminate, consolidate, and restructure several of its major professional programs. It proposed to focus resources and cut administrative expenses by eliminating schools of public health, library science, architecture, and urban planning and by consolidating some of their curriculum, students, and faculty in other programs. After an outcry from the public health community and its supporters, the initial proposal has been revised, for example, to continue the School of Public Health, albeit on a scaled-back basis (Mercer, 1994).

and often controversial position. They have made major contributions to university influence and prestige and simultaneously created significant tensions (Shapiro, 1994). With their considerable budgets, staffs, and reputations, these centers sometimes provoke resentment as well as concerns that university ideals are compromised by the exigencies of professional education. Bulger (1993) also points to cultural tensions: "The health professional schools on the academic health center campus are involved with teaching and research, and in addition actually do something with their students, whereas most programs in the rest of the university do not lead to efforts in the field of action for which the faculty are held responsible" (p. 204).

In addition to the general pressures on the university as described above, academic health centers face additional challenges deriving from the restructuring of the health care delivery and financing system. Chapter 6 describes these challenges and argues that dental schools may be either an asset or a liability in this environment.

SCHOOLS AT RISK

As noted in Chapter 1, one inspiration for this study was the decision by six universities—all private—to close their schools of dentistry in the 1980s and 1990s (see Table 1.1). Several more schools—some private, some public—have been given mandates by their universities to improve or risk closure.

What puts a dental school at high risk?[2] The committee's investigations pointed to several factors. *Financial* issues were repeatedly described as critical. Dental education was cited as an expensive enterprise that is or may become a drain on university resources. On average, current-year expenditures for the average dental school are about $1 million more than current revenues. *Uncompetitive patient care programs* may become an increasing liability in the future. The *declining size and quality of the applicant pool* during the 1980s played a

---

[2]For discussions of specific schools, see Elliott, 1988; Fritz, 1988; Wotman, 1989; and Stephens, 1993. Also relevant are the strategic analyses of schools that received support from the Pew National Dental Education Program (see, in particular, the February 1990 issue of the Journal of Dental Education; and Barker and O'Neil, 1992). For governmental assessments of the possible closure of public or private state-related schools, see Kentucky Council on Higher Education (1992) and Wisconsin Governor's Commission (1993).

role in some closures by threatening the tuition base and prestige on which private schools rely. *Faculty and alumni resistance to change* may feed impatience among university administrators. In some institutions, the comparative *isolation of dental schools within the university* has provided them with few allies or at least informed colleagues and has left them ill-prepared to counter proposals for "downsizing." Isolation also makes it difficult for the dental school to correct the misperceptions that caries are no longer a problem and that an oversupply of dentists makes continuation of most schools unnecessary. In addition to "cultural" isolation, some schools face geographic isolation from peer professional schools. Finally, the *limited involvement of some schools* in their surrounding communities leaves them without support from this potential constituency.

The above recitation lists factors that are, to varying degrees, both within and beyond the control of any dental school. Earlier chapters have discussed steps—including faculty practice plans, collaborative research, community health programs, and minority recruitment strategies—that should reduce the isolation of the dental school and serve other goals as well. From a dean's perspective, however, even the elements for which the school is held most accountable (e.g., faculty productivity) may not be easily amenable to change by management. As discussed elsewhere in this report, constraints include policies related to tenure and retirement age, shortages of qualified oral health researchers, and political disputes over expanded dental school services in the community. Because financing has been identified as such a crucial factor, the next section of this chapter considers the financial position and options of dental schools. It does not promise easy answers.

FINANCING DENTAL EDUCATION

In the committee's survey of dental school deans, financing stood out as a major issue. When asked to identify the most significant weaknesses of their schools, 47 out of 54 deans mentioned overall funding problems or specific funding problems related to overreliance on tuition. The senior university officials interviewed by the committee uniformly pointed to financing as their most immediate concern. The following discussion of dental school financing highlights selected data and issues, and the background paper by Douglass and Fein presents a more extensive analysis.

BASIC DATA

Overall, from 1985 to 1993, mean revenue per dental school increased from $14.0 million to $21.0 million for public schools and from $11.5 million to $18.9 million for private schools (ADA, 1994a). Both of these increases exceed the 34 percent increase in the Consumer Price Index for the same period.

Table 7.1 presents trend data showing changes in the proportion of dental school revenues from different sources from 1973 to 1991. The cutbacks in federal share and the increases in the state share of funding show up for both public and private schools. The proportion of state funds increased for private schools (including private state-related schools) from 8.3 percent in 1973 to 19.4 percent in 1981, but the figure had dropped back to 9.2 percent by 1991.[3] The proportion of state funds has also dropped for public schools in recent years, but these funds still comprise, on average, over half the revenues for these schools. Nearly half the revenues of private school derive from tuition.

For all dental schools in 1992, the average total expenditure per student was nearly $53,000, of which about 30 percent was recovered through tuition, student fees, and clinical revenues (Table 7.2). Behind these overall figures lie major differences between public and private schools. The average total expenditure per student was about $60,400 for public schools and $39,200 for private schools. The former recovered about 20 percent of these costs from student tuition and fees and clinic revenue compared to 64 percent for private schools. State appropriations account for most of this difference between public and private schools.

Variations in total expenditures per student vary even more dramatically at the level of the individual school. Excluding expenditures for sponsored research, the 1992 expenditures per stu-

---

[3]The figures for private schools include schools categorized as private state related. In general, these schools appear more similar to each other in expenditures, staffing, and tuition than they are to public schools. In rank order, the six private state-related schools received approximately 55, 30, 26, 20, 9, and 3 percent of their revenues from state appropriations in 1993 (ADA, 1994a). Of the 13 private schools not categorized as state related, six received from 0.16 to 2.16 percent of their revenues from state appropriations. Among public schools, revenues from state appropriations ranged from 27 to 75 percent of total revenues. From 1993 to 1994, one private state-related school closed, and another changed its classification to private.

TABLE 7.1 Sources of Dental School Revenue as Percentage of Total Revenue

Source	1973	1975	1977	1979	1981	1983	1985	1987	1989	1991
All Schools										
State	36.0	37.9	45.9	47.6	49.5	46.6	45.1	44.4	45.2	42.4
Federal	29.9	27.6	19.1	16.1	13.2	10.1	12.2	10.1	10.9	10.5
Tuition	17.3	16.6	17.3	19.3	19.9	23.5	23.1	22.3	21.0	22.0
Clinic	9.1	10.4	11.2	11.8	12.8	13.4	13.5	13.8	13.8	15.3
Other	7.7	7.5	6.5	5.3	4.6	6.4	6.1	9.3	9.0	9.9
Public Schools										
State	53.2	53.6	61.6	64.1	66.0	64.7	62.7	61.6	60.2	57.6
Federal	26.5	24.2	17.0	14.9	12.3	9.9	11.8	10.4	10.8	10.4
Tuition	8.2	7.9	8.0	8.6	8.7	10.5	10.3	10.0	10.0	10.4
Clinic	6.4	7.7	8.4	9.3	10.2	11.3	11.5	11.6	11.7	13.4
Other	5.6	6.6	5.0	3.1	2.8	3.6	3.8	6.4	7.2	8.2
Private Schools										
State	8.3	12.5	18.3	18.7	19.4	16.5	15.3	13.2	11.8	9.2
Federal	35.3	33.0	22.8	18.1	15.0	10.2	12.8	9.7	11.0	10.7
Tuition	32.0	30.7	33.7	37.8	40.4	45.1	44.8	44.7	45.5	47.3
Clinic	13.5	14.7	16.1	16.2	17.5	17.0	16.9	17.8	18.5	19.2
Other	10.9	9.1	9.1	9.2	7.7	11.2	10.2	14.6	13.2	13.5

SOURCE: Adapted from American Association of Dental Schools, 1993b.

dent ranged from $26,300 in one medium-sized private school to $91,600 in one small public school.

One explanation for the differences between public and private schools is that public schools are generally smaller, averaging just under 300 students per school, whereas private schools average just over 400 students. This means that fixed and semi-fixed costs are spread across a smaller student base. Private schools average 5.46 students per faculty member compared to 3.87 for public schools.

Do variations in expenditures per student indicate that private schools are more efficient than public schools? Beyond the size variable, the committee lacked the information to make such a determination. True educational costs per student are not easy to determine, and the committee found no in-depth empirical analyses of the actual costs of dental education. Likewise, a 1993 report from the Josiah Macy, Jr., Foundation found no recent analyses of the cost of medical education (Ginzberg et al., 1993). In fact, the only systematic in-depth study identified in the Carnegie re-

TABLE 7.2 Dental School Expenditures and Revenues per Student, 1977-1991 (in dollars)

School	1977	1981	1986	1989	1990	1991	1992
All Schools							
Total expenditures per DDSE	17,463	23,927	36,568	47,198	49,628	51,447	52,804
Average resident tuition and fees	2,824	4,933	7,556	8,867	9,427	10,106	10,690
Clinic revenue per DDSE	1,768	2,213	3,522	4,165	4,645	5,016	5,515
Remaining cost per student	12,871	16,781	25,490	34,166	35,556	36,325	36,599
Percentage of total cost not recovered in tuition, fees, or clinic revenue	73.7%	70.1%	69.7%	72.4%	71.6%	70.6%	69.3%
Public Schools							
Total expenditures per DDSE	20,412	27,349	41,776	54,419	57,037	59,226	60,366
Average resident tuition and fees	1,442	2,241	3,783	4,813	5,106	6,074	6,188
Clinic revenue per DDSE	1,553	1,870	3,166	3,901	4,336	4,800	5,341
Remaining cost per student	17,417	23,238	34,827	45,705	47,595	48,352	48,837
Percentage of total cost not recovered in tuition, fees, or clinic revenue	85.3%	85.0%	83.4%	84.0%	83.4%	81.6%	80.9%
Private Schools							
Total expenditures per DDSE	13,617	18,937	28,972	34,876	36,663	37,833	39,157
Average resident tuition and fees	4,808	8,702	13,297	15,962	16,990	18,090	19,443
Clinic revenue per DDSE	2,046	2,715	4,041	4,629	5,185	5,395	5,819
Remaining cost per student	6,763	7,520	11,634	14,285	14,488	14,348	14,309
Percentage of total cost not recovered in tuition, fees, or clinic revenue	49.7%	39.7%	40.2%	41.0%	39.5%	37.9%	36.2%

NOTE: DDSE = D.D.S. undergraduate equivalent. The American Dental Association equivalency formula counts advanced specialty student as equal to 1.7 of a predoctoral (D.D.S.) student and an allied dental professions student as equal to 0.5 of a predoctoral student.

SOURCE: American Dental Association, Council on Dental Education, annual reports.

port was a study conducted by the Institute of Medicine (IOM, 1973) in the early 1970s.[4]

One problem in determining true costs for education is allocating costs for jointly produced services such as teaching and patient care. Another problem arises when schools use residents in their advanced general dentistry or specialty programs to instruct predoctoral students. Moreover, in comparing costs across schools, one would—ideally—want a "quality-adjusted" measure of output that would indicate whether higher cost is associated with better student performance, for example, in licensing examinations and in practice. In addition, because schools may differ in the abilities of students recruited, one would want to know the "value added" by different schools.

Table 7.3 compares sources of revenues for dental and medical schools. It shows that dental schools rely more on tuition and fees (22 versus 4 percent) and less on faculty practice income (15 versus 42 percent).[5] The latter difference reflects the significant—but vulnerable—contribution of Medicare and Medicaid reimbursements for graduate medical education.

Variations in the cost of dental education are replicated in costs for dental hygiene education. The average cost in dental hygiene tuition and fees is approximately $4,500 at community colleges, $5,800 at technical institutes, $7,000 for four-year colleges, and $10,000 for dental school and university-based programs (Solomon et al., 1992). At private universities, tuition may exceed $20,000. Dental hygiene programs are relatively costly for educational institutions compared with many other allied health professions programs. Allied health education is, in general, expensive for institutions because it is faculty intensive, often demands expen-

---

[4]The 1973 IOM study worked from a statistical sample of 14 medical schools and relied in part on data derived from diaries "in which the faculty members logged their time by activity—education, research, and patient care." For joint activities such as teaching and patient care, the faculty estimated the time allocated to each aspect. The data were converted into estimates of instructional costs and costs for patient care and research associated with education. Extrapolating from the 1973 study, the authors of the 1993 report estimated that the 1990 inflation-adjusted costs for educating a medical student averaged $38,000 with a range of $21,000 to $56,000. However, the average cost derived by dividing instructional and department research costs was $68,000. The authors do not offer an explanation for the differences in the two approaches.

[5]Comparisons between medical and dental schools should be treated as provisional because of possible differences in definitions and reporting conventions not known to the committee.

TABLE 7.3   Sources of Income and Revenue for Dental Schools and Medical Schools, 1990-1991 (in $millions)

	Dental		Medical	
	$ Amount	% of Total	$ Amount	% of Total
Operating Revenue				
State	426.1	42.4	2,714	12.9
Federal	10.9	1.1	104	0.5
Tuition	221.2	22.0	876	4.2
Clinic/services	153.2	15.3	8,848	42.1
Endowment earnings	12.6	1.3	403	1.9
Gifts	16.3	1.6	448	2.1
Indirect cost recovery	24.8	2.5	1,385	6.6
Parent university	NA	NA	189	0.9
Other	25.8	2.6	880	4.2
Total operating revenue	890.9	88.7	15,847	75.4
Nonoperating revenue				
Sponsored education, research and training				
Nongovernment	22.5	2.2	1,039	4.9
Federal	71.7	7.1	3,211	15.3
State/local	7.2	0.7	239	1.1
Financial aid revenue				
Nongovernment	4.2	0.4	196	0.9
Federal	2.8	0.3	142	0.7
State/local	5.2	0.5	332	1.6
Total nonoperating revenue	113.6	11.3	5,159	24.6
Total revenue	1,004.6	100.0	21,006	100.0

NOTE: NA = not available. Parent university support may be in the form of reduced physical plant expenditures, overhead, administrative, and other noncash benefits.

SOURCE: American Dental Association, 1992d and Jolin et al., 1992.

sive space and equipment, and involves administrative and supervisory costs to arrange and oversee off-site clinical activities. Thirteen university-based hygiene programs have closed since 1982 (one of which was transferred to another university), and two others are being phased out (ADHA, personal communication, May 23, 1994).

ISSUES AND STRATEGIES

Dental education, like medical education, is distinguished from professional fields such as law and business by the costs incurred in providing students with extensive clinical experience. In addition, for dental schools, most of these costs are borne directly. Rather than relying on separate university-owned or affiliated hospitals as medical schools do, each dental school has its own large clinic dedicated to the clinical education of predoctoral students. The operation of these clinics subjects dental schools to financial requirements ranging from new government regulations to major technological innovations. The cost of these clinics is not shared with other users. Moreover, a substantial portion of expensive clinical faculty time is devoted to the unevenly paced and somewhat unpredictable task of reviewing the work of individual predoctoral students on individual patients. As medical schools move from hospital to outpatient settings for education, they too are encountering conflicts between the demands of patients (and payers) for fast, timely care and an educational process that has its own pace and scheduling requirements.

Contributing further to the financial pressures on dental schools are the expenses associated with many of the proposals for improvements in curriculum and instruction discussed in Chapter 4. For example, problem-based instruction involves higher faculty-to-student ratios and higher initial investments for developing instructional materials and training faculty. Similarly, student exposure to more varied patient care settings, generally off-campus, tends to add to costs and subtract from patient care revenues. Increased reliance on computers may cut some instructional costs by substituting less expensive machines for more expensive faculty, but computers are frequently a supplement, allowing more sophisticated instruction with substantial startup and ongoing maintenance costs.

The financial problems facing dental schools are not merely the concern of the schools and their universities but also the concern of the profession and of society generally. In Chapter 1, the committee stated as one its guiding principles that *"a qualified dental work force is a valuable national resource, and support for the education of this work force has come and must continue to come from both public and private sources."* That principle, unfortunately, does not translate easily into practice. Financial survival requires that dental schools demonstrate their contributions to their parent institutions and to the public. Schools that fail to do so are vulnerable even if their financial situation is not critical. Schools that succeed will have better allies in times of crisis.

OPTIONS

No grand solution to the financial problems of dental schools is on the horizon, and no single strategy or combination of strategies will fit all schools. Important as it is for every school to be concerned about mechanisms for cutting costs and increasing revenues, there is no general blueprint for doing this. Although some strategies such as trying to increase efficiency in student clinics are generally applicable, each school also should search its environment for unique or atypical opportunities. These opportunities might include a rapidly growing state population or a new policy commitment to oral health services for disadvantaged populations. Research-intensive schools may benefit from patents or royalties on new dental materials, instruments, and pharmaceuticals.

For most schools, a strategy for improving the school's financial position will consist of many modest steps. Occasionally, however, one step may dominate, for example, when a state decides to commit significant resources to upgrade a school through investments in both physical and human resources. The steps more generally available to schools include the creation or expansion of faculty practice plans; the pursuit of sponsored research; the development of more efficient learning strategies; the expansion of continuing education programs; the cultivation of alumni contributions and special gifts; and the consolidation or merger of courses, departments, and programs to reduce overhead costs.

When asked about the usefulness of various strategies for increasing funding, dental school deans showed commonalities as well as variations in their responses. A substantial majority of deans believed that increased state funding, expanded enrollment, and increased tuition were *unlikely* sources of additional revenues. Nonetheless, four deans cited increased state funding as a highly useful strategy, and three cited increased tuition. The revenue-increasing strategies cited by the deans as *most useful* included increases in sponsored research, alumni contributions, and patient care revenues from postdoctoral general dentistry programs. Again, a handful of deans had contrary views. On the cost-cutting side of the financial equation, no single strategy was identified by a majority of deans as having high utility for decreasing costs, possibly because the strategies were seen as having already achieved much of their potential.

Any financial strategy has its pluses and minuses, and each school's environment will make the calculus somewhat different. It is also clear that a financial problem as viewed from one perspective may be a solution when viewed from another. For example, dental schools and universities have viewed tuition increases as a way of offsetting declining revenues from other sources. The problems that this solution creates for students (see Chapter

4), however, place limits on its unconstrained use. In any case, no strategy should be adopted without careful analysis of its implications for the education, research, and patient care missions of the dental school.

In the aggregate, the combination of modest steps outlined above may be sufficient, but the committee recognized that they may not be. Thus, a more fundamental process of rethinking the most costly elements of dental education and experimenting with alternative strategies is needed. This rethinking requires more financial expertise and more detailed data than was feasible for this broadly focused study. The committee recognizes that dental schools acting alone may provide too small a market at this stage to interest those developing innovative technologies (e.g., sophisticated, specialized computer software) and that consortia-based ventures can be administratively and financially precarious. Moreover, experimentation with these or equivalent changes would likely require negotiation with accreditation and, possibly, licensure bodies. Despite these difficulties, the committee would hope to see new projects that bring together expertise from dental, business, computer science, and education schools or programs to rethink specific high cost components of traditional education. These could be built upon the example of past strategic development projects in dental schools, notably, those supported by the Pew National Dental Education Program (Barker and O'Neil, 1992).

Information Base and Cost Analyses

The foundation for a sound financial strategy is a formal cost analysis of programs and services. Such analyses are necessary for a sophisticated and accurate understanding of operational costs and of the opportunities for reducing these costs and managing resources more efficiently.

To cite an example, the dental school of Indiana University participated in a prototype effort to design and test an economic model of its activities (Lovrinic et al., 1993). The goals were (1) to determine production costs for the program's major products (e.g., students or graduates); (2) to identify opportunities to restructure and reduce costs; (3) to assess the cost impact of operational or policy changes; and (4) to help clarify how the program contributes to major missions of the university. The school was able to compare direct to total costs for graduates; identify costs devoted to instructional activity in lectures, labs, and clinics; compare clinic income to direct costs; and test alternative means of eliminating or consolidating activities. The data helped convince administrators and faculty to consolidate several departments, student clinics, and graduate-level courses without cutting educational programs. Costs for shared courses (e.g., between the medical and dental schools) and for support units (e.g., library and personnel office) were also examined to see whether they were reasonable for the benefits provided or whether different cost allocations needed to be negotiated.

In the committee's survey of deans, deans of private schools were more likely than public school deans to report formal cost analyses. This might reflect a greater need for and commitment to tight cost management, which might, in turn, contribute to their lower cost per student of private schools.

Faculty Practice Plans

Most dental schools see the creation or expansion of faculty practice plans as an important revenue-producing strategy. Although the specifics vary, faculty practice plans typically help schools to increase salaries for clinical faculty and thereby make them more competitive with the earnings of private practitioners. In addition, these plans have probably allowed schools to retain some experienced clinical faculty during a period of substantial enrollment declines and loss of faculty to private practice.

A recent survey of U.S. and Canadian dental schools revealed that 25 out of 32 responding schools with faculty practice plans used practice income to supplement faculty salaries, and 12 schools said that they used the income to provide or supplement faculty insurance or other benefits (Shnorkian and Zullo, 1993). Typically, about 10 percent of gross practice plan revenues was distributed to the dental school (i.e., the dean's office and the participating departments).

Faculty practice, if not overemphasized, has another, perhaps more significant advantage for some dental schools. That is, it involves full-time faculty in regular dental practice, an involvement that may make them more sensitive and credible role models for students. Such practice also may help build faculty credibility with the practitioner community. The committee heard repeatedly from practitioners that they or their colleagues do not see dental faculty as "real" dentists unless they provide regular patient care beyond that involved in the instruction and supervision of students. Faculty practice presumably provides an additional stimulus—and financial opportunity—for faculty to keep abreast of technical advances and to better judge when and if they should be incorporated in the predoctoral curriculum.

On the negative side, faculty practice plans have been criticized—particularly in the medical school—for deflecting faculty from their role as educators (Ginzberg et al., 1993). The survey cited above found predoctoral dental student involvement (primarily observation) in only 14 of the 39 schools reporting practice plans. Of the schools with advanced education programs, only 10 of 35 had a role for these students in practice plans. Because the revenues from faculty practice cover faculty compensation and other operating costs of the plan, practice plans do not generally provide significant additional resources for the educational and research missions of the school. The supplemental salaries available to clinical faculty can also create friction with nonclinical faculty.

Faculty practice plans can bring dental schools into conflict with community practitioners, especially in smaller towns and cities. In the survey cited above, half the responding schools with faculty practice plans said it was their perception that local practitioners viewed such plans as competitors (Shnorkian and Zullo, 1993). Half of these schools received 25 percent or less of their practice plan patients through referrals from community dentists.

Finally, requirements for up-front investments in physical plant and equipment may be obstacles to the creation or upgrading of practice plans. It also may take some time before a new plan even covers its overhead costs.

Student Clinics

Chapter 6 reported that student clinics, especially predoctoral clinics, generally run a deficit. Although reasons for the deficit derive primarily from the educational function of the clinics (e.g., the slow pace of student work, inability to charge market rates), deficits may, in some circumstances, be reduced. For example, some schools have improved the efficiency of student clinics through streamlining administrative practices such as those for scheduling patients, collecting fees, and keeping patient and student records. Clinic productivity may also be improved by having faculty deliver care that is beyond students' competency and assume primary responsibility for patient care. The dentist-attending model, similar to that in medicine, could work well if combined with teams that included beginning and advanced students. Even though payments may still be lower than those in private practice, schools may also be able to negotiate more favorable payment rules with state Medicaid programs for services provided by students. In addition, some schools may be able to participate with other parts of an academic health center in managed care plans for the university community (i.e., students, faculty, staff, and family members).

Curriculum Changes

Chapter 4 presents the case for curriculum reform including an overall reduction in clock hours and the restructuring or consolidation of some courses. To the educational motivation for reform can be added a financial motivation. As noted earlier, the existing model of dental education is expensive, partly because payments for patient care do not include the educational subsidy that Medicare provides to teaching hospitals. The existing model of dental education is also relatively unchanged from that of the 1930s and 1940s. New technologies such as computer-based instruction (including virtual reality simulators) and remote instruction have the potential to reduce costs while improving or maintaining educational outcomes. To simultaneously reduce costs and provide support to advanced education students, some preclinical education could be shifted from the faculty to these students, a practice common in other parts of the university.

Some curriculum changes may involve revenue losses or increased costs (e.g., to introduce problem-based learning or off-campus clinical opportunities), but offsetting savings can be sought elsewhere, for example, by removing redundant or outdated coursework or by reducing the number of separate departments or other organizational units. In some cases, however, tenure provisions will make any adjustments in faculty numbers or focus difficult.

To the extent that program development activities (e.g., designing computer simulations, developing cases for problem-based learning) can be successfully pursued by multi-institutional consortia and similar arrangements, per-institution costs should go down and product quality may very well benefit from collaboration. The same principle applies for other activities, for example, devising and conducting faculty development programs and creating software to inform and counsel students about their financial options and prospects.

Tuition

Although several committee members were concerned about the high tuition charged by many dental schools, the committee expected that a careful analysis of in-state and out-of-state tuition at a few state-sponsored schools would show that they are low compared to efficiently managed peer institutions. Such schools may have room to increase tuition if the return in educational benefits is clear. In 1992, 12 schools had in-state tuition of less than $5,000 per year, and an additional 10 schools were below $6,000. Out-of-state tuition averages about three times the in-state figure. For some public schools, tuition increases would require legislative approval. If tuition were raised, offsetting increases in financial aid might be necessary to preserve opportunities for economically disadvantaged applicants. At the other end of the tuition spectrum, high-tuition schools, as indicated elsewhere in this discussion, should be looking for educational efficiencies and other means of controlling the tuition burden on their students.

Sponsored Research

Although sponsored research is a relatively untapped revenue source for some schools, its main value is not financial rewards for the school but the creation of new knowledge and a more stimulating educational environment. In addition, research involvement tends to add more to dental school stature than any other faculty activity. On the negative side, faculty research involvement has—in common with faculty practice—been criticized as diverting attention from the education of students. Commercially sponsored research generates concerns about potential conflicts of interest. Adequate institutional oversight is essential to ensure that all research is properly conducted to advance knowledge. From a financial perspective, the real costs for conducting research must be accurately identified and recouped so that research activities are not unwittingly subsidized by other programs.

In any case, the pursuit of sponsored research is something of a zero-sum financial game across universities because significant expansions in the total revenue pool are unlikely. In the short term, the pursuit of sponsored research may also involve competition for a limited pool of research faculty. In addition, creating research capacity involves capital investments that may be impossible for some institutions in the foreseeable future.

Contributions and Gifts

Deans also mentioned alumni contributions as an important potential source of revenues. Although not cost free, the front-end costs of this strategy are relatively low compared to starting a faculty practice plan or creating a research capacity. A positive side effect (indeed, a condition) of an alumni strategy is improved ties with alumni that strengthen the school's political position and its ability to place graduates. On the negative side, the committee's site visits suggested that strong alumni can limit a school's flexibility to innovate.

Consolidation

Cost reduction through program consolidation or merger can be achieved in various ways. The discussion of curriculum efficiencies mentions consolidation to eliminate redundant or duplicative courses. Consolidation or merger of departments has been advocated both as a means of achieving administrative savings and as a strategy for increasing educational flexibility and innovation.

Similar arguments have been made for the consolidation of departments or programs across several schools within an academic health center or university. For example, the 1970 report by the Carnegie Commission on Higher Education noted that the "self-contained Flexner model" of internal basic science departments "leads to expensive duplication and can lead to some loss in quality" (cited in Fein, 1987, p. 71). A strategy mentioned to this committee on several occasions would merge basic science faculty into a single unit serving all health professions programs (if not the entire university). Three institutions with dental schools—the University of Texas Health Science Center at San Antonio, the University of Missouri at Kansas City, and Virginia Commonwealth University—have followed this model, but the last institution has recently dropped it. Compared to faculty merged under medical school control, the separate basic science unit might be somewhat more considerate of dental school interests.

In Chapter 4, one specific type of cross-school consolidation—incorporation of dentistry as a specialty within the medical school—has already been discussed. The emphasis in that discussion is on the character of future practice and its appropriate educational foundation. Financial savings are, in this committee's view, a minor rationale for this kind of consolidation, although savings in administration, student services, alumni programs, and other areas might be expected.

Regionalization of dental education focuses on dental education collectively not just on schools individually. In some cases, regionalization might involve a consolidation or merger of specific schools and their faculties and programs. Some of the key issues in such situations would be whether the strengths and weaknesses of the affected institutions are clearly identified, whether the expected benefits are being realistically assessed, and whether a merger strategy can resolve rather than exacerbate the problems. In other cases, regionalization might entail the closure of certain schools and a complex but not necessarily orchestrated reallocation of resources, some of which might flow to other dental schools and some of which might be retained by the university or the state that closed a school.

The major financial objective of regionalization is to achieve educational economies of scale. Dental education, research, and patient care involve relatively high fixed costs for clinic facilities and equipment, laboratories, and specialized staff. A shift from a larger number of small schools to a smaller set of large schools should, over time, reduce costs per student and per patient at the remaining schools. Such a shift probably would simultaneously reduce the number of schools competing for research or other funds[6] and increase the quality of the schools by concentrating academic talent that is currently spread thin, particularly in research. Consolidation of schools would, in many respects, be consistent with the "centers of excellence" strategy that is seen in other parts of the health care system and that is being promoted for research universities.

The arguments against a regionalization strategy are both substantive and practical. In the short term, consolidation may not save money. Consider, for example, an analysis of the implications of closing one of the two dental schools in Kentucky and shifting most or all of the closed school's enrollment to the remaining school (Kentucky Council on Higher Education, 1993; see also the council's 1992 report). This analysis (p. D-48) observed that the remaining school would experience substantial costs in "claiming or reclaiming, renovating, and equipping" the space required to nearly double its size and that additional costs would be incurred to relocate pro-

---

[6]For example, if a closed school had been receiving research funds from NIDR, those funds might stay with the parent institution if an investigator could finish his or her work elsewhere in the institution (e.g., the medical school). Alternatively, funds might follow an investigator to another school. In any case, the closed school would no longer compete for NIDR funds so funds would implicitly be reallocated to remaining competitors (which include investigators elsewhere in the parent institution).

grams displaced by such an expansion. In this particular case, some of the added costs would be offset by savings from the closed school (e.g., new construction costs forgone because expanding programs would be fitted into existing space).

Moreover, although the committee knows of no evidence on the point, it suspects that the economy of scale argument may not apply for dental schools beyond a certain size.[7] In schools beyond a certain size, faculty and students may also experience a loss of collegiality and freedom, and management structures may simultaneously become more oppressive and less efficient.

A reduction in the number of dental schools would bring a loss of diversity. It would also make future expansion of dental enrollments more difficult should that be judged desirable in the future. Absent compensatory actions, regionalization of schools might reduce access to care for some patients and would cost jobs in "losing" communities. Further, the vagaries of state politics offer no guarantee that the schools to be closed would be those with weaker educational, research, and service programs.

In addition, to the extent that consolidations were attempted across state borders, the distribution of expected costs and savings could create complications. Although a significant number of states do contract with out-of-state schools for positions for their students, the fungibility of state financial support for dental schools—a precondition for this strategy—is uncertain.

Where consolidation is not feasible, cooperation among dental schools in the same state or region may still permit some cost savings. For example, schools might work together to develop extramural sites for predoctoral and postdoctoral training or to make specialized programs at one school available to students from another. Accreditation standards should be flexible enough to recognize this kind of experimentation and cooperation.

UNIVERSITY AND STATE POLICIES AND PRIORITIES

The financial strategies considered and adopted by an individual dental school (or imposed on it) will be contingent to some degree on the financial and other policies of the parent university or academic health center. Some institutions, particularly private universities, operate under an "every tub on its own bottom"

---

[7]The literature on economies of scale in hospitals is suggestive but not necessarily generalizable (Zubkoff et al., 1978).

policy. That is, educational programs must be financially self-supporting except under special circumstances. Some universities explicitly subtract a percentage of initial program budgets and then reallocate the funds from this across-the-board "tax" to subsidize or upgrade selected university programs. Depending on the state's financial condition and priorities, public schools may face periodic dictates that they cut their total expenditures by particular amounts and in specific ways (e.g., across-the-board rather than targeted cuts). To the extent that states lack special policies for budgeting capital expenses, up-front investments on behalf of educational, research, or patient care missions or in support of long-term financial objectives may be compromised.

How the activities of a dental school correspond to state concerns can be crucial. For example, a 1993 analysis for the governor of Wisconsin (Wisconsin Governor's Commission, 1993) concluded that the most cost-effective way for the state to recruit an adequate supply of dentists overall was to contract with out-of-state schools to educate a defined number of Wisconsin residents rather than to continue to subsidize the existing private school in the state or to establish a new public school. The analysis, nonetheless, concluded that the contracting strategy was not desirable because the closure of the only dental school in the state would leave a major shortfall in services for the disadvantaged, especially in Milwaukee.

Although Wisconsin considered contracting with out-of-state schools and several states without dental schools do that, other states essentially maintain a "free-rider" philosophy, assuming or hoping that other schools or states will bear the cost of training their dentists. Eighteen states have neither an in-state school nor a financial commitment for out-of-state training. This free-rider stance has been rationalized by the argument that an oversupply of dentists exists and that other states will continue to train and export dentists. With the closure of schools, the significant drop in enrollments, and the decline in the ratio of dentists to the general population, some dental schools eventually may be able to negotiate new agreements with noncontributing states. An alternative to this voluntary cost-sharing strategy might be a national policy for health professions education that recognized the limitations of state-based funding. Some proposals for health care reform have included a "trust fund" to support graduate medical education through a tax on health insurance premiums, although it is not clear that action will be taken on any of these proposals. Other issues aside, this trust fund concept would not address the public good and state equity issues in predoctoral education.

PUBLIC AND PRIVATE SCHOOLS

The committee's view that dental education is a national resource deserving of both public and private support does not specifically address the situation of the nonprofit, private dental school. All six schools that closed in the last decade were private, and some other private schools are now at risk. How important is it that some private institutions be preserved? Is it important enough to warrant some public subsidy?

In considering this question, the committee had to rely on perceptions and philosophies rather than empirical evidence about the value added by private schools to the nation's system of dental education. Certainly, private institutions such as Columbia, Northwestern, and the University of Pennsylvania stand out in the historical record of dental education. More recently, private schools initiated several of the curriculum innovations cited in Chapter 4. Yet, many public schools also have an impressive record of achievement and innovation.

Ultimately, the committee's conclusion that a place for private institutions should be preserved rested on its conviction that a diversity of sponsorship and funding sources is desirable. In principle, such diversity can promote creativity, shelter challenges to conventional wisdom, help generate additional resources for testing new ideas, and diffuse power, including the power of the purse. Private schools may, for example, have greater flexibility and independence than state institutions. They also have provided opportunities for students whose states lacked a dental school and whose admission was limited by public schools in other states. For these reasons, the committee believes that public funding may, during difficult periods, be necessary and justifiable for private institutions. Public funds already flow to private institutions in many forms, including reimbursement for services to vulnerable populations, special projects, and competitive awards for research, training, and similar programs. Although not in the form of direct state appropriations for dental education, these funds may, to some degree, stem from a recognition of the value of private schools.

STRENGTHENING THE DENTAL SCHOOL WITHIN THE UNIVERSITY

Strengthening the position of dental schools within the university—on an individual and a collective basis—will require commitment from many sources. Some of this commitment must come from within the dental school, and some must come from the university or the academic health center. Support from state and federal governments is crucial in the form of both financial resources and prudent policies related to both health and higher education. In the private sector, it is important that organized dentistry, alumni, and community practitioners work to resolve tensions with dental educators that detract from their shared goals of quality professional education and improved oral health. Private philanthropy will not provide ongoing support, but it can provide crucial resources for specific projects.

Risk reduction is not an overnight task, and some factors are less subject to a school's influence than others. This makes it all the more important that each school assess its own position and develop a strategic plan for reinforcing its position within the university. Although the specifics will vary from school to school, this strategic plan should generally include an analysis of the university's circumstances and expectations, an assessment of the dental school's objectives and of its strengths and weaknesses, and an identification of steps for building on strengths and correcting weaknesses.

The three preceding chapters on the education, research, and patient care missions of the dental school have suggested specific strategies for modifying some of the factors that place schools at risk. They include improving the competitiveness of patient care programs in the community and building educational and research linkages with other parts of the university and academic health center. The middle section of this chapter considers financial strategies for improving the dental school's position. The following discussion focuses on leadership and service to the university.

LEADERSHIP AND THE CHALLENGE OF CHANGE

Calls for better leadership may seem pro forma. They are, nonetheless, hard to forgo despite recognition that effective leadership, especially leadership to be exercised in difficult times, is not an easily purchased commodity or a readily created talent.

One difference between the Flexner (1910) and Gies (1926) reports in the early years of this century and more recent examinations of medical and dental education lies in the strong emphasis of the latter on leadership and decisionmaking (see, for example, Association of American Medical Colleges, 1992; Pew Health Professions Commission, 1993; Ridky and Sheldon, 1993). Although Gies pleaded for university officials to upgrade dental schools and argued that lack of educational vision and understanding was a problem among deans (many of whom were expected at the time to continue in private practice), he did not focus on leadership as an issue in its own right.

From its visits to dental schools and other activities, the committee came away with a strong sense that individual leadership from dental school deans was moving some schools down paths not otherwise possible. The characteristics of these individuals could not be studied in any depth, but no single style or personality type appeared to dominate. Important qualities appeared to include an active engagement with—but not simple capitulation to—the university and the external environment; a strong commitment to change tempered by intelligent appreciation of uncertainties and opposing arguments; and an evident dedication to the good of the school and those it serves.

Leadership for change sometimes involves an expectation that a dean appointed to preside over dramatic restructuring will have a limited tenure rather than retiring from the position. Part of the explanation is "burnout," the physical and emotional demands of reconstituting an institution. Another part of the explanation is that those who effect the changes outlined in preceding chapters may create animosities that must be assuaged by a subsequent leader.

Dental educators have leadership roles that stretch well beyond the dental school. These roles include educating university, community, and state leaders about the continued seriousness of oral health problems, the disparities in oral health status, the projected downturn in the dentist-population ratio, and the challenges of oral health research. Dental school leaders can point to improvements in dental school applicants, as well as student and faculty contributions to the community in the form of patient care and other activities, and they can participate in the governance of the larger institution. Such strategies can help attract support from higher levels of the university or academic health center.

Beyond the dental school, the highest levels of the university must also provide leadership that is sensitive to the particular circumstances of dental schools. The position of many U.S. dental schools is aptly summed up by the provost of a major state university in the "challenge of excellence" that he set in 1986 for the institution's dental school: "[The school] faces challenges and pressures today which are unlike any we have seen in recent history. . . . if there was ever a component of the University which had to learn how to respond to a world of change, it is [this school]" (Duderstadt, cited in Wotman, 1989, p. 700).

This provost exercised leadership by backing his challenge with organizational and other resources. These included a "transition team" modeled on others used by the university in similar situations; interim positions for most of the school's administrators; recruitment of new leadership from outside; a more flexible budgeting structure with incentives for income generation by faculty and for early retirement for other faculty; pressure and direction for the reorganization of 18 departments into 6; and redefinition of appointment, promotion, and tenure policies.

In several schools visited by the committee, the academic health center, the university, or a state body had initiated intensive reviews of the dental school. The study's survey of deans showed that more than a third had faced such a review (Table 7.4). The results varied but many included recommendations that the financial position, research productivity, and program quality be improved through changes in leadership, structure, and policies. In some cases, the continued survival of the dental school was made contingent on measurable movement in the recommended directions.

The deans rated their university administration as relatively more supportive than their faculty of changes the deans wanted to undertake (Table 7.5). This is not surprising, given that the burdens of change—reorganization, financial cutbacks, and increased work loads—are likely to be experienced most acutely by faculty.

TABLE 7.4 Number of Dental Schools Subjected to Intensive Review over the Last Five Years

No. of Schools	Category
Excluding reviews related to institutional or programmatic accreditation, has your school been subject to intensive review in the last five years by any of the following? *Check as many categories as apply.*	
40	a. Dental school at own initiative
9	b. Parent academic health center (AHC) administration
18	c. Parent university administration
2	d. AHC governing board
4	e. University governing board
11	f. State legislature

SOURCE: Institute of Medicine and American Association of Dental Schools, 1994.

TABLE 7.5 Deans' Perceived Sources of Support for Changes in Educational Programs

Weighted Rank	Source

How would you rate the following as sources of support for changes you believe need to be undertaken in your educational programs?

1	a.	University administration
6	b.	University governing board
8.5	c.	Academic health centers (AHC) governing board
5	d.	AHC administration
8.5	e.	Accreditation standards
12	f.	Requirements of licensure examinations
2	g.	Clinical faculty
4	h.	Basic science faculty
3	i.	Alumni
11	j.	Organized dentistry
7	k.	Community groups
10	l.	State legislature

SOURCE: Institute of Medicine and American Association of Dental Schools, 1994.

During its site visits and other activities, the committee often heard faculty described as resistant to change. The survey, however, showed that deans nonetheless rated faculty and alumni as more supportive than, for example, state legislators or organized dentistry. The truth may be that faculty, by virtue of their critical numbers and responsibilities, are at once the greatest supporters of and obstacles to change.

SERVICE TO THE UNIVERSITY

Chapter 1 described the service mission of the dental school. Conceived broadly, it includes service to the university as well as service to patients and communities. Service in this sense is a form of leadership exercised in behalf of the university community as a whole by faculty, administrators, and even students of component parts of that community. Participation in university senates, ad hoc committees, and similar activities is sometimes exciting, sometimes tedious but, overall, essential for the governance, vitality, and sense of connection that binds the individual threads of today's complex universities together.

If service to the university benefits the university, it is must also be emphasized that it benefits those who serve. When dental school administrators and faculty participate in university life, they build relationships and respect, develop facility in the peculiar world of academic politics, position themselves to influence decisions, and gain skill in communicating and even translating outside norms to their colleagues within the dental school. Participation in university affairs also offers the chance to learn more about academic management and to pick up ideas from others.

FINDINGS AND RECOMMENDATIONS

Dental schools must remain part of universities. The committee started with this premise, and its investigations into the future of dental education have reinforced it. To fulfill and improve their basic missions of education, research, patient care, and service, dental schools need the intellectual vitality, organizational support, and discipline of universities and academic health centers.

Several factors make dental schools vulnerable as parts of universities. Risk factors include relatively high direct costs for education and patient care, low research and scholarly productivity, academic and professional isolation, uneven student quality, and resistance to change. Uncompetitive patient care programs are becoming a threat.

Universities and academic health centers vary in their involvement in the community, so opportunities for dental schools to support university service in the community or even initiate their own programs will also vary. Two opportunities mentioned elsewhere in this report include patient care (Chapter 6) and educational outreach to minority youth (Chapter 9).

Although education at all levels faces financial constraints ranging in severity from routine to critical, dental education faces particular problems given its relatively high costs, specialized needs, and in many cases, deliberate decisions to reduce enrollments. Although some might like to think that there is some kind of "silver-bullet" solution to financial problems, the committee suggests that this is unrealistic. The easy steps have generally been taken.

Most schools will have to rely on some combination of difficult or tedious actions, including program consolidation, further reductions in operating costs, and persistent efforts to raise funds from alumni, government, industry, and other sources. The committee recognizes the challenges posed to dental schools of designing, implementing, and monitoring financial strategies in ways that minimize harm and provide support to the educational, research, and patient care missions of dental schools.

Each school will need to tailor its own strategy to sustain and improve its position within the university and academic health center. A strategic plan that focuses on both financial and nonfinancial issues is an important starting point.

To consolidate and strengthen the mutual benefits arising from the relationship between universities and dental schools, each dental school should work with its parent institution to

• **prepare an explicit analysis of its position within the university and the academic health center;**

• **evaluate its assets and deficits in key areas including financing, teaching, university service and visibility, research and scholarly productivity, patient and community services, and internal management of change; and**

• **identify specific objectives, actions, procedures, and timetables to sustain its strengths and correct its weaknesses.**

To ensure that dental education and services are considered when academic institutions evaluate their role in a changing health care system, the committee recommends that dental schools coordinate their strategic planning processes with those of their academic health centers and universities.

To provide a sound basis for financial management and policy decisions, each dental school should develop accurate cost and revenue data for its educational, research, and patient care programs.

Because no single financing strategy exists, the committee recommends that dental schools individually and, when appropriate, collectively evaluate and implement a mix of actions to reduce costs and increase revenues. Potential strategies, each of which needs to be guided by solid financial information and projections as well as educational and other considerations, include the following:

• **increasing the productivity, quality, efficiency, and profitability of faculty practice plans, student clinics, and other patient care activities;**

• **pursuing financial support at the federal, state, and local levels for patient-centered predoctoral and postdoctoral dental education, including adequate reimbursement of services for Medicaid and indigent populations and contractual or other arrangements for states without dental schools to** support the education of some of their students in states with dental schools;

• rethinking basic models of dental education and experimenting with less costly alternatives;

• raising tuition for in- or out-of-state students if current tuition and fees are low compared to similar schools;

• developing high quality, competitive research and continuing education programs; and

• consolidating or merging courses, departments, programs, and even entire schools.

SUMMARY

The integration of dental education into the university has been both a major accomplishment and an ongoing challenge. This chapter has identified risk factors that make dental schools vulnerable. Collectively and individually, dental schools should assess their strengths and weaknesses within universities or academic health centers and develop strategic plans to reduce risk factors. They need to see that their contributions to the missions of the university are both real and recognized. This will require leadership from within the dental school, reinforcement from the university, and support from the practitioner community.

8

Dental Schools, the Profession, and the Public

Chapter 7 considers dental schools in their universities and academic health centers. This chapter shifts the view to the profession and the public. It focuses on two issues—institutional accreditation and professional licensure. The next chapter considers a third related topic of public importance, the supply of dental personnel and services.

Accreditation and licensure involve, respectively, private standard-setting activities and government regulations whose primary explicit purpose is to protect the public from poorly trained, incompetent, or unethical dental practitioners. Individually and together, these two processes account for many of the tensions between dental schools and the profession. When dental school deans were asked what recommendations from this committee would have greatest positive impact, changes related to accreditation and licensure headed the list.

Accreditation and licensure are components of a broad social strategy to ensure the quality of dental care. In examining the patient care mission of dental schools, Chapter 6 discussed basic concepts of quality assurance and improvement. Other quality-related mechanisms, for example, risk management strategies required by malpractice insurers, are not considered in this report, nor are a variety of other regulations and quasi-regulatory practices such as those intended to control communicable diseases, protect workers, and inform consumers. These regulations may involve substantial costs for practitioners and schools.

Chapter 2 briefly reviews the historical context of accreditation and licensure, highlighting the controversies that have marked their birth and development. This chapter examines current issues and debates. The background paper by Guarino provides additional information.

ACCREDITATION

The accreditation of U.S. dental educational programs is a private function with a public purpose. As expressed in the mission statement adopted by the Commission on Dental Accreditation in 1989, the purpose of accreditation is "to ensure the quality of dental and dental-related education" (CDA, 1993a). If effective, accreditation

- protects the public welfare by ensuring that dental school graduates are appropriately prepared to provide oral health services;
- ensures students that their educational program meets basic educational standards;
- guards public funds from use in support of inferior programs; and
- assists educational programs in achieving—and improving on—minimum standards.

In theory, accreditation is voluntary. In practice, it has become a virtual requirement for schools because graduation from an accredited school is a prerequisite for dental licensure in most states, although some states have special provisions for licensing those who have graduated from foreign dental schools. The debates about accreditation focus on whether it is effective, whether its benefits outweigh its costs, how its ratio of benefits to costs can be improved, whether it hinders innovation and flexibility, and whether it is unduly dominated by narrow vested interests. These debates take place in the context of larger debates about the proper role of accreditation and the dozens of organizations that accredit various educational institutions and other service organizations such as hospitals and home care agencies (CDA, 1993b; Wolff, 1993; Weiss, 1994). The typical university faces dozens of accrediting organizations. Not only do these accreditation processes impose significant costs, but they may be viewed as a form of self-interested lobbying on behalf of the disciplines in question. Beyond the educational arena, questions about the independence of credentialing organizations and their effectiveness in ensuring quality are a staple of the debate over procedures for ensuring the quality of care in hospitals and other health care organizations (IOM, 1990e).

STRUCTURE AND PROCESS

Organizations

A single organization, the Commission on Dental Accreditation (CDA), is responsible for accrediting dental education programs. Through five committees, it accredits programs in general dentistry education, dental specialty education, and allied dental education. The latter category includes dental hygiene, dental assisting, and dental laboratory technology programs. In addition to predoctoral programs in general dentistry, the CDA examines two advanced education in general dentistry programs and advanced programs in the eight recognized dental specialties. In total, the CDA accredits approximately 1,300 education programs (Table 8.1).

Although autonomous, the commission is an agency of the American Dental Association (ADA), which houses, staffs, and funds it. Its membership breaks down as follows: four members each from the ADA, the American Association of Dental Examiners (AADE), and the American Association of Dental Schools (AADS); two members from the general public; two from recognized dental specialty organizations (as a group); and one member each from the dental student body, the American Dental Hygienists' Association, the American Dental Assistants' Association, and the National Association of Dental Laboratories.

The Commission on Dental Accreditation formulates and revises accreditation standards, establishes procedures for applying those standards, and determines accreditation status for individual pro-

TABLE 8.1 Number of Programs Accredited by Commission on Dental Accreditation

No. of Accredited Programs:

54	Predoctoral dental programs
421	Specialty programs[a]
325	General practice residency/advanced general dentistry programs
233	Dental assisting programs
212	Dental hygiene programs[a]
41	Dental laboratory technology programs
1,286	Total number of programs accredited as of January 1994

[a]Includes accreditation eligible programs.

SOURCE: CDA, 1994a-c.

grams. It appoints consultants to assist with these activities and maintains a formal process for the appeal of its decisions. Accreditation decisions are based on periodic on-site reviews and regularly collected quantitative data that are intended to assess both the educational process and its outcomes (graduate dentists).

The commission and its accrediting programs are recognized by two national organizations, the U.S. Department of Education (USDOE), a government agency, and the Commission on Recognition of Postsecondary Accreditation (CORPA), a newly established private group.

The USDOE recognizes accrediting organizations that meet specified criteria that reflect the interest of Congress in ensuring the quality of educational programs supported by federal funds. One of the government's major concerns has been high default rates on student loans, particularly in some technical and vocational areas.

CORPA was created after its predecessor organization, the Commission of Postsecondary Accreditation, dissolved in 1993. The debate surrounding this event highlighted questions about whether accreditation is a "reliable indicator of an institution's quality or accountability" (Wolff, 1993, p. B1). The new organization, CORPA, has a seven-member governing body. A Committee on Recognition will review accrediting organizations before granting recognition. CORPA has adopted many procedures of its predecessor organization including its provisions for recognition, calendar of recognition, and required interim reports and deferrals. The Commission on Dental Accreditation has accepted the invitation of CORPA to become a member.

Process

Dental accreditation is unlike medical accreditation in two major respects. First, the Commission on Dental Accreditation differs from the Liaison Committee on Medical Education, the comparable body for medical education, in that it accredits postgraduate programs. In medicine, the Accreditation Council for Graduate Medical Education accredits residency training programs using 23 Residency Review Committees for each of the recognized medical specialties.

Second, CDA also accredits programs in dental hygiene, dental assisting, and dental laboratory technology. Programs for some other allied health professions, for example, occupational therapy and physical therapy, are accredited by independent bodies. Until July 1994, the Committee on Allied Health Education and Accreditation, an umbrella organization, accredited programs in 25 fields (e.g., medical laboratory technology and medical record administration). A successor organization, the Commission for the Accreditation of Allied Health Education Programs, is expected to include 40 organizations and 17 of its predecessor's accreditation review committees.

The process of dental accreditation is complex and time consuming, designed to involve all major parties. In overview, the major steps for the accreditation of D.D.S. or D.M.D. programs include the following:

- Development of standards
  Selection of expert panels (and consultants)
  Development of draft standards
  Review by interested parties followed by revisions
  Open hearing followed by revisions
  Preliminary publication for comment followed by revisions
  Approval by entire commission
  Publication and distribution
  Effective date
  Updating as indicated

- Cyclic accreditation of each school (every seven years)*
  Self-study (initiated one year prior to site visit)
  Site visit
  Preliminary decision and report
  Review by site visit team and revisions
  Review by school and response
  Consideration of responses and any changes in school
  Hearing and appeal processes
  Final decision

- Monitoring
  Annual survey of all schools
  Reports, revisits, and reevaluation of conditionally or
    provisionally approved schools

As of May 1993, the CDA specified 250 standards (or "must" statements) for dental schools in eight broad areas: administration, financial resources and facilities, faculty and staff, students, curriculum, patient care and clinic management, research, and outcomes. The curriculum area is the most extensive. The stan-

---

*Every five years for programs in oral and maxillofacial surgery.

dards and their accompanying discussion (which includes many "should" statements that do not constitute standards) vary greatly in specificity (CDA, 1993a). In addition to the commission's 27-page listing of accreditation standards, the self-study manual and other supporting material provide further detailed descriptions of the documentation that is needed to demonstrate compliance with the standards.

Given the breadth of the commission's responsibilities for dental school accreditation, it is not surprising that the typical site visit involves a large team of visitors. In contrast to the usual four-person survey team for medical accreditation, the average survey team for a dental school has fifteen members including five consultants for the predoctoral program and one consultant for each advanced education or allied education program. The AADS estimates that accreditation costs an individual school from more than $200,000 to more than $300,000 including the self-study, site visit, and response (AADS, 1993c). Most of the cost involves faculty time.

ACCREDITATION DECISIONS

The Commission on Dental Accreditation has established three categories of accreditation results: approval, conditional approval, and provisional approval. The first category applies to programs judged to have achieved or to have exceeded published requirements, and it implies that a program has no serious deficiencies or weaknesses. Conditional approval applies to programs that have identified deficiencies or weaknesses that are considered correctable within a set period of time. This category allows an institution's graduates to meet requirements associated with state licensure and board certification. Provisional accreditation likewise allows an institution to meet these requirements, but it indicates that a program has a number of serious deficiencies and that significant improvement in the program must occur within one year.

In 1994, fifty-three programs were fully approved, and one was provisionally accredited (CDA, 1994a). The commission makes public an institution's overall accreditation status. Confidentiality is, however, maintained for most information including the self-study documents, site visit reports, institutional responses to site visits, progress reports, surveys, exit interviews, on-site communications, and proceedings of meetings.

ISSUES AND DEBATES

The criticisms of dental school accreditation are both substantive and procedural (see, for example, AADS, 1993c; Hutchison, 1993; Pew Health Professions Commission, 1993; ten Pas, 1993). In the committee's survey, a majority of dental school deans expressed concern that government regulatory agencies or other outside forces were influencing the accreditation process or affecting the independence of the CDA. In addition, 14 disagreed and 12 were neutral on the statement that the current process helps ensure entry-level competency. Ten deans did not agree that candidates for state licensure should be graduates of accredited programs.

Accreditation has been such a significant concern to dental educators that the AADS has planned a major study of accreditation (House of Delegates Resolution 24-93-H). Nonetheless, as critical as dental educators have been of aspects of the accreditation process, it is important to note that the AADS itself has conceded that "if one were to start over to design an accrediting body for dental education, . . . the basic features of that accrediting body . . . might not be all that dissimilar from what exists currently" (AADS, 1993c, p. 27). Even a purely internal program of quality assurance and improvement would make many similar demands on schools for information, analysis, and faculty participation.

The Commission on Dental Accreditation has, in recent years, made numerous changes in its processes and standards. It has, for example, shifted the accreditation cycle from ten to seven years. The organization has been recognized for its efforts by USDOE, particularly in the area of calibrating its processes, committees, and consultants.

Effectiveness and Quality

A major issue in the debate about accreditation is the lack of evidence that it is effective in identifying substandard schools or improving educational quality and, concomitantly, that it protects students from deficient education or the public from deficient dental care. The problem of evidence has at least two parts: (1) linking educational programs to outcomes, in particular, competency of graduates, and (2) identifying educational processes, methods, or structures (e.g., faculty organization, data systems, accounting procedures) that are desirable in and of themselves.

The high rates of failure on regional examinations, cited below in the discussion of licensure, are invoked in critiques of the accreditation process as well as in critiques of the dental schools themselves. The argument is that if accreditation were ensuring a basic level of quality overall, failure rates should be lower in general and no school should see half or more of its licensure applicants failing regional clinical examinations. This argument assumes the validity and reliability of the licensure examinations, which are questioned later in this chapter.

Of the 54 dental schools, 53 are accredited without qualification. As noted earlier, detailed accreditation results are not published. Committee members—based on their own involvement in the process—seconded complaints made during site visits and other meetings that substandard programs were allowed to continue despite identified (but not public) deficiencies that are both serious and persistent. The CDA does not encourage closure of schools that do not improve, arguing that such a strategy would be "contrary to the spirit of accreditation" (CDA, 1993b, p. 5). This position is consistent with the commission's mission statement and with the models of continuous quality improvement now widely endorsed (if not successfully applied) in U.S. industry and health care. Such a position is, arguably, inconsistent with enforcing a minimum standard of quality to protect students and the public generally, a process that may require more decisive action for institutions with persistent problems.

Cost and Benefit

Overall, critics of the current accreditation process argue that its costs in time, money, and aggravation are excessive for its positive results. The aggravation factor is highlighted colorfully in the remark that "we will not make it into the 21st Century without killing each other off unless . . . we find the correct manner to relook at accreditation" (Formicola, 1993, p. 214). The cost of the process is indicated by an estimate from the dental school of the University of Maryland that the direct and indirect costs of its 1981 site visit exceeded $200,000 (Linthicum and Moreland, 1981).

The Commission on Dental Accreditation recognizes that the accreditation process makes heavy demands on institutions, and this committee commends its efforts to streamline the process and reduce its costs. The organization hopes to increase the use of electronic data transfer to collect information more quickly and inexpensively. The commission also is helping to develop materials that individual schools can use in assessing student competency and outcomes.

Innovation and Flexibility

Dental accreditation has been criticized for being inflexible, overly prescriptive, insufficiently independent of dental society leadership, and too focused on process and structure. It is said, thus, to stifle innovation. Further, the current system is criticized as being too little concerned with outcomes. It places excessive burdens on satisfactory schools while inadequately protecting students and the public from unsatisfactory programs. Even if accreditation results were valid, the confidentiality of accreditation results for specific dental schools raises questions about how well the process can protect students and the public.

In response to the argument that accreditation standards and processes are inflexible and stifle innovation, the Commission on Dental Accreditation argues that its standards are designed to allow for considerable flexibility. Its work to devise outcome assessments reflects its interest in methods for better evaluating innovative as well as traditional educational programs. Dental schools have, in fact, initiated a number of innovative programs over the years independently and with the assistance of organizations such as the Pew Foundation (Barker and O'Neil, 1989, 1992). The committee heard, however, that some of the schools had faced opposition from accreditors that had created time-consuming and stressful delays in implementing program innovations. For example, efforts to give students some leeway from the traditional "lockstep" curriculum by instituting special focus tracks encountered concerns that the tracks amounted to early specialization, which is restricted under current standards stating that "specialization must not be permitted until the student has achieved a standard of minimal clinical competency in all areas necessary to the practice of general dentistry."

Governance and Representation

Accreditation is, like various other professional standard-setting processes, sometimes criticized as a self-serving mechanism for professional control and protection from competition. For example, a recent suit against the accrediting activities of the American Bar Association (ABA) charged that the ABA process imposed "costly and unnecessary standards that protect the financial interests of professors, law librarians and standardized-test services" (Slade, 1994, p. A19). That the Commission on Dental Accreditation operates under the auspices of the ADA raises questions about its autonomy in an area characterized by considerable tension between elements of organized dentistry and dental schools.

The issue of independence is also an acute concern for allied dental personnel. The argument can be made that accreditation by an organization dominated by dentists protects dentists as much as it ensures the appropriate education of allied personnel. Allied dental groups and those involved with dental specialties also question their representation and influence in the process of accrediting allied and specialty programs. The committee heard oral and written testimony citing the lack of a separate, impartial, arm's-length accreditation commission. Only one hygienist sits on the Commission on Dental Accreditation, most of whose other members are dentists. The CDA committee that is responsible in the first instance for drafting accreditation standards for dental hygiene programs currently includes four hygienists, one public member, and three dentists (a dentist is always the chair). Site visit teams for dental hygiene programs generally have a majority of hygienists. Previous reviews of standards for dental hygiene did not address the changes requested by dental hygiene professionals, for example, required coursework in gerontology (ADHA, 1993).

LICENSURE

Licensure provides dentists and dental hygienists with legal authority to practice. Initial licensure involves an extensive set of requirements including written and clinical examinations. Continued licensure is largely a matter of filing forms and paying fees, although most states also require documentation of attendance at continuing education courses. Continued competency is not routinely assessed, but egregious errors or misconduct can bring discipline from state licensing bodies.

Dental licensure is distinctive in two respects. First, the requirement for a state or regional clinical examination distinguishes dentistry and dental hygiene from most other health professions. Physicians, for example, take national written examinations but face no clinical examination at either the national or the state level. In medicine, the last clinical examination element—suturing pig carcasses—was dropped 30 years ago (Foti, 1992). Some nonhealth professionals, for example, lawyers and engineers, may face special state or local examinations related to particular state laws or to geophysical conditions (e.g., earthquake zones).

Second, dental licensure is distinctive in requiring clinical examinations that use live patients who may be subjected to irreversible treatments. Some medical specialty organizations, in their certification examinations, use individuals trained to simulate patient problems. Candidates are evaluated on their interviewing, diagnosis, and treatment planning skills, but they do not actually treat these "patients." In optometry, the National Board of Examiners in Optometry (NBEO) began in 1989 to administer a "live performance examination," which is now accepted by 24 states (NBEO, 1993). (Many state optometry boards continue to administer their own clinical examinations.) The NBEO examination involves no therapeutic or irreversible interventions and appears to subject patients to very minor risks from the diagnostic procedures. The board recruits the patients for the examinations, which are held in a small number of cities. In addition, some states require allied professionals in audiology and related fields to demonstrate skills using live patients, but no therapeutic or irreversible procedures are required (S. Larson, American Speech Language Hearing Association, personal communication, July 1994).

STRUCTURE AND PROCESS

General Licensure

In the United States, licensure is a state responsibility, generally one that is delegated to an appointed board supported by a staff of government employees. Boards vary in the extent to which they include other oral health professionals. Some include representatives of the general public. The National Practitioner Data Bank and the American Association of Dental Examiners collect information on disciplinary actions against dentists taken by state boards, hospitals, or professional organizations.

For a dentist, initial licensure in a state typically requires the following: (1) graduation from an accredited U.S. dental school; (2) successful completion of a two-part national written examination; (3) successful completion of written and clinical examinations administered by the state or other designated organization (e.g., a regional board); and (4) a "jurisprudence" examination to check familiarity with specific state practice law. Other requirements (e.g., criminal background checks) may also be imposed.

All states accept the national written examination conducted by the Joint Commission on National Dental Examinations, which operates under the auspices of the ADA. This examination consists of two parts: Part I tests knowledge of the basic biomedical sciences; Part II tests knowledge of dental sciences. To take Part II, a candidate must have passed the first part of the examination.

Twelve states require their own clinical examinations. The other 38 states and the District of Columbia accept the results of one or more of four regional examination boards. The regional boards and the states that recognize their examinations are listed in Table 8.2.

TABLE 8.2 States Participating in Regional Dental Testing Agencies, January 1994

Central Regional Dental Testing Service

Colorado	Nebraska
Illinois	North Dakota
Iowa	South Dakota
Kansas	Wisconsin
Minnesota	Wyoming
Missouri	

Northeast Regional Board of Dental Examiners

Connecticut	New Jersey
District of Columbia	New York
Illinois	Ohio
Maine	Pennsylvania
Maryland	Rhode Island
Massachusetts	Vermont
Michigan	West Virginia
New Hampshire	

Southern Regional Testing Agency

Arkansas	Kentucky
Georgia	Tennessee
Illinois	Virginia

Western Regional Examining Board

Alaska	Oklahoma
Arizona	Oregon
Idaho	Texas
Montana	Utah
New Mexico	

Nonparticipating States (administer their own examinations)

Alabama	Louisiana
California	Mississippi
Delaware	Nevada
Florida	North Carolina
Hawaii	South Carolina
Indiana	Washington

NOTE: Under certain conditions, states (e.g., Illinois) may accept examination results from more than one regional organization.

SOURCE: American Dental Association, 1994d.

Once an individual is licensed in a single state, the procedures for obtaining a license in other states vary considerably (USDHHS, OIG, 1993). More than half the states permit credentialing under some circumstances; that is, they allow individuals currently licensed in another state to become licensed without a new state or regional clinical examination. These states may, however, require that a previous written or clinical examination be taken within the preceding five years and that the candidate have been in active practice for a specific period prior to applying for credentials. The credentialing process may also include interviews, background checks, evidence of continuing education, letters of reference, reviews of patient case reports, and other requirements. Some state boards have never exercised their credentialing authority. A few states require "reciprocity," that is, they accept credentials only from states that do likewise (AADE, 1992).

In an effort to promote agreement on licensing requirements for out-of-state dentists, the ADA and AADE convened a national conference in 1992. One result was a paper on guidelines for valid and reliable examinations (ADA and AADE, 1992). These guidelines set forth a conceptual and methodological framework for analysis and included data from the ADA's 1990 Survey of Dental Services, a 1990 examination of the clinical content of licensure examinations, and special surveys of dental schools and testing agencies. The recommendations from this conference have influenced the efforts of two of the four regional licensing boards to develop a common clinical examination (AADE, 1993b). In addition, the ADA issued a general set of guidelines for credentialing requirements (ADA, 1992a).

Specialty Licensure

Although all states license general dentists, only 16 license specialists (ADA, 1993d; see background paper by Guarino).[1] Most of these 16 states administer their own specialty examination, and all require specialists to have a general dentistry license as

---

[1]The ADA Principles of Ethics and Code of Professional Conduct state that dentists "who choose to announce specialization should . . . and shall limit their practice exclusively to the announced special area(s) of dental practice." Specialty groups argue that they violate their ethics in practicing general dentistry on a real patient during a legally required but otherwise irrelevant and unnecessary clinical licensing examination.

well. States that license by credentials may accept general or specialty licenses from other states. States that do not have specialty examinations or licensure by credentials require specialists coming from other states to pass their general clinical licensure examination. Practicing specialists who pass a general dentistry examination are subsequently precluded by law from practicing general dentistry.[2]

In addition, eight specialty areas recognized by the ADA have formal, voluntary certification processes. (As described earlier, the Commission on Dental Accreditation oversees accreditation of advanced specialty education programs.) The recognized specialties are dental public health, endodontics, oral and maxillofacial surgery, oral pathology, orthodontics, pediatric dentistry, periodontics, and prosthodontics. The ADA has established rules and monitoring procedures for the recognition of specialties and for the certifying boards associated with them. Certification generally requires graduation from an accredited program of advanced specialty education, a specified number of years of practice experience in the specialty area, and passage of an examination, which may include an oral examination and a clinical component.

ISSUES AND DEBATES

With few exceptions, even strong critics of current policies for dental licensure recognize a legitimate public interest in having a formal process for granting people the right to practice dentistry based on some evidence of competency. Where defenders and critics divide is on what constitutes evidence of competency, who should judge it, how often it should be demonstrated, and whether live patients should be used in examinations (see, for example, Friedland and Valachovic, 1991; ADA, 1992c; AADS, 1993c; ADA, 1993c; Dugoni, 1993; Gaines, 1993; Hutchison, 1993; USDHHS, OIG, 1993; and the background paper by Guarino). Other disagreements focus on the effects licensure has on the educational process, the mobility of practitioners, and the geographical availability of services.

In addition to the criticisms discussed further below, specialty organizations also criticize requirements that specialists obtain

---

[2]By way of comparison, states, with few exceptions, do not license or certify medical specialists (Stromberg, 1992).

general dentistry licenses even when they do not plan to practice general dentistry and are, in fact, legally precluded from doing so. For example, the committee heard testimony that "it is senseless to require a . . . specialist to perform dental procedures on a licensing examination which he or she has not done in the past twenty years and has no intention of doing so in the future" (AAO, 1993, p. 25). In the same vein, "how is the public interest protected when a specialist is examined in an area of care he/she will not practice" (AAOMS, 1993).

Evidence of Competency

On the issue of what constitutes public evidence of competency, the major dividing line is between those who believe that a freestanding clinical examination is necessary and those who believe that competency is adequately demonstrated by a combination of dental school graduation, passage of national written examinations, and completion of a year in a certified residency program (AMA, 1994). This latter approach is termed the medical model, although some details vary from state to state. The content of the national written examinations is the subject of ongoing discussion and critique, but few seriously challenge the continued use of these tests for dental licensure.

Those who support a separate clinical examination in dentistry typically argue that, at a minimum, (1) a dental school diploma is no guarantee of competency; (2) a written examination is an insufficient measure of competency; (3) residency programs are too variable for residency experience to serve as an adequate measure of competency; and (4) public safeguards in medicine, such as hospital procedures for granting practice privileges and hospital peer review, are less generally applicable to dentists. To the committee, supporters of the clinical examination also cited legal and financial pressures on dental schools that might compromise their ability to ensure the competency of their graduates. As evidence of problems, they cite the initial failure rates on regional board examinations displayed in Figure 8.1 for the 1993 Northeast Regional Examination Board (NERB) examinations.

In addition, in testimony to this committee the Central Regional Dental Testing Service (CRDTS) expressed concern that the limited clinical experience of dental students was showing up in their examinations as poor test results. CRDTS also pointed to poor results in the discipline of periodontics and urged better faculty training in assessment methodologies.

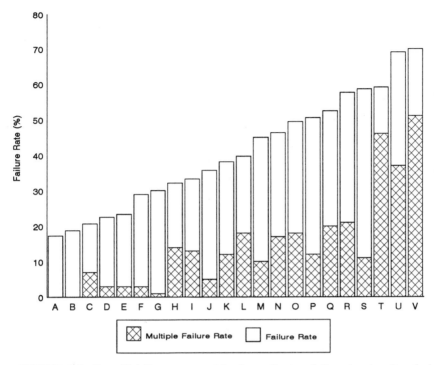

FIGURE 8.1 Overall failure rate on Northeast Regional Examination Boards by school. SOURCE: Northeast Regional Board of Dental Examiners, Inc., 1993.

In contrast, critics of current licensure arrangements argue that the clinical licensure examination is itself a flawed measure of competency. The examination (1) is intrinsically too narrow in scope to constitute a valid assessment of an applicant's ability to provide comprehensive patient care proficiently; (2) subjects applicants to capricious or at least highly subjective and unreliable evaluations despite procedures to calibrate the evaluations of individual examiners; and (3) varies in content across states and regions in ways that cannot be justified by documented regional differences in patient needs or effective practice. A uniform national examination (discussed further below) would answer the third criticism but would not by itself overcome other criticisms. As long as live patients are used in an examination, variations in the testing "material" will make it particularly difficult to standardize and monitor assessments.

To critics, the inadequacy of the clinical examination—not the schools—is revealed every year in the variable failure rates from region to region and state to state. To Damiano et al. (1992, p. 72), this variability suggests that "factors other than the ability of the candidates influence exam outcomes." Deans and faculty complain that "extremely competent applicants frequently" fail initial clinical examinations (Hutchison, 1993). The fact that most of those who fail eventually pass, without any required remedial work, reinforces concerns about the inadequacies of the examinations. Other criticisms, as described below, focus not on the validity of the clinical examination but on ethical shortcomings in using live patients.

Although state, regional, and national examining organizations have made efforts to improve the validity and reliability of examinations, fundamental problems remain. Too little is known about the outcomes of dental practice and variations in that practice. As in medicine and other health professions, this knowledge gap raises questions about the content of professional education and performance assessments of all kinds.

Locus of Responsibility

Those who reject the medical model for licensure may still differ on the question of who should judge competency. One subgroup argues that a state-level judgment of clinical competency is required. The other supports a uniform regional if not national clinical examination and generally supports a credentialing process for licensed dentists who move to a new state.

As heard by this committee, the stated "public interest" arguments for a state-level examination are that (1) regional examinations as designed, as administered, or both cannot be trusted as a measure of competency; (2) the National Practitioner Data Bank, other clearinghouses, and dental boards in other states cannot be trusted to identify incompetent practitioners; and (3) special state circumstances require state-specific measures of competency. On occasion, the committee heard that some state examiners have a stake in working closely and cooperatively with dental schools in the state to ensure that students are prepared to pass the examination.

The committee also heard more dubious arguments for state clinical examinations. One is that "we've always done it this way, and it is too much trouble to ask state boards to give up this power." The other is that "we will be overrun by out-of-state dentists attracted by our lifestyle or economy." The latter argument is rarely stated officially for legal reasons. The case law on licensure recognizes protection of the public as a rationale for regulation but rejects protection from competition as a basis for policy (Stromberg, 1992; see background paper by Guarino, 1994). Nonetheless, it is telling that requirements for state clinical examinations are concentrated in southern and western states such as Florida and California that have mild climates and fast-growing populations.

Live Patient Examination

Many critics of the clinical examination focus their harshest criticism on the continued use of live patients. These criticisms cite such problems as (1) inappropriate delays in treatment because patient problems are "saved" for the examination rather than treated promptly; (2) unnecessary or duplicative X rays and other evaluative procedures; (3) incomplete and otherwise inappropriate patient care that violates the normal expectation of competent, comprehensive, and continuous care, especially when patients undergo irreversible procedures or must return after the procedure to another state; and (4) recruitment under questionable circumstances (e.g., for money, without true informed consent). Further, in exposing patients to such risks or harms, the clinical examination inevitably involves applicants and examiners in unethical practices. It also subjects participants, including sponsors, evaluators, and applicants, to unacceptable legal risks. These problems are intensified when patients are recruited for examinations that require travel to a distant site, a frequent situation for dentists seeking licensure in a new state.

State and regional examiners have been moving to limit their use of live patients in the clinical examination. Still, many defend the practice on grounds that typodonts or manikins do not adequately represent "real-world circumstances" either physiologically or behaviorally. Indeed, concern about the sterility and artificiality of written examinations has led medical specialty groups to consider how "standardized patients" (often actors) might be used to assess diagnosis and treatment planning skills for purposes of specialty certification. Although no changes have occurred in the examinations required for initial medical licensure in the United States, an "objective structured clinical examination" using standardized patients has been tested in Canada for possible inclusion in national licensure requirements. The rationale is that it is important to evaluate "behavioral performance . . . by observing 'what is being done' rather than finding out if the practitioner 'knows how to do it'" (Martini, 1988, p. 1057).

Educational Process

Clinical licensing examinations (both regional and state) are said to undermine dental education by distorting the curriculum, stifling innovation, and complicating faculty recruitment. Schools understandably want their students to pass the examinations; thus, to varying degrees, faculty "teach to the examination." One result is that procedures that are covered on the examination may receive more attention than warranted by their relevance to current patient needs and may thereby divert time from other, more relevant topics. To the extent that a school feels that it must prepare students for more than one examination, the problem is multiplied.

The committee often heard that clinical examinations still focus too much on prosthetic exercises that very few dentists currently perform themselves. The schools must devote extra curriculum time to procedures that could otherwise be allocated for new or more common services. Until and unless each state or regional clinical examination is revised to reflect new and more effective technologies, schools may make uncomfortable compromises in the curriculum. For example, the gold-foil procedure (a kind of restoration) was long criticized as an "out-of-date" requirement. This procedure has finally been eliminated entirely or made optional in state and regional examinations, but only after years of lobbying—and largely wasted curriculum time.

Faculty recruitment may also be complicated by state licensure requirements. In a case discussed during a visit to one university, an oral surgeon recruited from another region failed to pass the general dentistry clinical examination administered by the state board. Once he finally passed the exam, he was then barred from practicing general dentistry because he was a specialist. The clinical examination requirement in such cases appears both burdensome and irrelevant to the public interest.

Those who defend the clinical examination typically argue that critics overstate their case and that little would change in the curriculum if the clinical examination were eliminated. That is, teaching to the exam probably enters into the rigidity of curriculum as only one factor among many, including accreditation, faculty self-interest, alumni pressure, and the financial cost of change. To the extent that the examinations are off-target, educators and examiners could work together to improve them.

Continued Competency

Although most states have requirements for continuing education, none, according to the U.S. Department of Health and Human Services, Office of Inspector General (1993, p. 9), requires "any assessment of what a dentist actually learned from a course." Some states examine competency of licensed, out-of-state dentists on a one-time basis by requiring them to be reexamined through a state clinical examination or requiring reexamination if a past examination dates back more than five years. None of these states, however, requires periodic reexamination for in-state dentists.

Those who favor periodic assessment of competency argue that state boards do not satisfactorily monitor continued competency and that required continuing education is inadequate because courses are too variable in content and impact. (Issues related to continuing education are discussed in Chapter 4.) Within dentistry, the American Association of Oral and Maxillofacial Surgery has adopted a recertification process that is scheduled to begin in 1998 (AAOMS, 1993).

In the future, periodic reviews of competency may become increasingly feasible and acceptable with the growth of sophisticated electronic communication and computer-based patient records. Such assessments would have to be relatively unobtrusive and inexpensive as well as valid. (See discussion of the Dental Interactive Simulations Corporation below.) To the extent that assessments are designed to help improve performance rather than punish poor practice, they are more likely to be welcomed.

Dentist Mobility and Access to Care

Clearly, dentists in many parts of the United States view clinical examination requirements for out-of-state dentists as a barrier to mobility. Some also cite the potential adverse effect on access to care (Pew Health Professions Commission, 1993). The Inspector General of the U.S. Department of Health and Human Services reported instances in which state licensure requirements discouraged National Health Service Corps dentists from staying in underserved areas (USDHHS, OIG, 1993). However, the Inspector General's 1993 report stated that "we found no data, nor any studies, to indicate that licensure-by-credentials policies have much overall bearing on the access to dental services in underserved areas" (p. 10). Other factors such as isolation, family preferences, and earnings potential appear more significant.

Issues in the Licensure of Dental Hygienists

Most of the issues raised above also are raised with respect to hygienists. Dental hygienists too are concerned about the variability of state licensure requirements, reliability and validity problems with clinical examinations, and the appropriateness of using live patients during examinations. In addition, the scope of practice permitted under state laws has provoked considerable controversy among hygienists. Most of the controversy focuses on provisions regarding supervision. A sizable minority of states requires that dentists directly supervise certain hygienists' services (i.e., they must be physically present). This limits the opportunity for hygienists to provide routine hygiene services in nonoffice settings such as nursing homes. At least nine states forbid the employment of more than two hygienists in a dental office (ADHA, 1993). A 1993 analysis by the staff of the Federal Trade Commission suggested that such restrictions should be examined for their anticompetitive effects (Wise, 1993).

In principle, training, competency, and patient or societal needs should inform practice acts; in actuality, they are heavily shaped by economic interests of the dominant professional groups. Critics of licensing policies for dental hygiene note that the majority of state boards members are dentists (IOM, 1989a). On a few state licensing boards, the dental hygiene member or members may vote only on matters relating to hygiene, whereas the public or consumer member has full voting privileges (ADHA, 1994).

OPTIONS

In the course of its study, the committee identified three options for improving the current process of entry-level dental licensure. They were to (1) continue the current system with incremental steps to remedy deficiencies; (2) intensify efforts currently under way to move toward a uniform national clinical examination accepted by all states and away from unreasonable restrictions on professional mobility; or (3) adopt the medical model and eliminate the state or regional clinical examination.

The line between incremental and major changes is not precise. For purposes of this discussion, incremental change focuses primarily on continued efforts to improve the validity, reliability, and relevance of competency assessments for a variety of educational, quality improvement, and other purposes. To call these efforts incremental is not to imply that they are unimportant.

Major change would involve at least two additional steps. First, the use of live patients would be reduced and eventually eliminated. Second, a uniform clinical examination would be accepted by all state licensing authorities.[3] This step would be an extension of those that led to the regional examination organizations.

One initiative that would support both incremental and major change is a technology-oriented effort to improve competency assessments organized by the Dental Interactive Simulations Corporation or DISC (Foti, 1992). The product of the effort is also called DISC. Members of the nonprofit corporation include the AADE, AADS, ADA, CRDTS, NERB, Southern Regional Testing Association, and Western Regional Examination Board. Notable for their absence are the state boards of California, Florida, and North Carolina, which do not participate in regional examination boards.

DISC proposes a "computer software program that uses high-quality images and video to represent real patients . . . [with extensive] intraoral images . . . [and links] to a knowledge base that would support instant [information] retrieval, cross-referencing, glossaries, images, animations, and motion video features" (Foti, 1992, p. 5). The simulated patients could be "questioned," "treatments" could be ordered, and consequences evaluated. All candidates being assessed would be evaluated on their handling of the same case. Patient variability would not complicate examination findings, although reliable evaluation of results would still be an issue. The difficult search for complex or special patients as test subjects would be avoided.[4]

If the technology and processes on which these and other initiatives are based prove valid, reliable, and acceptable to both

---

[3]Although the committee did not consider specific procedures, the uniform clinical examination can be viewed as somewhat similar to the third step of the U.S. Medical Licensing Examination. The first two steps are administered nationally, but the third step is to be administered by individual state licensing authorities. "Step 3 will assess whether an examinee possesses the medical knowledge and understanding of biomedical and clinical science considered essential for the unsupervised practice of medicine" (AMA, 1994). States can require a postgraduate training year as an eligibility requirement for the third step.

[4]At this time, this $11 million-plus project is in its early stages and needs substantial additional funding for developmental work. A comparable project in medicine, which is sponsored by the National Board of Medical Examiners, has proceeded much further with the aid of a $4 million grant from the W.K. Kellogg Foundation.

regulators and educators, it is likely that dental schools will be employing much the same technology and procedures to evaluate student competency during the course of their predoctoral education. This should narrow the gulf between examiners and educators and should facilitate movement toward the medical model, perhaps in a form that brings examiners into the schools.

Those who would eliminate clinical exams and adopt the medical model were supported by the Pew Health Professions Commission, which recommended that "graduates should be granted entry-level licensure based upon graduation from an accredited dental school, successful completion of the national board examinations, and completion of a postdoctoral training program" (Pew Health Professions Commission, 1993, p. 54). That commission also endorsed relicensure and recertification based on continued competency.

The options for relicensure involve two distinct issues (1) the treatment of dentists relocating from one state to another and (2) the assessment of continued competency for all practitioners. For relocating dentists, the options are essentially to continue the current system or to persuade all states to adopt some form of credentialing including background checks and similar requirements but not a repeated clinical examination. For all dentists, the options are, again, to continue the present system or to move toward some periodic reassessment of competency as some specialty groups are doing.

FINDINGS AND RECOMMENDATIONS

ACCREDITATION

Although the current process for accrediting dental education programs has many positive features, it is in need of significant revision. The accreditation process is too expensive, too focused on procedural details, and too inhospitable to educational innovation. Although the specifics of accreditation assessment are not made public, the committee believes that the process tolerates some inferior educational programs. The standards may be too low or their application may be too permissive or both.

Accreditation reform should focus on standards and methods (1) that will identify and improve those schools that are not educating their students effectively or ethically and (2) that will not allow persistently poor performance. At the same time, excessively detailed assessments of structures and processes should be trimmed.

Improvements in methods of assessing educational outcomes are as central to accreditation reforms as they are to improvements in predoctoral education, entry-level licensure, and assessment of continued competency. Thus, cooperation and coordination among responsible organizations in each of these arenas should be established to avoid conflicting strategies and costly duplication of effort. Improvements in the processes for collecting information—particularly those based on electronic transfer of data—likewise will produce multiple benefits and should be coordinated.

The committee understood and sympathized with concerns expressed about self-regulation, but it believed that the major alternative—a federal accreditation process—would not, on balance, solve (and, in fact, might worsen) most current problems including costliness, inflexibility, and questionable effectiveness. The committee, however, does believe it prudent that dental accreditors and educators be prepared to respond constructively to reasonable demands for increased public accountability and information. The committee supported the goal of better information for the public, but members were split about recommending extensive disclosure of accreditation results. Most believed that the current process needed improvement first. Some believed that disclosure would promote defensiveness and work against cooperative and candid analyses of educational deficits and strategies for correcting them.

The committee agreed that after steps are taken to improve the validity and reliability of licensure and accreditation processes, the AADS, AADE, and CDA should investigate the relationships among accreditation results, school-wide pass rates on national written examinations and on regional or state clinical licensure examinations, student grades, and graduates' subsequent performance in practice. They should then review current policies limiting public disclosure of institution-level information about student performance on licensure examinations and should study the advantages and disadvantages of making more accreditation information public.

To protect students and the public from inferior educational programs and to reduce administrative burdens and costs, the committee recommends that the Commission on Dental Accreditation involve concerned constituencies in a sustained effort to:

• expand the resources and assistance devoted to schools with significant deficiencies, and decrease the burden imposed on schools that meet or exceed standards;

• increase the emphasis on educational outcomes rather than on detailed procedural requirements; and

• develop more valid and consistent methods for assessing clinical performance for purposes of student evaluation, licensure, and accreditation.

LICENSURE

The dental community has begun important steps to improve the validity, reliability, relevance, and fairness of competency assessments for dental professionals. Many of the deficiencies or uncertainties that characterize licensure processes also characterize evaluations within dental schools and health care organizations. Further improvements in assessment methodologies will benefit both dental education and practice. One major problem in assessing current licensure processes is the lack of research on their effectiveness in protecting patients from inept practitioners.

Although states can be criticized for occasional parochialism and inefficiency, they are a reasonable locus of responsibility for professional regulation. The relevant task is not to construct a new national licensure system but rather to minimize deficiencies in the present system and to involve all major parties in the process of change.

In the view of this committee, the most important deficiencies are concentrated in a few areas: the use of live patients in clinical licensure examinations; variations in the content and relevance of clinical examinations; unreasonable barriers to movement of dentists and dental hygienists across state lines; inadequate means of assessing competency after initial licensure; and practice acts that unreasonably restrict the use of appropriately trained allied dental personnel. In addressing these problems, the committee suggests that a task force of the relevant organizations of dental examiners, educators, consumers, and others should be created to devise demonstration projects to test alternative regulatory policies and mechanisms. Possible anticompetitive features of current statutes and regulations should also be examined carefully.

To improve the current system of state regulation of dental professionals, the committee recommends that the American Association of Dental Examiners, American Association of Dental Schools, professional associations, and state and regional boards work closely and intensively to

• develop valid, reliable, and uniform clinical examinations and secure acceptance of the examinations by all state

licensing boards as replacements for state or regional clinical examinations and as complements to current National Dental Board Examinations;

• accelerate steps to eliminate examinations using live patients and replace them with other assessment methods, such as the use of "standardized patients" for evaluating diagnosis and treatment planning skills and simulations for evaluating technical proficiency;

• strengthen and extend efforts by state boards and specialty organizations to maintain and periodically evaluate the competency of dentists and dental hygienists through recertification and other methods;

• remove barriers to the movement of dental personnel among states by developing uniform criteria for state licensure except in areas where variation is legitimate (e.g., dental jurisprudence); and

• eliminate statutes and regulations that restrict dentists from working with allied dental personnel in ways that are productive and consistent with their education and training.

SUMMARY

Debates about accreditation and licensure are among the most divisive in dentistry. Greater agreement on reliable and valid methods for assessing clinical competency in all settings would reduce tensions as would greater agreement on the clinical skills that need assessment. Both would pave the way for state acceptance of uniform clinical examinations and for less procedurally oriented accreditation standards.

9

A Dental Work Force for the Future

What characteristics should the dental work force of the twenty-first century have? Do we now have or are we facing an oversupply or undersupply of dental personnel and services? Anxiety about these issues played a major role in the birth of this study, and the "supply question," as the committee came to call it, was a continuing theme in the public hearing, site visits, and other committee activities. As examined in this chapter, the supply question has several elements. How many dentists and allied dental professionals does the country now have, and what numbers are projected for the future? What will the demand and need for dental services be in the future, and how certain are the answers? Are the composition and distribution of the dental work force satisfactory? Should enrollments in dental schools be increased, decreased, or held steady? The last question was a particular concern of community practitioners and dental society leaders, who referred often to a perceived "busyness" problem (more accurately, the lack of busyness) that resulted from the training of too many dentists after dental schools increased enrollments during the 1970s.

This chapter reviews work force trends and projections for dental practitioners and examines the strengths and limitations of models for work force forecasting. It assesses prospects for an over- or undersupply of dental services and personnel and makes recommendations about work force policies. The chapter is premised on the principle stated in Chapter 1 that *a qualified dental work force is a valuable national resource.* Its future is too important to be determined solely by the isolated decisions of individual universities and states.

Earlier sections of this report have also touched on work force issues. Chapter 2 briefly reviews the shift from the 1960s to the 1980s from concerns about an undersupply of dental practitioners to worries about an oversupply. Expansionist policies were adopted and then abandoned in favor of policies of neutrality or contraction. One legacy of the policy turnaround is a set of structures and processes for collecting work force and other data and forecasting future supplies and requirements for dental and other health professionals and services.

Chapter 5 discusses the oral health research work force and notes the shortage of qualified researchers. It cites the recent report of the Office of Science and Engineering Personnel of the National Research Council. That report concluded that at least 200 graduates per year were needed to meet the need for oral health researchers, and it noted that this is roughly four times the current production. The recommendation in Chapter 4 for an increase in the number of general dentistry residencies was intended not to increase the supply of generalists but rather to improve their qualifications.

WORK FORCE TRENDS AND PROJECTIONS

DENTISTS

Numbers and Projections

More than 140,000 dentists are in active practice in the United States, and the ratio of dentists to population currently stands at approximately 56:100,000 persons. Forecasts of the numbers of dentists are generally consistent in predicting that the absolute number of dentists in the United States will peak around the year 2000 and then level off before beginning a gradual decline (AADS, 1989; ADA, Bureau of Economic and Behavioral Research, 1991; USDHHS, PHS, 1992). These projections are depicted in Figure 1.2 in Chapter 1. Because the U.S. population continues to grow, the ratio of dentists to the general population will drop earlier and more sharply, falling by 2010 to a estimated level of less than 50:100,000 (or approximately 2,000 people per dentist).

The projections in the dentist work force reflect the combined effect of the retirements of dentists trained in peak enrollment years and the reduced enrollments of more recent years. As reported earlier, six schools have closed during the last several years, and a majority of the remaining schools have cut enrollments. According to one reckoning, the total enrollment decrease is *equivalent to the closure of 20 average-sized dental schools* (Consani, 1993).

The cuts in dental school enrollments have primarily affected the supply of generalist dentists. The *number* of specialty training positions has not increased absolutely, but the *ratio* of such positions to dental school graduates has increased. Thus, the proportion of dentists who are specialists is projected to increase from about 15 percent in 1985 to more than 25 percent by the second decade of the next century. Despite this growth, general practice still prevails in dentistry, in sharp contrast to the situation in medicine in which more than two-thirds of all physicians are specialists (Kindig et al., 1993).

In its survey of deans, the committee found that three-quarters of those surveyed felt that the supply of dentists today is about right. However, nearly two-thirds believed that the country would be undersupplied with dentists in 15 years (Table 9.1). A majority of respondents reported that the supply of dental hygienists and formally trained dental assistants was too low currently and pro-

TABLE 9.1 Deans' Responses to Supply Questions in Institute of Medicine and American Association of Dental Schools Survey

For the following questions, please indicate your opinion.

Too Low	About Right	Too High	Not Sure	Question
7	42	3	2	The supply of dentists in the U.S. today is _____.
34	16	2	1	The supply of dentists in the U.S. 15 years from now is likely to be _____.
4	7	0	3	The supply of dental hygienists in the U.S. today is _____.
38	8	1	5	The supply of dental hygienists in the U.S. 15 years from now is likely to be _____.
39	7	0	7	The supply of formally trained dental assistants is _____.
34	16	2	1	The supply of formally trained dental assistants and dental hygienists in the U.S. 15 years from now is likely to be _____.

SOURCE: Institute of Medicine and American Association of Dental Schools, 1994.

jected that the supply of these allied personnel would be too low in the year 2008.

Regional Variations and Shortage Areas

Regional data show considerable variation in dentist-to-population ratios. Figure 9.1 shows trends for three regions. For the New England and the Middle Atlantic regions, the number of active dentists per 100,000 population is projected to remain 10 to 15 dentists more than the national average through 2020, although each ratio is declining (AADS, 1989). In contrast, the dentist-to-population ratio for the Pacific region is expected to move from above to below the national average by the turn of the century while the ratio for the South Atlantic is expected to rise to the national average by 2010. Variations across and within states are even greater than regional variations. In 1993, Alabama had 41 dentists per 100,000 population whereas Connecticut had 73 per 100,000 (or 2,439 persons per dentist in Alabama and 1,370 in Connecticut).

In FY 1993, 1,069 areas were designated as dental health professional shortage areas, and these areas collectively were short 2,087 full-time equivalent dentists (J. Rosetti, personal communication to M. Allukian, April 4, 1994). The Department of Health and Human Services has defined a shortage area as one with a ratio of 5,000 or more people per dentist. It has defined 3,000 people per dentist as a target.

A recent U.S. General Accounting Office (GAO) study found that health professional shortage areas in urban counties report greater needs for full-time general dentists (GAO, 1994) whereas those in rural counties have a greater need for part-time positions (GAO, 1994). Many rural shortage areas would move off the shortage list if they added less than half of a full-time position. Recruiting individuals for part-time practice in shortage areas is, however, particularly difficult.

Composition of Work Force

Dentistry used to be a profession of white males, but that is changing. The proportion of women in the dental work force has grown dramatically since women began entering dental schools in substantial numbers in the 1970s. In 1970, 2 percent of first-year dental students were female compared to 38 percent in 1990. Although only about 10 percent of all dentists are female, nearly 20

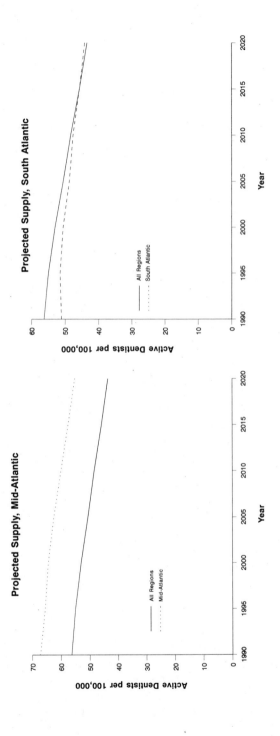

258

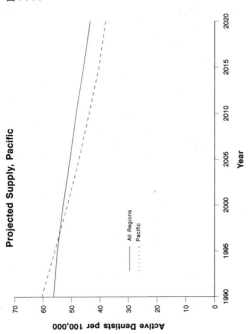

Projected Supply, Pacific

All Regions
Pacific

FIGURE 9.1 Trends in supply of dentists for these regions, 1990-2020. SOURCE: American Association of Dental Schools, 1989.

percent of those under age 40 are female (ADA, CYP, 1992). With its relatively predictable and manageable work week, attractive financial returns, and moderate length of professional training (compared to medicine), dentistry has many attractions for women interested in both career and family. One drawback is state licensing requirements that complicate interstate moves for two-career couples. As noted in the preceding chapter, such requirements may make it more difficult for dentists to relocate to shortage areas.

The picture for unrepresented racial and ethnic minorities is less encouraging than it is for women. Another Institute of Medicine committee has defined underrepresented racial and ethnic minorities as African-Americans, Hispanics, and Native Americans—groups that are both underrepresented and characterized by a group history of deprivation (IOM, 1994b). Although incomplete American Dental Association (ADA) data on race and ethnicity suggest that perhaps 10 percent of all dentists and 30 percent of dentists under age 40 are minorities, *underrepresented* minorities make up less than half of this younger group (which is 30 percent Hispanic and 13 percent African-American) (ADA, CYP, 1992).

Since 1971, first-year African-American enrollments in dental school have stayed relatively steady, whereas Asian enrollments have increased substantially and Hispanic enrollments, modestly. As a result, African-Americans now represent less than 25 percent of minority enrollment compared to more than 50 percent in the early 1970s. Attrition rates for African-Americans are approximately twice the rates for whites and Hispanics (ADA, CYP, 1992). According to a 1994 report, African-Americans have not achieved overall population parity in dental school enrollments but are closer to educational parity (GAO, 1994). Population parity compares the percentage of African-Americans in dental schools to the group's percentage of the total population. On a population basis, African-American dental school graduates stood at 37 percent of parity for dental school graduates in 1991 compared 34 percent in 1980. (Full parity equals 100 percent.) Educational parity compares the percentage of the group in dental school to its percentage of the population of college graduates. For dental graduates, the educational parity figures for African-Americans stood at 80 percent in 1991 versus 76 percent in 1980, but for first-year enrollments, the comparable figures were 113 versus 93 percent, respectively. These figures underscore the importance of the strategies described later in this chapter for increasing the pool of college-educated minorities.

Work Force Requirements

Most dental work force models focus only on the supply of practitioners. The econometric model developed by the federal government's Bureau of Health Professions attempts to project prices and utilization, but it does not generate a specific comparison of future supply against future demand (or need) to generate an explicit projection of work force requirements. The background paper by Capilouto et al. notes that the model did not do well in predicting precise dentist supply requirements necessary to maintain stable prices.

The committee did not find specific quantitative projections of population "requirements" for dental personnel similar to those that have been developed for the physician work force (Feil et al., 1993; Wennberg et al., 1993; Weiner, 1994). This analytic disparity presumably reflects the greater concern of analysts and policymakers about a physician work force that is—compared to the dental work force—much larger, much more specialized, more expensive, and more routinely involved in more diverse practice sites and organizational systems. Most assessments of the physician work force point to a probable aggregate oversupply of physicians, particularly specialists, and most proposals for health care reform would shift the emphasis in medical education from specialists to generalist physicians (Feil et al., 1993; PPRC, 1994). Although there is argument on this point, some believe that the projected supply of generalist physicians is adequate to meet expected demands for care (if there is a continued move to health plans that limit the number of participating physicians) but that the supply of specialists is considerably in excess of what is needed (Weiner, 1994).[1] Proposals to limit the

---

[1]Some, however, note that medical directors of health maintenance organizations claim that today's generalist physicians are not adequately trained for practice in a managed care environment that limits the use of specialist physicians (Rivo et al., 1994). Other analysts argue that a clearer framework of definitions, data, and analyses is needed to guide physician work force planning in coming years (Kindig, 1994). For example, should work force policies focus on categorizing some specialties a priori as "generalist specialties" (e.g., family practitioners but not gynecologists) or on defining primary care competencies and training requirements and then evaluating how specialty programs fit these definitions (Rivo et al., 1994)? A number of analysts also argue that planners should attempt to define numerical requirements for generalists and specialists (recognizing the complexities of doing so) rather than to specify a percentage split between the two (PPRC, 1994).

number or proportion of specialist residency positions have provoked considerable controversy.

In dentistry, aggregate work force planning focuses more on predoctoral enrollments than on residency positions. Moreover, most of the concern about residencies focuses on increasing the number of general dentistry positions rather than cutting the absolute number of specialist positions or specifying a percentage split between generalist and specialist positions. One concern in assessing the adequacy of supply to meet requirements for oral health services is the work load of practitioners. ADA survey data (1992f) indicate that the average general dentist works 48 weeks a year and spends an average of 37 hours per week in practice (33.6 hours treating patients). The average appointment wait time was about seven days. One ADA analysis suggests that less than two-thirds of available "capacity in dentistry" has been used in recent years. That number was derived by assuming that all dentists could provide the volume of service provided by the top quartile of dentists (ADA, 1993a).

Similarly, a study comparing educational costs and incomes for professionals reported fewer hours worked annually for dentists than for primary care and procedure-based specialty physicians, lawyers, and business people with M.B.A. degrees (Weeks et al., 1994). For example, for professionals aged 36-45, annual hours worked were 1,613 for dentists (patient care hours only, generalists and specialists); 1,893 for lawyers; 2,520 for business people; 2,674 for primary care physicians (patient care only); and 2,730 for specialists (patient care only). Differences in data definitions and sources undoubtedly account for some of this variation, and professional interpretations of terms such as "patient care hours" may vary. Nonetheless, the numbers raise the possibility of some reserve capacity in the dental work force, although differences in work load may reflect different choices about lifestyle, income, and other factors that might limit the extent to which dentists would increase their work load in response in an increase in the demand for their services.

Whatever the national supply picture, state or regional circumstances may differ. As described in the background paper by Capilouto et al., some research has attempted to assess work force requirements within states based on information and judgments about supply, demand, and need. Several regional organizations exist to assist states with higher education planning and policy. These organizations, which include the Western Interstate Commission for Higher Education, the New England Board of Higher Education, and the Southern Regional Education Board, provide policymakers with region-specific work force analyses and comparisons (see, for example, Hebbeler, 1984 and McPheeters, 1987). With appropriate funding, health services researchers in dental schools could also undertake such regional or state studies.

ALLIED DENTAL PERSONNEL

In 1989, the American Dental Hygienists' Association (ADHA) reported 98,000 currently licensed and 71,540 actively practicing dental hygienists. The Bureau of Health Professions estimated that 201,400 dental assistants and 70,000 dental laboratory technologists were active in the work force in 1990 (USDHHS, PHS, 1992). Figure 9.2 shows historic trends in dental hygiene, dental assisting, and dental laboratory technology enrollments. Enrollments grew sharply in the late 1960s and most of the 1970s, then declined in the 1980s. Neither the growth nor the decline was, however, as sharp as that for dentists. Most of the deans surveyed by this committee believed that the current supply of dental hygienists and formally trained dental assistants was too low now and would still be too low in 15 years (see Table 9.1).

Although no government or private organization routinely makes formal projections of trends in the supply of hygienists, assistants, or laboratory technologists, the Bureau of Health Professions predicts the number of jobs that will be available for hygienists in the future. The bureau has projected that the number of hygienists' jobs would grow twice as fast as jobs for the dentists who employ them (IOM, 1989a). These estimates are derived from surveys of incorporated dentist offices and, thus, omit hygienists employed by unincorporated dentists. Moreover, because many hygienists may work in more than one office, the figures do not translate directly into statements about the number of employed hygienists.

FORECASTING MODELS AND THEIR LIMITATIONS

The background paper prepared for this study by Capilouto et al. examines models and data used by four organizations to project the supply, demand, and need for dentists. Two of these organizations, the American Dental Association and the American Association of Dental Schools, are private, and two, the Bureau of Health Professions and the Bureau of Labor Statistics, are agencies of the federal government. The proprietary or nonpublic ele-

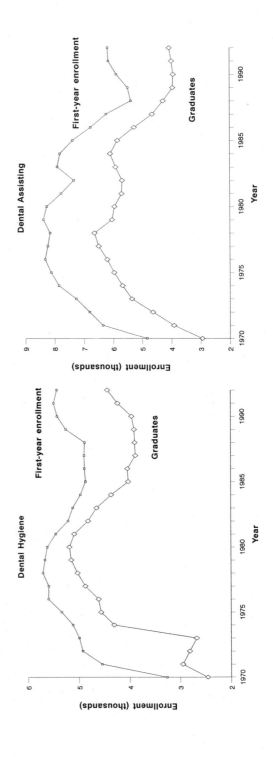

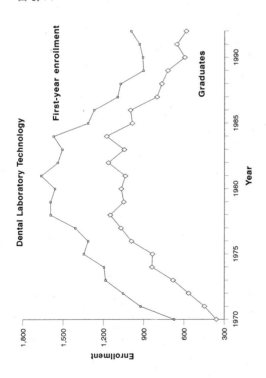

FIGURE 9.2 Enrollment trends in allied dental programs. SOURCE: Compiled in American Association of Dental Schools, 1993b.

265

ments of some models limited examination of their features. The following discussion draws heavily on this background paper.

Although the models agree in the *pattern* they forecast, the actual *numerical* predictions differ as shown in Table 9.2. Each model has tended in the past to produce estimates in excess of actual numbers. Such disagreement is not unique to these forecasts. A recent analysis of estimates of physician supply describes similar variations and concludes that there is "little scientific basis on which to claim that one projection is more credible than another" (Feil et al., 1993, p. 2863).

Forecasts may vary for several reasons including differences in data sources, definitions, choices of variables to include in models, and assumptions about those variables. Although models and data can be refined, uncertainty about the future is a given. Thus, the mechanical use of models and predictions (and, indeed, any planning and decisionmaking tool) is risky. Even when reasonably good data are available, they may be ignored. For example, the background paper by Capilouto et al. reviews data showing positive income trends for dentists compared with other professions, especially when inflation was considered. In contrast, the media have portrayed declining incomes due to a surfeit of dentists. Because perceptions do influence behavior, they may have to be considered in formulating assumptions for models or presenting their results.

TABLE 9.2 Projection of Active U.S. Dentists by Year of Published Prediction

Organization	Year Prediction Published	Year Predicted 1990	2000	2010	2020
American Association	1988	149,680	154,007	148,187	137,365
of Dental Schools	1989	140,699	142,379	137,197	133,214
American Dental	1988	149,970	156,611		
Association	1989	140,842	143,057		
(1990 Census)		(150,762)			
	1991	140,543	142,793	140,611	
Bureau of Health	1988	150,300	154,700	145,800	
Professions	1990	149,700	154,600	151,200	140,700
	1992	148,800	154,500	149,800	138,500

SOURCE: Table excerpted from Tables 3-5 of the background paper by Capilouto et al. Notes omitted.

Supply Estimates

For supply models, the major uncertainties involve assumptions about future dental school enrollments, graduation rates, and retirement from practice. In recent years, different models have projected declines in dental school enrollment ranging from less than 1 to approximately 5 percent per year and educational attrition rates ranging from 5 to 12 percent.

As an example of the prediction errors that can arise from incorrect assumptions, the 1978 Bureau of Health Professions overestimated supply because it incorrectly assumed that the decline in school enrollments would level off in the early 1980s. Because enrollments continued to drop instead, the resulting enrollment estimate was too high by 7,500 over an eight-year period. Similarly, none of the forecasts examined in the background paper by Capilouto et al. anticipated the sharp growth in numbers of international dental graduates admitted to advanced standing in several private dental schools, and current projections still do not account for this development. Thus, even though estimates of future supply are considered more reliable than estimates of demand or need, they are still subject to error. Sometimes accurate predictions result from offsetting errors in assumptions.

In addition, models focus on the supply of practitioners (or jobs) rather than on the supply of services. They tend not to incorporate information or assumptions about productivity (services per practitioner) that result from differences in practice styles, use of allied dental personnel, and other factors. Changes in such factors can significantly affect the supply of services available from the same number of dentists. As the background paper by Bader and Shugars notes, dentistry—like medicine—is characterized by significant unexplained variations in practice patterns.

Demand and Need Estimates

Demand is commonly defined as the willingness and ability to purchase a good or service whereas as need, in a clinical context, refers to phenomena that require clinical attention or treatment (Donabedian, 1973). Demand without need leads to overuse of medical services; need without demand leads to underuse of services. In principle, work force planning models that consider both demand and need for service are more appropriate than models that rely on simple practitioner-to-population ratios and statistical norms for establishing work force "requirements." In practice, such models are sufficiently subjective and vulnerable to changing events and data limitations that they are less useful as specific numbers than as means of illuminating supply-demand dynamics and helping plan for uncertainty.

The difficulties encountered in projecting current and future requirements for dental personnel and services include the subjectivity of dental diagnoses, the lack of evidence on outcomes and lack of agreement on appropriate interventions for different conditions, and the limited number of conditions for which any data are available. In addition, although the demand for dental services is sometimes measured by utilization of office visits, this measure does not reveal variations in the quantity and types of service that may be delivered during a visit. (For further discussion, see the background papers on oral health status by White et al. and on outcomes and effectiveness by Bader and Shugars.)

Projected into the future, estimates for demand and need encounter additional problems. In particular, the timing and impact of scientific or technological advances—the future equivalent of the fluoride "revolution" of the 1950s and 1960s—are not easily factored into estimation models. The technological basis for caries vaccine is, for example, on the horizon, but neither its introduction into practice, its acceptance by patients, nor its overall effectiveness can be predicted with any precision. Nor can it be readily predicted whether the preponderance of scientific or technical advances will involve relatively simple, demand-reducing preventive measures (similar to water fluoridation or childhood vaccinations) or whether they will stimulate demand for better therapies (e.g., tissue regeneration as treatment for periodontal disease).

To the extent that a scientific or technological breakthrough only gradually diffuses or changes the demand or need for a service or the way it is produced, routine processes for updating forecasting models and adjusting estimates would be timely enough to warn those who make or implement work force policies. In contrast, a breakthrough that diffuses rapidly and that quickly changes the demand or need for a service (or the way that service is produced) could catch planners and policymakers unprepared. In the background paper by Greenspan and elsewhere, the committee found no evidence suggesting such breakthroughs in caries or periodontal prevention or management.

Given a more than decade-long period in which health care reform was not an active policy issue, it was reasonable for demand forecasting models to ignore policy options for dental coverage that are now being actively debated. Some policies, notably the inclusion of dental benefits in a universally available benefit package, would likely increase demand for care. Other policies, such as the end of tax exclusions for employer-paid dental benefits, could decrease the demand for dental services. As final revisions were being made in this report, the prospects for health care reform in the next few years were quite uncertain.

In sum, the committee found a very mixed picture of the future adequacy of the supply of dental services. Some factors point to a shortage based on the declining ratio of dentists to the general population and the increasing elderly population (with more teeth at risk for dental problems than preceding generations). Extension of existing preventive measures (e.g., fluoridated water, dental sealants) could continue to reduce the need for restorative services in the younger population. Scientific and technological developments could, on balance, increase or decrease demand depending on the extent to which they favored prevention rather than more intensive treatment. Whether the availability of better treatments would translate into more demand for care would depend on the extent to which they required more time and the extent to which patients could afford to pay for them. The prospect for increased insurance coverage of dental services is uncertain, but an expansion of public or private coverage could increase demand, especially if additional efforts are made to reach those with significant unmet needs. The presence of reserve capacity in the current dental work force could, however, absorb some or all of any increased demand.

PLANNING FOR UNCERTAINTY

The desire of dental educators and public officials for technical models and analyses that provide specific quantitative estimates of the "right" size of the future work force is understandable. Educators and policymakers have no choice but to plan for the future and make choices that may affect the supply of dental services. Using historical experience and quantitative models of the future, they must assess trends, identify options, and project possible best and worst consequences of different actions given alternative future conditions.

Although forecasting models cannot provide firm bases for many important policy decisions, they are still useful monitoring and analysis tools.[2] They help planners and policymakers formulate alternative hypotheses about the future and assess how alternative strategies would fare under these different futures. The models also guide the monitoring and analysis of trend data and encourage analysts to be alert to events that might affect trends. For example, the closure of a large number of dental schools for financial reasons would require a reassessment of the future supply of oral health services and the appropriateness of compensating actions.

Continued investments by government agencies and private organizations in the forecasting models and analyses are prudent as are similar investments in the quality and scope of data used in the models. This, in turn, implies a *more sustained investment in a comprehensive oral health data infrastructure* than has been evident over the last decade. Although the committee recognizes the tensions that may arise in supporting information resources at the expense of other, more tangible health objectives, it believes that the former ultimately serves the latter.

THREE POSSIBLE FUTURES

Based on its review of work force models and projections and analyses of scientific, policy, and other trends, the committee concluded that there is not a compelling case for predicting either a oversupply or an undersupply of dental practitioners in the next quarter century. Recognizing, however, that educators and public officials must look to the future and consider options however uncertain the future appears, the committee considered three broad possibilities for the future supply of dental personnel and services and the ways that dental educators and policymakers might respond. The three possible futures are that the supply might be too high, too low, or within an acceptable range.

Prospects for an Oversupply of Dentists

A decade ago after the substantial increase in dental schools enrollments, the prospect of an oversupply of dentists was a ma-

---

[2]If forecasting models have their limits for planners and policymakers, so likewise the value of historical precedents is circumscribed. To cite a military analogy, historical experience is particularly useful in helping decisionmakers prepare to fight the last war.

jor concern for many in dentistry, and many of those interviewed for this study believed the current supply of dentists is too high. Population and educational trends described earlier assure that there will be fewer dentists relative to the population after the turn of the century. This ratio could nonetheless be "too high" under some circumstances, for example, unexpected, dramatic improvements in preventive strategies could change the picture.

Should an oversupply of dentists once again become a worry, strategies proposed to shrink the supply of physicians might apply to dentistry (Wennberg et al., 1993). These strategies include barriers to entry (e.g., further cuts in predoctoral enrollments and specialty residencies) and incentives for early retirement of employed dentists or relocation to underserved areas.

Prospects for an Undersupply of Dentists

As reported earlier, supply forecasts show a downturn in the dentist-to-population ratio, and a majority of dental school deans believe that a shortage of dentists is likely in the future. The committee was not convinced of this point, but it recognized that unexpected but not inconceivable events (e.g., independent actions by several universities to close their dental schools) could change the picture considerably—not only within a state or region but for the nation as a whole.

How might decisionmakers respond to projections of a future shortage? The traditional options have been to increase the supply of dentists or allied dental personnel or to increase work force productivity or both.

Increased Dental School Enrollments. Although concerned about a possible future shortage of dentists, few deans in the committee's survey believed that their school should increase its enrollment. Even fewer believed that they should cut enrollments. Some schools would, in any case, find it difficult to increase enrollments substantially without compromising student quality or incurring significant expansion costs.

The last broad increase in enrollments in health professions schools was spurred by increased federal and state funding, a simple replication of which seems highly unlikely given current fiscal stringency and past government experience with this strategy. Compared to most other fields, an increase in predoctoral dental school enrollments makes heavy demands for specialized and expensive physical space, and many schools that have cut enrollments say they have given up space to other university divisions that could not be easily reclaimed. Nonetheless, it is reasonable for dental educators to maintain some sense of the extent to which schools could collectively accommodate modest increases in enrollments should the need be convincingly demonstrated.

Increased Productivity of the Dental Team. The most frequently mentioned responses to any future excess of the demand for dental services over their supply involve the productivity of dental personnel. Although, as noted earlier, few data exist to document the point, it is likely that some dentists could considerably increase their individual output of services, for example, by working several more hours each week and seeing more patients. Although not all dentists would choose such a schedule, some surely would. Faced with high demand for their services, some dentists might also seek to free up time for medically needed care by encouraging fewer purely cosmetic services such as bleaching of teeth.

A broader productivity strategy focuses not just on dentists but on the entire dental team (AADS, 1993c; ADA, 1993g; ADHA, 1993). As described by one proponent (Nash, 1993), the "high-performance" dental team of the future would provide "new and challenging roles" for

• dental hygienists in treating periodontal disease and educating patients in and beyond the dental office;
• dental assistants in acting as dentist-extenders, especially for rehabilitative services;
• dental laboratory technicians in providing complete denture services; and
• dentists in providing the leadership that helps every member of the team to perform effectively.

These roles involve a mix of new responsibilities and old responsibilities more intensively exercised. Studies suggest that dentists trained to work with allied dental personnel are more productive and that allied personnel working in less restrictive delivery systems can provide high-quality care within their areas of competency (Burt and Eklund, 1992; Freed and Perry, 1992; see also the background paper by Tedesco).

A team strategy is not without problems, however (Bader et al., 1989; IOM, 1989a; DeVore, 1993; Pew Health Professions Commission, 1993; Robinson, 1993). First, as noted in Chapter 8, state practice acts limit the scope and efficiency of services that allied personnel can provide. For example, a sizable minority of states require that dentists directly supervise certain hygienist services (i.e., a dentist must be physically present when the services are provided). At least nine states forbid the employment of more than two hygienists in a dental office (ADHA, 1993). The restrictions on dental assistants (e.g., whether they can apply topical fluorides or pit-and-fissure sealants) vary greatly from state to state.

State practice acts are heavily shaped by the economic interests of the dominant professional groups (Starr, 1982; Friedland and Valachovic, 1991; Burt and Eklund, 1992). Efforts to increase the output of the dental "team" through better use of allied dental personnel were attempted in the 1970s but abandoned in the face of a threatened oversupply of dentists. Dentists remain wary of these strategies and might oppose policies to implement them even in the face of an evident shortage of services. Funding for innovative programs to build on the team strategies tested in the 1970s is virtually nonexistent at the federal level. In Chapter 4, the committee suggests further study of the role of existing and new categories of dental personnel in the context of a closer integration of medicine and dentistry.

A second problem with the team strategy is that many hygienist abandon the field after a few years (IOM, 1989a; Miller, 1990). Their reasons include boredom, unsatisfactory pay and benefits, limited opportunities for career advancement, and concern about workplace conditions that increase risk of infection. The ADHA has argued that the perceived shortage of hygienists (as revealed in the committee's survey of deans) is more accurately described as a failure to use the existing work force appropriately (ADHA, 1989, cited in ADHA, 1993). Although dental hygiene enrollments have recently increased, inadequate recruitment for a broad range of allied health fields is still a concern (IOM, 1989a; Pew Health Professions Commission, 1993). To be successful, a team strategy would have to deliver on its promises to allied dental professionals—including increased responsibilities and levels of decisionmaking commensurate with education.

A third issue is the variability in educational background, the declining proportion of university-trained hygienists, and possible shifts in the type of individuals recruited. Each of these factors raises questions about how well dental hygiene education prepares students for increasingly complex oral health problems and suggests that more, rather than less, education is necessary for dental hygienists to meet these challenges (Kraemer, 1985; DeVore, 1993). Similar questions apply for dental assistants.

In 1989, another Institute of Medicine (IOM, 1989a) committee
made several relevant and reasonable recommendations to strengthen
the dental hygiene and other allied health professions. Among
the group's recommendations were that

1. the Department of Health and Human Services should "convene an interagency task force . . . to work toward increasing the
amount and improving the quality of data needed to inform [deci-
sions] about the allied health occupations" (p. 4);

2. "students should be sought in less traditional applicant pools"
(p. 7) and "alternative pathways to entry-level practice . . . and
mobility between community college and baccalaureate programs"
should be encouraged whenever feasible" (pp. 7-8);

3. employers should "strive to increase the supply of allied health
practitioners . . . [through means including] increasing compensation and developing mechanisms for . . . prolonging their attachment to their fields" (p. 9); and

4. "flexibility in licensure" and reliance on "statutory certification" (pp. 11-12) should be accepted to the extent consistent with
the public interest.

It is worth observing that physicians or nurse practitioners might,
in principle, enlarge the supply of some oral health services, particularly as medical management of oral health problems becomes
more important. At this time, however, physicians do not appear
inclined by either education or interest to assume a larger role in
oral health services, a reluctance reinforced by the modest levels
of insurance for such services. Although this committee did not
systematically investigate how generalist or specialist physicians
might provide oral health services in the event of undersupply of
dental professionals, Chapters 3 and 4 of this report have called
for increased attention by physicians to oral health concerns.

Reducing the Use of Dental Care. Another set of responses to
an undersupply of dental services could target the utilization of
dental services. Reductions in service use could come through
cutting consumer demand for services, for example, by increasing
cost-sharing requirements in dental insurance plans or improving
health habits. Reductions could also be achieved by changing
provider behavior, for example, by instituting capitated payment
to providers to eliminate possible incentives for overtreatment of
insured patients.

Strategies targeting the demand for care or the provision of
services raise concerns, first, that they would affect both inappropriate *and* appropriate care and, second, that they would discrimi-

nate against poorer or less sophisticated patients and consumers. For example, increased insurance deductibles and coinsurance levels could prompt patients, especially those with lower incomes, to forgo both needed and unneeded services. Such concerns are not restricted to an "undersupply" scenario as current debates over strategies to contain health care costs attest. They reinforce the committee's call for intensified efforts to measure oral health outcomes and to distinguish clearly beneficial interventions from those that are harmful or ineffective.

Prospects for Supply in Balance with Requirements

A third possible projection is that the future supply of dental services would be essentially in balance with requirements for those services overall. In practical terms, this may seem similar to the committee's conclusion that it could not confidently predict either an oversupply or an undersupply of services. The major difference is that the latter conclusion reflects uncertainty rather than a positive judgment. The implications for policymakers are, however, essentially the same—that caution should govern steps to increase or decrease the future dental work force.

A projection of supply in balance with requirements still leaves a number of work force concerns for planners and policymakers. These include the geographical distribution of practitioners, the composition of the work force, and the productivity of dental personnel. The first two topics are discussed below; the last has been discussed earlier.

WORK FORCE DISTRIBUTION AND COMPOSITION

Geographic Distribution of Personnel and Services

The discussion to this point has emphasized the total supply of dental personnel, but the committee has indicated concern about two other important issues: geographic distribution of personnel and work force composition. Past policies to deal with maldistribution problems by increasing the overall supply of personnel have been abandoned because the increased supply of physicians has done little to reduce shortage problems in many rural and inner-city locales (GAO, 1994). Greater competition in health care might reduce the demand for services in oversupplied areas and propel more practitioners to relocate in shortage areas, but this remains to be demonstrated.

To attract health personnel to undersupplied areas, more targeted strategies have been developed. In Britain, for example, a negative incentive denies physicians a list of publicly insured patients (almost the entire population) if they locate in oversupplied areas such as London. The United States has tried positive incentives in the form of the National Health Service Corps (NHSC). The NHSC includes loan repayment features for health professionals that serve in designated shortage areas, and it encourages personnel to remain in these areas after their service period is finished. These strategies are attractive because they address both the shortage problem and the problem of student debt repayment. The General Accounting Office, however, concluded recently that the impact of these programs on underserved areas is difficult to establish (GAO, 1994). It found, however, that the increased total supply of primary care physicians and dentists in the past decade has not been accompanied by increases in "those urban and rural areas where the greatest shortages exist" (p. 2). The Department of Health and Human Services developed an oral health initiative in FY 1994 in response to Senate concerns about limited access to "primary care oral health services" and inadequate identification of affected areas and populations (U.S. Senate Appropriations Committee, 1994, p. 41). The GAO report concluded that "these actions are not likely to have much impact, at least in the short run" (1994, p. 2).

One problem with the NHSC and related programs is restricted funding. Of the 1,069 designated dental shortage areas in 1993, only 356 had been updated since 1988 and thereby made eligible for assistance through the NHSC (J. Rosetti, personal communication to M. Allukian, April 4, 1994). Moreover, the U.S. Health Resources and Services Administration has approved only 75 dental vacancies for loan repayment participants, and at the time information was provided to this committee, only 23 positions had been filled. One report states that there are no "ready" sites available for additional dental school placements (AADS, 1994c). Such sites have the equipment, salary, and staff to support an NHSC participant. One additional problem cited earlier is that many shortage areas call for part-time positions, and such positions are particularly difficult to fill.

REPRESENTATIVENESS OF THE WORK FORCE

As noted earlier, the composition of the dental student body and the dental work force has changed rather dramatically in some respects. In particular, the proportion of women and those of Asian background has risen sharply. The proportion of African-Americans has, in contrast, not grown. Recent declines in the number of African-Americans entering and completing college will make it difficult for dentistry and other professional and graduate programs to meet their recruitment goals for this group (New York Times, 1994). Hispanic and Native American populations are also underrepresented.

Since the 1960s, the health professions have focused on the objective and the problems of achieving racial and ethnic diversity, particularly in medicine, dentistry, and nursing. A recent ADA report focused specifically on minority and female representation in dentistry (ADA, 1992f), and another IOM committee recently examined the issue (IOM, 1994a). The latter report emphasized strategies to broaden the "pipeline" of minority students. The GAO figures on population versus educational parity for African-American enrollments in dental schools underscore the importance of increasing the flow of individuals academically prepared from their earliest educational experiences to choose a health professions career. Reform of science and math education from elementary through collegiate stages is a particularly crucial element of the pipeline strategy.

Among the set of supportive attitudes and mechanisms cited by the IOM (1994a, p. 66) study, mentoring was particularly recognized as a critical component with a "proven track record of helping minorities pursue their aspirations and achieve their career goals." To attract and support youths interested in the health professions, academic health centers should enlist the aid of corporations, other educational institutions, foundations, and government in developing mentoring programs; information networks; positive messages for talented students; and other projects. Another supportive step would be for universities to recognize "some level of community service among the criteria for academic recognition and advancement, in addition to the time-honored measures of scholarly and clinical achievement." Clearly, efforts to increase minority representation in dentistry must reach far beyond the dental school and involve practitioners, educators at all levels, policymakers, foundations, and corporations.

A recent California report also recommended a series of outreach programs and other actions to build a "strong educational pipeline" (University of California, 1993, p. ix). These steps included "working to bolster science curricula, developing feeder networks of health sciences high schools and undergraduate colleges, keeping health sciences professions within the financial reach of all students, and fostering a supportive learning environment within the health professions programs."

The committee on dental education was encouraged to see many dental educators recognizing and attempting to help implement strategies such as those described above. It notes, however, that medical schools are already attracting a very large percentage of minority science graduates (IOM, 1994a). Thus, recruitment aimed primarily at these graduates is not very promising if dental schools want to do more than "steal" applicants from other health or science careers. The problem of minority attrition after recruitment to dental school warrants particular attention.

FINDINGS AND RECOMMENDATIONS

After reviewing work force models and projections and their underlying assumptions, the committee found no compelling case, at this juncture, that the overall production of dentists will, in the next quarter century, prove too high or too low to meet public demand for oral health services. Accordingly, it found no responsible basis for recommending that total dental school enrollments should be pushed higher or lower.

However, even in the absence of compelling evidence that the nation faces either an oversupply or an undersupply of dentists, decisionmakers cannot abandon interest in either prospect. Scientific, economic, political, and other uncertainties warrant active surveillance and monitoring of developments that could change trends in supply, demand, or need. If a shortage in dental services is identified in the future, policymakers should look first to these options and increase enrollments at the predoctoral level only if these strategies prove insufficient.

In Chapter 4, the committee recommended that opportunities for advanced education in general dentistry be expanded, a step that would not affect the total supply of dentists but that would strengthen generalist practice. Chapter 5 endorsed increases in the oral health research work force.

The committee notes the persistence of dental professional shortage areas and the limited reach of federal programs to alleviate these shortages. The underrepresentation of African-Americans and certain other minorities in the dental work force is another continuing concern.

Because the prospects for a future oversupply or undersupply of dental personnel are uncertain and subject to unpredictable scientific, public policy, or other developments, the committee recommends that public and private agencies

• avoid policies to increase or decrease overall dental school enrollments;
• maintain and strengthen programs to forecast and monitor trends in the supply of dental personnel and to analyze information on factors affecting the need and demand for oral health care.

To respond to any future shortage of dental services and to improve the effectiveness, efficiency, and availability of dental care generally, educators and policymakers should

• continue efforts to increase the productivity of the dental work force, including appropriately credentialed and trained allied dental personnel;
• support research to identify and eliminate unnecessary or inappropriate dental services; and
• exercise restraint in increasing dental school enrollments unless other, less costly strategies fail to meet demands for oral health care.

To improve the availability of dental care in underserved areas and to limit the negative effects of high student debt, Congress and the states should act to increase the number of dentists serving in the National Health Service Corps and other federal or state programs that link financial assistance to work in underserved areas.

To build a dental work force that reflects the nation's diversity, dental schools should initiate or participate in efforts to expand the recruitment of underrepresented minority students, faculty and staff, including

• broad-based efforts to enlarge the pool of candidates through information, counseling, financial aid, and other supportive programs for precollegiate, collegiate, predoctoral, and advanced students; and
• national and community programs to improve precollegiate education in science and mathematics, especially for underrepresented minorities.

SUMMARY

Work force planning is a source of continual frustration for policymakers and educators. The failures or unintended consequences of past work force policies have left considerable wariness about proposed solutions to work force problems, and the limitations of forecasting models and data preclude confident predictions about the future. Another legacy of past policies is tension between the education and practice communities that extends beyond enrollment questions to complicate efforts to broaden and enrich the educational and patient care programs of dental schools. This chapter has argued for caution in changing dental school enrollments and for continued efforts to reshape the distribution and composition of the dental work force. It also has reinforced arguments in other chapters for increased effort to make more productive use of the entire dental team.

10

Summary and Conclusions

As the end of twentieth century approaches and the challenges of the twenty-first century approach, it is instructive to recall how the century opened for dental education—with an abundance of proprietary schools, a trade not fully transformed into a profession, a minuscule research and science base, a population beset by serious dental disease and resigned to tooth loss, and a limited set of treatments. During the twentieth century, dental health, practice, and education have been transformed. Oral health research has led to preventive, diagnostic, and management strategies that have greatly diminished the incidence and severity of dental disease. Independent proprietary schools have vanished amidst a series of educational reforms in student recruitment and qualifications, faculty responsibilities, and instruction in the basic, clinical, and behavioral sciences.

These changes flow in part from broader scientific and social developments including public policies to promote individual and community health. Beyond these influences, however, lies the dedication of several generations of dental practitioners, educators, researchers, and public officials to improving oral health through educational, professional, and scientific achievements. Because it is in the nature of reports such as this one to be critical, the committee wants to stress that it recognizes these contributions.

Some of the principles upon which these contributions have been founded remain solid, for example, dentistry's commitment

TABLE 10.1 Recapitulation of Guiding Principles

---

1. *Oral health is an integral part of total health, and oral health care is an integral part of comprehensive health care, including primary care.*

2. *The long-standing commitment of dentists and dental hygienists to prevention and primary care should remain vigorous.*

3. *A focus on health outcomes is essential for dental professionals and dental schools.*

4. *Dental education must be scientifically based and undertaken in an environment in which the creation and acquisition of new scientific and clinical knowledge are valued and actively pursued.*

5. *Learning is a lifelong enterprise for dental professionals that cannot stop with the awarding of a degree or the completion of a residency program.*

6. *A qualified dental work force is a valuable national resource, and support for the education of this work force must continue to come from both public and private sources.*

7. *In recruiting students and faculty, designing and implementing the curriculum, conducting research, and providing clinical services, dental schools have a responsibility to serve all Americans, not just those who are economically advantaged and relatively healthy.*

8. *Efforts to reduce the wide disparities in oral health status and access to care should be a high priority for policymakers, practitioners, and educators.*

---

to prevention. Others need to be reinvigorated, reformulated, or even replaced to prepare the profession for the future. Table 10.1 summarizes the key principles that guided this committee's work.

In considering the future of dental education, the committee had three basic tasks. One task was understanding and describing the current system and its evolution. A second task was trying to assess the forces that would shape dental practice and education in the future. The third was to draw conclusions about the reasonable and desirable steps that dental educators and others should take to capitalize on the positive opportunities before the profession and minimize the negative consequences of change.

Each of the preceding chapters has presented the results of the committee's work. This final chapter reviews the committee's findings about the key trends that will shape dental education and dental practice in the future, considers how the field is positioned to manage that future, and summarizes the committee's recommendations. A list of the formal recommendations is included in the summary at the beginning of this report.

TRENDS AND DEVELOPMENTS

The broad scientific, economic, social, and other forces that will shape dental practice are, for the most part, clear. Much less predictable are the magnitude, timing, scope, and details of developments in each area and the complex ways such developments may interact.

The scientific and demographic context of dental practice will undoubtedly continue to change. These changes will result from

- new scientific and technological advances (e.g., better understanding of the oral effects of various diseases and their treatment, increasing availability of pharmacological methods of preventing or treating oral diseases, and telecommunication tools to support diagnostic and other consultations);
- the continued impact of past scientific developments (e.g., water fluoridation and other uses of fluorides that have reduced the incidence of caries in children and changed the mix of oral health problems they present as adults);
- increased research on the outcomes of alternative preventive, diagnostic, and treatment strategies, as well as more evidence-based guidelines for appropriate dental practice; and
- an increase in the number and proportion of older patients who not only will have chronic problems and complicating medical conditions but also will be more highly educated, and possibly have higher expectations and demands for dental care, than their predecessors.

In addition, the management and conduct of dental practice will be altered by other social, economic, political, and technological developments that may or may not include legislative reform of the health care system. With or without federal action, the health care system is restructuring itself in ways that will affect dental practice and dental education. It appears that the pace of change for dentistry may be slower in some respects, but the directions are reasonably clear. The future will bring

- continued creation and diffusion of sophisticated information management technologies that will allow individual patient care, practice costs, and other variables to be tracked and assessed more readily;
- ongoing evolution of expectations and methods for assessing and improving the quality and efficiency of care provided in ambulatory settings;
- intensified pressure for control of health care costs;
- further growth of managed care and integrated care systems as a prevalent if not dominant method of organizing and administering medical and other health services; and
- greater emphasis on the contributions of health care to community as well as individual well-being.

Dental education will also be affected by changes in the university environment. Financial pressures on educational institutions undoubtedly will persist, although their severity may vary over time and across schools. Universities—and government policymakers—will continue to reevaluate their programs—adding, deleting, and restructuring them. Procedural changes in areas such as financial management, information systems, tenure, evaluation of educational outcomes, and accreditation may make life more difficult for educators in some ways and easier in others. Academic health centers will be under stress from the same changes in health care organization and financing that will affect dental schools, and in some respects, the impact of these changes may be more traumatic for medical schools and university hospitals than for dental schools. Overall, the world of higher education is likely to become less stable and thus more unpredictable and stressful for its constituent parts.

The implications of these trends and prospects for dental practice and dental education are clearer in some areas than in others. Dental schools and the dental community generally will see continued demands for greater professional accountability and evidence of effectiveness from public and university officials, institutional purchasers of dental services, managed care organizations, organized consumer or patient groups, and students. Relatedly, traditional practice and education will be challenged by a renewed focus on the dental practice team, multidisciplinary health care, and practice beyond the office setting. Dental practitioners will be relying more on medical management of a broad range of oral health problems, treating more patients who have chronic or complex medical problems, and undertaking a greater proportion of complex surgical and restorative services. For the majority of the population, however, the emphasis will continue to be on individual and community-based preventive and primary care services.

Much less clear is how changes in technology, demography, public policy, and health care organization will interact to affect the supply, demand, and need for oral health services. Although educators have no choice but to plan for the future and make choices that may affect the supply of dental services, this planning must account for uncertainty and consider alternative futures.

Further, although oral health status will continue to improve, it is not clear whether the society will commit the resources needed to reduce disparities in oral health status. Even if relatively inexpensive new preventive strategies were to emerge in the next few years, the problems—untreated caries, periodontal disease, and tooth loss—that now characterize disadvantaged groups will create continued needs for care for many years to come. These groups have been a traditional source of patients for dental school clinics, but dental school efforts to extend their services into the community are vulnerable to public budget-cutting. Resource constraints also dictate less than optimal treatment in many cases. In theory, health care reform that extends coverage to dental services could give poor patients more choices, but the immediate prospects for such reform seem dim.

The difficult debate over health care reform in 1993 and 1994 illustrates both the short- and the long-term uncertainties facing those responsible for dental education and work force policies. Although important policy changes may be slow in coming, they could occur relatively quickly. The dental community should be cognizant of this possibility. Accordingly, it should be ready to explain the role of oral health in total individual and community health to those who develop health care policy, be organized to evaluate the implications of possible policy changes, and be prepared to take action to preserve the integrity of the oral health of the nation and the educational, research, and patient care missions of the dental school.

STRENGTHS AND WEAKNESSES

How are dental schools and dental professionals situated when it comes to responding constructively to the scientific, organizational, financial, and other challenges outlined above? Answering this question requires a look at the current strengths and weaknesses of the field.

The strengths of dental education and the dental profession are, in the committee's view, both significant and in need of constant protection. These strengths include

• a tradition of, and continuing commitment to, prevention and general practice that have helped achieve significant improvements in oral health;

• a valuing of oral health and a reservoir of trust in the population, despite a "fear of the dentist's chair" that is both cliché and reality;

• a core of educators, researchers, and practitioners dedicated to educational progress and advances in oral health;

• a surrounding community of educators, health professionals, and public officials that supports the search for more effective and efficient educational strategies, on the one hand, and more effective and efficient health care, on the other; and

• a research and development establishment that produces a steady stream of technological and scientific advances.

Still, dental education, like any other enterprise, suffers from a myriad of problems ranging from minor irritants to potentially disabling conditions. The major weaknesses of concern to the committee fall in several areas. The mission of education is undermined by curricula and faculty that have become out of touch with the needs of students and prospective practitioners, patients, or communities. The mission of research is frustrated by the small numbers of qualified researchers and the limited acceptance by clinical faculty of the importance of research and scholarship. The mission of patient care has been subservient to that of education, leaving most dental schools ill-prepared to attract patients in a world marked by increasing competition, organizational integration, and managed care.

Further, each mission is weakened by dental schools' isolation from the intellectual and organizational life of the university, from the broader research community, and from the larger health care system. This isolation puts dental schools at risk within the university. Other risk factors include relatively high costs for education and patient care, low research productivity, uneven student quality, and resistance to change. Uncompetitive patient care programs are becoming a financial threat to schools.

Dentistry has been relatively slow to support outcomes research, to investigate the rationale for practice variations, and to demand proof of cost-effectiveness for new technologies. In a broader health care environment increasingly concerned about the effectiveness of health services, this stance is a liability.

In addition, tensions between the academic and practice communities too often impede efforts to revise educational standards, rationalize professional licensure, and improve community health. Politically, much of organized dentistry views distance from health care reform as a way of insulating the profession from demands for change and accountability. To a worrisome degree, dental education lacks strong allies to sustain it in the face of high costs and constrained resources.

DIRECTIONS FOR THE FUTURE

Stated in very broad terms, the committee envisions a future for dental education based on four propositions. First, dentistry will and should become more closely integrated with medicine and the health care system on all levels: research, education, and patient care. Second, to prepare both their students and their schools for change, dental educators will need to teach and display desirable models of clinical practice. Third, securing the resources essential for educational improvement and, indeed, survival will require that dental schools demonstrate their contributions to their parent universities, academic health centers, and communities through achievements not only in education but also in research, technology transfer, and community and patient service. Fourth, to prepare for the future, the dental community—educators, practitioners, regulators, and policymakers—will benefit from continued testing of alternative models of education, practice, and performance assessment for both dentists and allied dental professionals.

In developing specific recommendations, the committee attempted to be both principled and pragmatic. That is, it tried to be neither so idealistic that its recommendations would be of little use to real-world decisionmakers nor so fixated on the practical difficulties of change that it would provide no direction, motivation, or benchmarks to help decisionmakers move through difficulties toward desired goals. Still, the following recommendations individually or collectively may strike some as weighted toward the idealistic and others as weighted toward the status quo. If, however, a 10- to 20-year horizon is accepted as necessary and reasonable for the more demanding recommendations, then the possible and the ideal draw closer together.

Similarly, as the committee concluded in several instances, the case for some recommendations may not be robust when grounded in a single objective but may be convincing when supported by benefits on multiple fronts. In particular, a number of the education financing recommendations promise only modest economic benefits but would, if implemented, strengthen clinical education and research.

The recommendations reflect the principles that guided the committee, its findings about the current status and future prospects of dental schools and its broad judgments about directions for dental education. These judgments attempt to balance idealism, realism, and prudence. They are not, however, a blueprint for the future. Such a blueprint would have required confident predictions about the pace and direction of key scientific, economic, and social changes, and the committee either found current knowledge insufficient to warrant such confidence or disagreed about what the predictions should be. In addition, the committee did not reach consensus on some policy matters. Finally, the committee believes that no single blueprint is appropriate for all dental schools or all policymaking organizations.

ORAL HEALTH STATUS AND SERVICES

The committee emphasized four broad objectives for the effective use of health resources to advance the nation's oral health. These objectives are to

1. *improve our knowledge of what works and what does not work* to prevent or treat oral health problems;
2. *reduce disparities* in oral health status and services experienced by disadvantaged economic, racial, and other groups;
3. *encourage prevention* at both the *individual level* (e.g., feeding practices that prevent baby-bottle tooth decay, reduced use of tobacco) and the *community level* (e.g., fluoridation of community water supplies and school-based prevention programs); and
4. *promote attention to oral health* (including the oral manifestations of other health problems) not just among dental practitioners but also *among primary care providers, geriatricians, educators, and public officials.*

Dental education can play a central role in each of these areas. In particular, dental educators should be involved in basic science, clinical, and health services research to distinguish effective and ineffective oral health services, to clarify oral disease patterns and trends and the factors affecting them, and to develop cost-effective strategies likely to help those with the poorest health status and those with limited access to oral health services. Such strategies should include both technologies and new ways of organizing and delivering services to reach underserved populations. In their outreach activities, dental educators and practitioners should continue to encourage physicians, nursing home personnel, public officials, and others to be alert to oral health problems among those whom they serve and to provide information about good oral health habits.

Public support is critical if disparities in health status and access to oral health services are to be reduced. This committee therefore recommends that all parts of the dental community work together to secure more adequate public and private funding for personal dental services, public health and prevention programs, and community outreach activities, including those undertaken by dental school students and faculty.

In their efforts to improve oral health status, both educators and policymakers are hampered by inconsistent and insufficient information on oral health status and services. Thus, this committee recommends a stronger public commitment to the regular collection and analysis of data on oral health status and services;

the formulation and implementation of outcomes research agenda; and the translation of knowledge into clinical advice for practitioners and patients.

THE MISSION OF EDUCATION

In terms of education, the problem is not so much consensus on directions for change but difficulty in overcoming obstacles to change. Agreement on educational problems is widespread. The curriculum is crowded with redundant or marginally useful material and gives students too little time to consolidate concepts or to develop critical thinking skills. Comprehensive care is more an ideal than a reality in clinical education, and instruction still focuses too heavily on procedures rather than on patient care. Linkages between dentistry and medicine are insufficient to prepare students for a future of patients with more medically complex problems and more medically oriented strategies for prevention, diagnosis, and treatment. The basic and clinical sciences do not adequately relate the scientific basis of oral health to clinical practice. Lack of flexible tenure and promotion policies or of resources for faculty development limits efforts to match the faculty to educational needs. Despite progress, an insensitivity to students' needs is still a concern. All of these weaknesses undermine efforts to prepare students for lifelong learning.

Agreement on the obstacles to educational change is also strong. Obstacles include a lack of specific information on course content, limited evaluation of educational outcomes, financial constraints, university policy restrictions, and faculty conservatism.

In the hope of stimulating movement toward generally held goals, the committee proposes that each dental school develop a plan and timetable for curriculum reform. It urges closer integration of dental and medical education and more experimentation with new formats for such integration. Using excellent practice in the community as a model, dental school clinics should seek to be more patient centered and efficient and to provide students with a greater volume and breadth of clinical experience. All dental graduates should have the opportunity for a year of postgraduate education with an emphasis on advanced education in general dentistry.

THE MISSION OF RESEARCH

Research is a fundamental mission of dental education, but too many dental schools and dental faculty are minimally involved in research and scholarship. A commitment to research in dental schools is important because research builds a knowledge base for improving the effectiveness and efficiency of oral health services; enriches the educational experience for students; reinforces the school's role as a disseminator of validated practice advice to dental practitioners; and strengthens the stature of dentistry within the university and in the broader community.

The committee recognizes the problems facing schools that are trying to build or maintain a strong research program, most notably, limited funding and a dearth of capable researchers. The expansion of the oral health research work force is an important priority.

Dental schools will differ in how they define the specifics of their research priorities, but all schools need to formulate a program of faculty research and scholarly activity that meets or exceeds the expectations of their universities. To build research capacity and resources, as well as foster relationships with other researchers, it is important for dental schools to pursue collaborative research opportunities that start with the academic health center or the university and extend to industry, government, dental societies, and other institutions able to support or assist basic science, clinical, and health services research. Throughout this report, the committee has tried to point out opportunities for dental school faculty to participate in clinical, behavioral, and health services research that will support the missions of education and patient care and will help improve voluntary and governmental oversight of the profession.

THE MISSION OF PATIENT CARE

The typical dental clinic, put simply, is not patient centered. Current trends in health care delivery and financing are requiring academic health centers to compete for patients and inclusion in managed care plans of various sorts. Whether the patient care activities of the dental school add or subtract from the overall institution's market position is likely to be an issue in its future. At a minimum, financial viability is likely to require that schools put more emphasis on efficiency, quality, and accountability for care from the *patient's* perspective.

Over the long term, the committee believes that dental schools have no ethical or practical alternative but to make their programs more patient centered as well as more economically viable and to develop the programs and the data needed to assess and document the quality and efficiency of care. They will have to ensure that their activities and objectives are compatible with those of their parent institutions.

THE DENTAL SCHOOL IN THE UNIVERSITY

To fulfill and improve their basic missions of education, research, patient care, and service, dental schools need the intellectual vitality, organizational support, and discipline of universities and academic health centers. In return, dental educators must contribute to university life, especially through research, scholarship, and efficient management of educational and patient care programs. More generally, leaders in dental education and practice should work together to diminish the divisions that may undermine public and private support for dental schools and oral health.

The closure of several dental schools has, however, made the vulnerability of their relationship to the university clear. Reduction in the factors that put dental schools at risk in the university is not an overnight task, and some factors are less subject to a school's influence than others. This makes it all the more important that each school assess its own position and develop a specific plan for analyzing and reinforcing its position within the university.

Although education at all levels faces financial constraints ranging in severity from routine to critical, dental education faces particular challenges given its relatively high costs and specialized needs. For most schools, financial health will not be achieved through a single grand solution. Rather, some combination of more modest and difficult steps will be necessary. Schools will need to develop better cost and revenue data if they are to design steps that match their particular problems and characteristics and minimize harm to their educational, research, and patient care missions.

ACCREDITATION AND LICENSURE

Accreditation and licensure are components of a broad social strategy to ensure the quality of dental care by protecting the public from poorly trained, incompetent, or unethical dental practitioners. They also account for many of the tensions between dental schools and the profession. The dental community has taken important actions to improve licensure and accreditation processes, but further work is needed.

The accreditation process remains too focused on process and too inhospitable to educational innovation. The committee believes that the process tolerates some inferior educational programs, although data to document this are not publicly accessible. Accreditation reform should focus on standards and methods that will identify and improve those schools that are not educating their students effectively or ethically, and that will not allow persistently poor performance. At the same time, excessively detailed assessments of structures and processes should be trimmed. In addition, dental accreditors and educators should be prepared to respond constructively to reasonable demands for increased public accountability and information.

In the view of this committee, the most important deficiencies of dental licensure are concentrated in a few areas: the use of live patients in clinical licensure examinations; variations in the content and relevance of clinical examinations; unreasonable barriers to movement of dentists and dental hygienists across state lines; practice acts that unreasonably restrict the use of appropriately trained allied dental personnel; and inadequate means of assessing competency after initial licensure.

The committee understood and sympathized with concerns expressed about self-regulation of dental education and parochial state regulation of the profession. It concluded, however that it is neither practical nor necessary to construct new national systems for licensure and accreditation. Rather, the committee urges dental leaders to cooperate to achieve greater uniformity in licensing, minimize barriers to professional mobility, and revise laws that limit dentists from working more productively with allied dental personnel. A uniform national clinical examination (one that does not include real patients) should be developed for acceptance by each state. Voluntary accreditation should focus on dental schools with significant deficiencies and reduce administrative burdens on other schools.

Improvements in methods of assessing educational outcomes are as central to accreditation reforms as they are to improvements in predoctoral education, entry-level licensure, and assessment of continued competency. Thus, cooperation and coordination among responsible organizations in each of these arenas should be established to avoid conflicting strategies and costly duplication of effort. Improvements in the processes for collecting information—particularly those based on electronic transfer of data—likewise will produce multiple benefits and should be coordinated.

DENTAL WORK FORCE

The dental community is characterized by much anxiety and disagreement about whether the nation faces a future shortage or a future oversupply of dental services. The committee found no compelling evidence that would allow it to predict either outcome with sufficient confidence to warrant recommendations that dental school enrollments be increased or decreased. On the one hand, the ratio of dentists to the general population is declining, and the coverage of dental services under expanded public or private health insurance could substantially increase the demand for such services, especially if additional efforts are made to reach those with significant unmet needs. On the other hand, the current dental work force appears to have reserve capacity that could be mobilized through better use of allied dental personnel, improved identification and elimination of care with little or no demonstrated health benefit, and more efficient delivery systems. Scientific and technological developments could increase or reduce overall need and demand depending on whether they promoted prevention or expensive treatment.

In the face of uncertainty, the committee believes it is prudent to continue monitoring trends in the supply of dental personnel and developing better understanding of their productivity, of the appropriateness of dental services, and of the factors that impede access to dental care. This course will require a more sustained investment in a comprehensive oral health data infrastructure than has been evident over the last decade.

To respond to any future shortage of dental services and to improve the effectiveness, efficiency, and availability of dental care generally, educators and policymakers should continue efforts to increase the productivity of the dental work force, including appropriately credentialed and trained allied dental personnel, and to support research to identify and eliminate unnecessary or inappropriate dental services.

Two persistent work force problems involve dental shortage areas and minority representation in the future. The National Health Service Corps (NHSC) and other federal or state programs link financial assistance to practice in underserved areas and also help relieve the serious problem of high student debt. The shrinkage in dental positions in the NHSC should be reversed. Building a dental work force that reflects the nation's diversity will require broad-based efforts to reduce attrition among predoctoral students and to enlarge the pool of candidates for dental school admission through information, counseling, financial aid, improved precollegiate education in science and mathematics, and other supportive programs for precollegiate and collegiate students.

FROM RECOMMENDATIONS TO ACTION

From the beginning, this committee was quite aware that reports like this one are far from self-implementing. Indeed, one goal of this report has been to stimulate renewed efforts to implement reforms that have long been recommended and are even more urgently needed today. Members of this committee look forward to discussing the report's analyses and recommendations with many groups, and they hope to see the creation of task forces and similar groups to turn those recommendations that require collective responses into specific, workable action plans. Such groups may be organized both within and across leadership organizations such as the American Association of Dental Schools, the American Association of Dental Examiners, the American Dental Association, the American Dental Assistants' Association, and the American Dental Hygienists' Association. Given its discussions with leaders of these groups, the committee trusts that activities like these will be organized in the months following publication of this report.

Many of this report's recommendations explicitly recognize that dental educators, regulators, researchers, and practitioners will have to work together with an understanding that they are investing in the well-being of their profession and their communities. Further, the dental community collectively will have to enlist support from university and public officials and from other health professionals, a task that current tensions sometimes make difficult.

Individually, each dental school will find itself in a different position with respect to the problems, opportunities, and directions identified here. Each school will need to tailor a strategy that reflects its objectives and resources—but does not simply capitulate to obvious difficulties. Notwithstanding differences in their individual circumstances, dental schools will gain by sharing ideas and strategies for solving common problems.

Finally, the committee recommends that the Institute of Medicine convene a conference or workshop to bring interested parties together, within a year after this report's publication to assess the initial impact of this report. The agenda would include the responses of different organizations, discussion of initial individual or collective steps to implement recommendations, and suggestions about follow-up strategies. If the spirit of cooperation among dental leaders that led to this study persists, that gathering should find that this effort has begun to make a constructive contribution to the health of the profession and the public.

References

Ad Hoc Working Group on Research-Intensive Universities and the Federal Government. *In the National Interest: The Federal Government and Research-Intensive Universities.* Washington, D.C.: National Science Foundation, 1992.

Agency for Health Care Policy and Research (AHCPR). *Bibliography of Dental Health Services Research.* Rockville, Md.: AHCPR, 1990.

Albanese, M.A., and Mitchell, S. Problem-Based Learning: A Review of Literature on Its Outcomes and Implementation Issues. *Academic Medicine* 68:52-81, 1993.

American Academy of Pediatric Dentistry (AAPD). Testimony presented at a public hearing of the Institute of Medicine Committee on the Future of Dental Education, Washington, D.C., September 26-27, 1993.

American Association for Dental Research (AADR). Testimony presented at a public hearing of the Institute of Medicine Committee on the Future of Dental Education, Washington, D.C., September 26-27, 1993.

American Association of Dental Examiners (AADE). *Composite.* Chicago, Ill.: AADE, 1992.

AADE. *Criteria and Mechanisms for Continued Competency.* Chicago, Ill.: AADE, 1993a.

AADE. Testimony presented at a public hearing of the Institute of Medicine Committee on the Future of Dental Education, Washington, D.C., September 26-27, 1993b.

American Association of Dental Schools (AADS). *Manpower Project Report No. 2.* Washington, D.C.: AADS, Manpower Committee, January 1989.

AADS. *Survey of Dental Seniors: Summary Report, 1992.* Washington, D.C.: AADS, 1992.

AADS. AADS 70th Annual Session and Exposition. Education, Research, Practice: Going Forward in Harmony. *Journal of Dental Education* 57(2):79-197, 1993a.

AADS. *Deans Briefing Book: Academic Year, 1992-93.* Washington, D.C.: AADS, 1993b.

AADS. Testimony presented at a public hearing of the Institute of Medicine Committee on the Future of Dental Education, Washington, D.C., September 26-27, 1993c.

AADS. *Expansion of Postdoctoral General Dentistry Training: Meeting National Need and Demand.* Washington, D.C.: AADS, February 15, 1994a.

AADS. *Facts, Figures, and Recommendations Regarding the National Health Service Corps and Oral Health Initiative.* Washington, D.C.: AADS, April 1994b.

AADS. *Survey of Clinic Fees and Clinic Revenue: Summary Report, 1992-93.* Washington, D.C.: AADS, 1994c.

AADS, Accreditation Council for Continuing Dental Education. *Standards and Guidelines for Accreditation of Dental School Continuing Education Programs.* Washington, D.C.: AADS, Accreditation Council for Continuing Dental Education, 1992.

AADS and W.K. Kellogg Foundation. *Advanced Dental Education: Recommendations for the 80s.* Washington, D.C.: AADS, September 1980.

American Association of Oral and Maxillofacial Surgery (AAOMS). Testimony presented at a public hearing of the Institute of Medicine Committee on the Future of Dental Education, Washington, D.C., September 26-27, 1993.

American Association of Orthodontists (AAO). Testimony presented at a public hearing of the Institute of Medicine Committee on the Future of Dental Education, Washington, D.C., September 26-27, 1993.

American Association of Public Health Dentistry. Testimony presented at a public hearing of the Institute of Medicine Committee on the Future of Dental Education, Washington, D.C., September 26-27, 1993.

American Association of University Professors (AAUP). 1940 Statement of Principles on Academic Freedom and Tenure with 1970 Interpretive Comments. *Policy Documents and Reports.* Washington, D.C.: AAUP, 1990.

American Board of Dental Public Health (ABDPH). Testimony presented at a public hearing of the Institute of Medicine Committee on the Future of Dental Education, Washington, D.C., September 26-27, 1993.

American Dental Association (ADA). *Report of the Special Higher Education Committee to Critique the 1976 Dental Curriculum Study.* Chicago, Ill.: ADA, 1980.

ADA. *Guidelines for Licensure.* Chicago, Ill.: ADA, 1992a.

ADA. Report of the Provider Recognition Program Special Committee. *1992 Annual Reports and Resolutions.* Chicago, Ill.: ADA, 1992b, pp. 141-178.

ADA. Resolution 89H-1992; adopted by the 1992 ADA House of Delegates. *Transactions of the ADA*, 1992c.

ADA. *Supplement 6: Analysis of Dental School Finances 1991-92.* Chicago, Ill.: ADA, 1992d.

ADA. *Supplement 7: Dental School Curriculum, Clock Hours of Instruction Summary Report* Chicago, Ill.: ADA, 1992e.

ADA. *The 1991 Survey of Dental Practice: General Characteristics of Dentists.* Chicago, Ill.: ADA, 1992f.

ADA. *Annual Report, Allied Dental Education, 1991/92.* Chicago, Ill.: ADA, 1993a.

ADA. *Dental School Trend Analysis, 1992/93.* Chicago, Ill.: ADA, 1993b.

ADA. *Report to Joint Commission on National Dental Examinations.* Chicago, Ill.: ADA, 1993c.

ADA. *Requirements for Recognition of Dental Specialties and National Certifying Boards for Dental Specialists* (approved 1983). Chicago, Ill.: ADA, 1993d.

ADA. *Supplement: Dental School Admissions 1992/93.* Chicago, Ill.: ADA, 1993e.

ADA. *Supplement: Dental School Faculty and Support Staff 1992-93.* Chicago, Ill.: ADA, Department of Educational Surveys, 1993f.

ADA. Testimony presented at a public hearing of the Institute of Medicine Committee on the Future of Dental Education, Washington, D.C., September 26-27, 1993g.

ADA. *1993/94 Analysis of Dental School Finances.* Chicago, Ill.: American Dental Association (ADA) Survey Center, 1994a.

ADA. *1993/94 Dental School Curriculum, Clock Hours of Instruction: Summary Report.* Chicago, Ill.: ADA Survey Center, 1994b.

ADA. *Facts on Licensure.* Chicago, Ill.: ADA, 1994c.

ADA, Bureau of Economic and Behavioral Research. *Annual Report to the American Dental Association House of Delegates.* Chicago, Ill.: ADA, Bureau of Economic and Behavioral Research, 1991.

ADA, Commission on the Young Professional. *A Portrait of Minority and Women Dentists.* Washington, D.C.: Decision Demographics, 1992.

ADA, Continuing Education Recognition Program (CERP). *List of Recognized Continuing Education Providers, Fall 1993.* Chicago, Ill.: ADA, 1993a.

ADA, CERP. *Standards and Procedures.* Chicago, Ill.: ADA, 1993b.

ADA, Council on Dental Education (CDE). *Dental Education in the United States 1976.* Chicago, Ill.: ADA, Council on Dental Education, 1977.

ADA, Department of State Government Affairs. *Continuing Education Requirements of State Dental Boards: Dentists and Auxiliaries.* Chicago, Ill.: ADA, Department of State Government Affairs, July 29, 1994.

ADA and AADE. *Guidelines for Valid and Reliable Dental Licensure Clinical Examinations.* May 1992.

American Dental Hygienists' Association (ADHA). Testimony presented at a public hearing of the Institute of Medicine Committee on the Future of Dental Education, Washington, D.C., September 26-27, 1993.

ADHA. *State Dental Board Composition.* Chicago, Ill.: ADHA, January 1994.

American Fund for Dental Health. *Oral Health 2000 News* 1(1):1, 1992.

American Medical Association (AMA). *Attributes to Guide the Development of Practice Parameters.* Chicago, Ill.: AMA, 1990a.

AMA. *Legal Implications of Practice Parameters.* Chicago, Ill.: AMA, 1990b.

AMA. *Directory of Practice Parameters.* Chicago, Ill.: AMA, 1991.

AMA. Appendix C: Medical Licensure Requirements. In *Graduate Medical Education Directory.* Chicago, Ill.: AMA, 1994.

American Student Dental Association. Testimony presented at a public hearing of the Institute of Medicine Committee on the Future of Dental Education, Washington, D.C., September 26-27, 1993.

Anderson, O.W. *The Uneasy Equilibrium: Private and Public Financing of Health Services in the United States, 1875-1965.* New Haven, Conn.: United Printing Services, 1968.

Angell, M., and Kassirer, J.P. Setting the Record Straight in the Breast Cancer Trials. *New England Journal of Medicine* 330:1448-1449, 1994.

Antczak-Bouckoms, A. Issues Related to Quality and Effectiveness of Existing, New and Emerging Oral Health Delivery Mechanisms. Presentation for a conference on Oral Health for Aging Veterans, Department of Veterans Affairs and Foundation for Health Services Research, Washington, D.C., November 30-December 2, 1993.

Association of Academic Health Centers (AAHC). *Human Resources for Health: Defining the Future.* C.M. Evarts, P.B. Bosomworth, and M. Osterweis, eds. Washington, D.C.: AAHC, 1992.

AAHC. *Academic Health Centers: Missions, Markets, and Paradigms for the Next Century.* J.P. Howe III, M. Osterweis, and E.R. Rubin, eds. Washington, D.C.: AAHC, 1994.

Association of American Medical Colleges (AAMC). *ACME-TRI Report: Educating Medical Students.* Washington, D.C.: AAMC, 1992.

AAMC. *Academic Medicine and Health Care Reform: Roles for Medical Education in Health Care Reform.* Washington, D.C.: AAMC, 1994.

Association of State and Territorial Dental Directors. Testimony presented at a public hearing of the Institute of Medicine Committee on the Future of Dental Education, Washington, D.C., September 26-27, 1993.

Audet, A., Greenfield, S., and Field, M. Medical Practice Guidelines: Current Activities and Future Directions. *Annals of Internal Medicine* 113:709-714, 1990.

Bader, J.D. A Review of Evaluations of Effectiveness in Continuing Dental Education. *Mobius* 7:39-48, 1987.

Bader, J.D. Guest Editorial: The Emergence of Appropriateness-of-Care Issues. *Journal of Dental Research* 71(3):502-504, 1992.

Bader, J.D., and Shugars, D.A. Variation, Treatment Outcomes, and Practice Guidelines in Dental Practice. *Journal of Dental Education.* In press.

Bader, J.D., Rubinstein, L., Friedman, J., et al. Task Force on Innovation in Dental Hygiene Curricula. *Journal of Dental Education* 53:(12):731-737, 1989.

Bailit, H.L. *Environmental Issues in Dentistry: Reflections on the Practice of Dentistry in the 21st Century.* Durham, N.C.: Pew Health Professions Commission, 1987.

Bánóczy, J. The Evolution of Dental Education—-A European Perspective. *Journal of Dental Education* 57(8):634-636, 1993.

Barker, B.D., and O'Neil, E.H. Shaping the Future Profession: A New Tableau for Dental Education. *Journal of Dental Education* 56(4):229-235, 1992.

Batalden, P.B., Nelson, E.C., and Roberts, J.S. Linking Outcomes Measurement to Continual Improvement: The Serial "V" Way of Thinking About Improving Clinical Care. *Journal of Quality Improvement* 20(4):167-180, 1994.

Baughan, L.W., Hagan, B.A., and Dishman, M.V. Student Evaluation in the Comprehensive Care Setting. *Journal of Dental Education* 57(3):239-243, 1993.

Baum, B.J., Burstone, C.J., Dubner, R., et al. Advances in Diagnosis and Detection of Oral Diseases. *Advances in Dental Research* 3(1):7-13, 1989.

Baumol, W. J. *Private Affluence, Public Squalor.* Economic Research Reports. New York: C.V. Starr Center for Applied Economics, 1992.

Bepko, G. The Future of Promotion and Tenure for Dental School Faculty—A View from the University. *Journal of Dental Education* 55(10):681-688, 1991.

Berry, J. Parameters Project Ends in '91 House. *ADA News* 22(20):1,11,14, 1991.

Blackburn, R. Faculty Development: Policies and Practices. *Journal of Dental Education* 55(10):665-667, 1991.

Bland, C.J., and Ridky, J. Human and Organizational Resource Development. In *Managing in Academics: A Health Center Model.* J. Ridky and G.F. Sheldon, eds. St. Louis, Mo.: Quality Medical Publishing, 1993.

Blauch, L.E. *A Course of Study in Dentistry: Report of the Curriculum Survey Committee, American Association of Dental Schools.* Chicago, Ill.: American Association of Dental Schools, 1935.

Blumenthal, D., and Meyer, G.S. The Future of the Academic Medical Center Under Health Care Reform. *New England Journal of Medicine* 329:1812-1814, 1993.

Boyer, E. *Scholarship Reconsidered: Priorities of the Professoriate.* Princeton, N.J.: The Carnegie Foundation for the Advancement of Teaching, 1990.

Bradford, M. Dental Plans Filling a Need. *Business Insurance* December 21, 1992, p. 18.

Brook, R. Practice Guidelines and Practicing Medicine: Are They Compatible? *Journal of the American Medical Association* 262:3027-3030, 1989.

Brown, L.J. Trends in Tooth Loss Among U.S. Employed Adults from 1871 to 1985. *Journal of Dental Education* 125(5):533-549, 1994.

Bulger, R.J. Dental Education and the 21st Century. *Journal of Dental Education* 57(3):203-207, 1993.

Burner, S.T., Waldo, D.R., and McKusick, D.R. National Health Expenditure Projections Through 2030. *Health Care Financing Review* 14(1):1-29, 1992.

Burt, B.A., and Eklund, S.A. *Dentistry, Dental Practice, and the Community.* Philadelphia, Pa.: W.B. Saunders Company, 1992.

Bush, V. The Endless Frontier. Washington, D.C.: National Science Foundation, 1945.

Butters, J.M., Williams, J.H., and Abbott, L.J. Quality Assessment/Assurance Activities in U.S. Dental Schools. *Journal of Dental Education* 55(9):565-569, 1991.

Capilouto, E., Capilouto, M.L., and Ohsfeldt, R. A Review of Methods Used to Project the Future Supply of Dental Personnel and the Future Demand and Need for Dental Services. *Journal of Dental Education.* In press

Caplan, D.J., and Weintraub, J.A. The Oral Health Burden in the United States: A Summary of Recent Epidemiologists. *Journal of Dental Education* 57(12):853-862, 1993.

Caplan, D.J., Hollister, C., McKaig, R., Watkins, C., and Weintraub, J.A. Assessment of Oral Disease and Oral Health Status. Report prepared for the American Association of Dental Schools. University of North Carolina, Chapel Hill, December, 1992.

Carey, R.M., Wheby, M.S., and Reynolds, R.E. Evaluating Faculty Clinical Excellence in the Academic Health Sciences Center. *Academic Medicine* 68(11):813-817, 1993.

Carnegie Commission on Higher Education. *Higher Education and the Nation's Health: Policies for Medical and Dental Education.* New York: McGraw-Hill, 1970.

Carnegie Council on Policy Studies in Higher Education. *Progress and Problems in Medical and Dental Education.* San Francisco, Calif.: Jossey-Bass Publishers, 1976.

Centers for Disease Control (CDC). *Fluoridation Census.* Atlanta, Ga.: CDC, 1993.

Chambers, D.W. It's So Hard to Have a Dialogue with Yourself. *Journal of Dental Education* 56(6):380-383, 1992a.

Chambers, D.W. The Continuing Education Business. *Journal of Dental Education* 56(10):672-679, 1992b.

Clarkson, B.H., and Kremenak, N.W. The Value of Research Experience for Undergraduate Dental Students. *Journal of Dental Education* 47(4):276-278, 1983.

Coggeshall, L.T. *Planning for Medical Progress Through Education.* Evanston, Ill.: Association of American Medical Colleges, 1965.

Cohen, D.W., Cormier, P.P., and Cohen, J.L. *Educating the Dentist of the Future: The Pennsylvania Experiment.* Philadelphia, Pa.: University of Pennsylvania Press, 1985.

Cohen, D.W., Galbally, J., and Garfunkel, A.A. The Future of Dental Education. *Current Opinion in Dentistry* 1(4):451-459, 1991.

Commission on Dental Accreditation (CDA). Accreditation Standards for Dental Education Programs. Chicago, Ill.: ADA, May 1993a.

CDA. Testimony presented at a public hearing of the Institute of Medicine Committee on the Future of Dental Education, Washington, D.C., September 26-27, 1993b.

CDA. Listing of Accredited Predoctoral Dental Education Program. Chicago, Ill.: American Dental Association, January 1994a.

CDA. Listing of Advanced Specialty and General Dentistry Education Programs. Chicago, Ill.: American Dental Association, January 1994b.

CDA. Listing of Dental Assisting, Dental Hygiene, and Dental Laboratory Technology Education Programs. Chicago, Ill.: American Dental Association, January 1994c.

Consani, J.W. Presentation at a meeting of the Institute of Medicine Committee on the Future of Dental Education, Washington, D.C., September 27, 1993.

Corbin, S.B., and Kohn, W.G. The Benefits and Risks of Dental Amalgam: Current Findings Reviewed. *Journal of the American Dental Association* 125:381-388, 1994.

Council on Dental Education (CDE), American Dental Association. Requirements for the Approval of a Dental School. *Journal of the American Dental Association* 28:151-156, 1941.

Damiano, P.C., Shugars, D.A., and Freed, J.R. Clinical Board Examinations: Variation Found in Pass Rates. *Journal of the American Dental Association* 123:68-73, 1992.

Davis, D., and Parboosingh, J. "Academic" CME and the Social Contract. *Academic Medicine* 68(5):329-332, 1993.

Davis, D.A., Thomson, M.A., Oxman, A.A., et al. Evidence for the Effectiveness of CME: A Review of 50 Randomized Controlled Trials. *Journal of the American Medical Association* 268:1111-1117, 1992.

Dawes, C. Editorial: Should Dentists Be Doing What They Do. *Journal of Dental Research* 70:1221, 1991.

DePaola, D.P. The Basic Sciences: What Is Left After the Facts Are Forgotten? *Journal of Dental Education* 50(8):487-493, 1986.

DePaola, D.P. Impact of Dental Science on Dental Education: Past and Future. *Advances in Dental Research* 3(1):83-84, 1989.

Detmer, D.E., and Finney, M.D. The Academic Health Center: Issues and Leadership. In *Managing in Academics: A Health Center Model.* J. Ridky and G.F. Sheldon, eds. St. Louis, Mo.: Quality Medical Publishing, Inc., 1993.

DeVore, L.R. Allied Dental Education: Past, Present, and Future. *Journal of Dental Education* 57(8):611-615, 1993.

Dirksen, T.R. A Research Training Program for Dental Faculty. *Journal of Dental Education* 56(6):393-395, 1992.

Dodge, W.W., Dale, R.A., and Hendrickson, W.D. A Preliminary Study of the Effect of Eliminating Requirements on Clinical Performance. *Journal of Dental Education* 57(5):667-672, 1993.

Donabedian, A. *Aspects of Medical Care Administration: Specifying Requirements for Health Care.* Cambridge, Mass.: Harvard University Press, 1973.

Douglass, C. and Fein, R. Financing Dental Education. *Journal of Dental Education.* In press.

Douglass, C.W., and Fox, C.H. The Emerging Field of Oral Pharmaceuticals. *Journal of the American Dental Association* 125:2S-4S, 1994.

Douglass, C.W., Jette, A.M., Fox, C.H., et al. Oral Health Status of the Elderly in New England. *Journal of Gerontology: Medical Sciences* 48(2):M39-M46, 1993.

Dugoni, A.A. Licensure—A House Divided. *Journal of Dental Education* 57(10):770-771, 1993.

Dummett, C.O. *The Growth and Development of the Negro in Dentistry in the United States.* Chicago, Ill.: The Stanek Press, 1952.

East, T.D., Morris, A.H., and Wallace, C.J., et al. A Strategy for Development of Computerized Care Decision Support Systems. *International Journal of Clinical Monitoring and Computing* 8:263-269, 1992.

Eddy, D. Variations in Physician Practice: The Role of Uncertainty. *Health Affairs* 3:74-89, 1984.

Eddy, D. Practice Policies—What Are They? *Journal of the American Medical Association* 263:877-880, 1990.

Eddy, D. (in collaboration with the Council of Medical Specialty Societies). *A Manual for Assessing Health Practices and Designing Practice Policies: The Explicit Approach.* Philadelphia, Pa.: American College of Physicians, 1991.

Edelstein, B.L. The Medical Management of Dental Caries. *Journal of the American Dental Association* 125:31S-39S, 1994.

Eisenberg, J.M. *Doctors' Decisions and the Cost of Medical Care: The Reasons for Doctors' Practice Patterns and the Ways to Change Them.* Ann Arbor, Mich.: Health Administration Press, 1986.

Eisenberg, J.M. Clinical Economics: A Guide to the Economic Analysis of Clinical Practices. *Journal of the American Medical Association* 262:2879-2886, 1989.

Elliott, R.W. Anatomy of the Demise of Georgetown Dental School. *Journal of the American College of Dentists* 55(2):6,8-11, 1988.

Enarson, C., and Burg, F.D. An Overview of Reform Initiatives in Medical Education: 1906 Through 1992. *Journal of the American Medical Association* 268(9):1141-1143, 1992.

Feil, E.C., Welch, H.G., and Fisher, E.S. Why Estimates of Physician Supply and Requirements Disagree. *Journal of the American Medical Association* 269(20):2859-2863, 1993.

Fein, R. Medical Education: Impact of the Social Sciences on a Changing

Delivery System. In *Flexner: 75 Years Later. A Current Commentary on Medical Education.* C. Vevier, ed. Lanham, Md.: University Press of America, 1987.

Feldman, C.A., Baumritter, A., Levy, J., et al. Impact of Phase I Pew National Dental Education Program on U.S. Schools of Dental Medicine. *Journal of Dental Education* 55(5):307-315, 1991.

Flexner, A. *Medical Education in the United States and Canada: A Report to the Carnegie Foundation for the Advancement of Teaching.* Boston, Mass.: D.B. Updike, The Merrymount Press, 1910.

Formicola, A.J. The Dental Curriculum: The Interplay of Pragmatic Necessities, National Needs, and Educational Philosophies in Shaping Its Future. *Journal of Dental Education* 55(6):358-364, 1991.

Formicola, A.J. Where to Next? The Issues in Dentistry from the Perspective of a Dental Educator. *Journal of Dental Education* 57(3):212-214, 1993.

Foti, S.K. Mighty Machine: Will D.I.S.C. Drive the Profession? *Academy of General Dentistry Journal* 5-10, November 1992.

Fox, P.D., and Wasserman, J. Academic Medical Centers and Managed Care: Uneasy Partners. *Health Affairs* 12(1):85-93, 1993.

Freed, J.R., and Perry, D.A. *Access, Utilization and Quality of Independent Dental Hygiene Practices.* March 18, 1992.

Friedland, B., and Valachovic, R.W. The Regulation of Dental Licensing: The Dark Ages? *American Journal of Law and Medicine* 17(3):249-270, 1991.

Fritz, M.E. The Closing of the D.D.S. Program at Emory University. *Journal of the American College of Dentists* 55(2):7,12-17, 1988.

Gaines, J.H. Licensure. *Journal of Dental Education* 57(3):221-222, 1993.

Garrison, R.S. Traditional Patient Care Model Response. *Journal of Dental Education* 57(5):343-345, 1993.

Genco, R.J. Pharmaceuticals and Periodontal Diseases. *Journal of the American Dental Association* 125:11S-19S, 1994.

General Accounting Office. *Health Professions Education: Role of Title VII/VIII Programs in Improving Access to Care is Unclear.* GAO/HEHS-94-164. Washington, D.C.: United States General Accounting Office, 1994.

Gibson, Jr., W.A. Supporting Student Research at the Administrative Level. *Journal of Dental Education* 57(4):298-300, 1993.

Gies, W.J. *Dental Education in the U.S. and Canada: A Report to the Carnegie Foundation for the Advancement of Teaching.* New York: Carnegie Foundation for the Advancement of Teaching, 1926.

Gift, H.C., and Frew, R.A. Sealants: Changing Patterns. *Journal of the American Dental Association* 112:391-392, 1986.

Gift, H.C., and Newman, J.F. How Older Adults Use Oral Health Care Services: Results of a National Health Interview Survey. *Journal of the American Dental Association* 124:89-93, 1993.

Ginzberg, E., Ostow, M., and Dutka, A.B. *The Economics of Medical Education.* New York: Josiah Macy, Jr. Foundation, 1993.

Gray, C.F. Discussion Summary: Symposium on Required Postdoctoral Education Programs in General Dentistry. *Journal of Dental Education* 51(6):320-321, 1987.

Greenspan, J.S. Current and Future Prospects for Oral Health Science and Technology. *Journal of Dental Education*. In press.

Guarino, K.S. Licensure and Certification of Dentists and Accreditation of Dental Schools. *Journal of Dental Education*. In press.

Guerini, V. *A History of Dentistry: From the Most Ancient Times Until the End of the Eighteenth Century*. Philadelphia, Pa.: Lea & Febiger, 1909.

Halpern, S.A. Professional Schools in the American University. In *The Academic Profession: National, Disciplinary and Institutional Settings*. B.R. Clark, ed. Berkeley, Calif.: University of California Press, 1987, pp. 304-330.

Handelman, S., Meyerowitz, C., Iranpour, B., et al. Evaluation of Advanced General Dentistry Education. *Special Care in Dentistry* 13(S4):176-185, 1993.

Harrington, M.S. Organizational Characteristics of Dental Schools Associated with Research Productivity. *Journal of Dental Education* 51(10):583-588, 1987.

Harris, R.R. *Dental Science in a New Age: A History of the National Institute of Dental Research*. Rockville, Md.: Montrose Press, 1989.

Harris, S.E. *The Economics of Health Care: Finance and Delivery*. Berkeley, Calif.: McCutchan Publishing Corporation, 1975.

Hasler, J.F., and Hall, H.D. Faculty for Comprehensive Care Programs. *Journal of Dental Education* 48(6S):40-42, 1984.

Hebbeler, E.L. *Dental Education and Supply of Dentists: Policy Issues of the Eighties*. Atlanta, Ga.: Southern Regional Education Board, 1984.

Hein, J.W. Fostering Research Activity in Academic Dentistry: Comments on the National Scene. *Journal of Dental Education* 47(4):239-243, 1983.

Hendrickson, W.D., Payer, A.F., Rogers, L.P., et al. The Medical School Curriculum Committee Revisited. *Academic Medicine* 68(3):183-189, 1993.

Heyssel, R.M. *The Academic Medical Center: Old Responsibilities and New Realities*. Richard and Hinda Rosenthal Lectures at the Institute of Medicine, Washington, D.C., April 1990.

Hoffman-Axhelm, W. *History of Dentistry*. Chicago, Ill.: Quintessence Publishing Company, 1981.

Hogness, J.R. Prospects for Dental Education. *Journal of Dental Education* 46(3):129-134, 1982.

Hollinshead, B.S. *The Survey of Dentistry: The Final Report, Commission on the Survey of Dentistry in the United States*. Washington, D.C.: American Council on Education, 1961.

Hollister, M.C., and Weintraub, J.A. The Association of Oral Status with Systemic Health, Quality of Life, and Economic Productivity. *Journal of Dental Education* 57(12):901-912, 1993.

Honan, W.H. Wary of Entrenchment in the Ranks, Colleges Offer Alternatives to Tenure. *New York Times*, Wednesday, April 20, 1994a, p. B13.

Honan, W.H. New Law Against Age Bias on Campus Clogs Academic Pipeline, Critics Say. *New York Times*, Wednesday, June 15, 1994b, p. B9.

Horn, S., and Hopkins, D. *Clinical Practice Improvement: A New Technology for Developing Cost-Effective Quality Health Care*. New York: Faulkner and Gray, 1994.

Horner, H.H. *Dental Education Today*. Chicago, Ill.: University of Chicago Press, 1947.

Howell, J.D. Lowell T. Coggeshall and American Medical Education: 1901-1987. *Academic Medicine* 67(11):711-718, 1992.

Huber, R.M. *How Professors Play the Cat Guarding the Cream: Why We're Paying More and Getting Less in Higher Education*. Fairfax, Va.: George Mason University Press, 1992.

Hunt, L.R. Presentation to the Institute of Medicine Committee on the Future of Dental Education, Washington, D.C., September 27, 1993.

Hutchinson, R.A. Perceptions on Accreditation and Licensure. *Journal of Dental Education* 57(3):215-217, 1993.

Iglehart, J.K. The American Health Care System: Teaching Hospitals. *New England Journal of Medicine* 329:1052-1056, 1993.

Institute of Medicine (IOM). *Cost of Education of the Health Professions*. Washington, D.C.: National Academy Press, 1973.

IOM. *A Manpower Policy for Primary Health Care*. Washington, D.C.: National Academy of Sciences, 1978.

IOM. *DHEW's Research Planning Principles: A Review*. Washington, D.C.: National Academy Press, 1979.

IOM. *Public Policy Options for Better Dental Health*. Washington, D.C.: National Academy Press, 1980.

IOM. *Medical Education and Societal Needs: A Planning Report for the Health Professions*. Washington, D.C.: National Academy Press, 1983.

IOM. *Community Oriented Primary Care: A Practical Assessment. Volume I. The Committee Report*. Washington, D.C.: National Academy Press, 1984.

IOM. *Assessing Medical Technologies*. Washington, D.C.: National Academy Press, 1985.

IOM. *Allied Health Services: Avoiding Crises*. Washington, D.C.: National Academy Press, 1989a.

IOM. *Controlling Costs and Changing Patient Care? The Role of Utilization Management*. B. Gray and M. Field, eds. Washington, D.C.: National Academy Press, 1989b.

IOM. *Effectiveness Initiative: Setting Priorities for Clinical Conditions*. Washington, D.C.: National Academy Press, 1989c.

IOM. *Clinical Practice Guidelines: Directions for a New Program*. M.J. Field and K.N. Lohr, eds. Washington, D.C.: National Academy Press, 1990a.

IOM. Educating Dentists for the Future: Summary of a Planning Meeting, Washington, D.C., June 27, 1990b.

IOM. *Effectiveness and Outcomes in Health Care: Proceedings of an Invitational Conference.* K.A. Heithoff and K.N. Lohr, eds. Washington, D.C.: National Academy Press, 1990c.

IOM. *Funding Health Sciences Research: A Strategy to Restore Balance.* F.E. Bloom and M.A. Randolph, eds. Washington, D.C.: National Acadmy Press, 1990d.

IOM. *Medicare: A Strategy for Quality Assurance.* Vol. 1. K.N. Lohr, ed. Washington, D.C.: National Academy Press, 1990e.

IOM. *Guidelines for Clinical Practice: From Development to Use.* M.J. Field and K.N. Lohr, eds. Washington, D.C.: National Academy Press, 1992.

IOM. *Access to Health Care in America.* M. Millman, ed. Washington, D.C.: National Academy Press, 1993a.

IOM. *Assessing Health Care Reform.* M.J. Field, K.N. Lohr, and K.D. Yordy, eds. Washington, D.C.: National Academy Press, 1993b.

IOM. *Employment and Health Benefits: A Connection at Risk.* M.J. Field and H.T. Shapiro, eds. Washington, D.C.: National Academy Press, 1993c.

IOM. *Balancing the Scales of Opportunity: Ensuring Racial and Ethnic Diversity in the Health Professions.* M.E. Lewin and B. Rice, eds. Washington, D.C.: National Academy Press, 1994a.

IOM. *Careers in Clinical Research: Obstacles and Opportunities.* W.N. Kelley and M.A. Randolph, eds. Washington, D.C.: National Academy Press, 1994b.

IOM. *Definition of Primary Care: Interim Report.* M. Donaldson, K. Yordy and N. Vanselow, eds. Washington, D.C.: Institute of Medicine, 1994c.

IOM. *Health Data in the Information Age: Use, Disclosure, and Privacy.* M.S. Donaldson, and K.N. Lohr, eds. Washington, D.C.: National Academy Press, 1994d.

IOM and AADS. Survey of Deans of United States Dental Schools. Unpublished analysis, January 1994.

Isman, R.E. Integrating Primary Oral Health Care into Primary Care. *Journal of Dental Education* 57(12):846-852, 1993.

Jeffcoat, M.K., and Clark, W.B. Research, Technology Transfer, and Dentistry. *Journal of Dental Education.* In press.

Jolin, L.D., Jolly, P., Krakower, J.Y., and Beran, R. U. S. Medical School Finances. *Journal of the American Medical Association* 268:1149-1155, September 2, 1992.

Jonas, H.S., Etzel, S.I., and Barzansky, B. Educational Programs in U.S. Medical Schools. *Journal of the American Medical Association* 270:1061-1068, 1993.

Jones, J.A., and Levinson, P., with Gibson, G. Overview of VA Oral Health Services and Eligibility. Presentation for Conference on Oral Health for Aging Veterans, Department of Veterans Affairs and Foundation for Health Services Research, Washington, D.C., November 30-December 2, 1993.

Kalkwarf, K.L. Dental Faculty Tenure. Relationship of the Dental Faculty to the University Tenure System. *Journal of the American College of Dentistry* 53(3):14-19, 1986.

Kantor, M.L., ed. Symposium Proceedings, Clinical Decision Making in Dentistry. *Journal of Dental Education* 56(12):788-878, 1992.

Kaste, L.M., Marianos, D., Chang, R., et al. The Assessment of Nursing Caries and Its Relationship to High Caries in the Permanent Dentition. *Journal of Public Health Dentistry* 52:64-68, 1992.

Keefe, M.M. Dental Benefits Market Has Evolved but Where Is it Headed? *Employee Benefit Plan Review* 48(9):24-26, 1994.

Keller, J.C., Seydel, S.K., Kremenak, N.W., et al. The Development of a Dental Student Research Program. *Journal of Dental Education* 57(5):369-372, 1993.

Kennedy, J.E. Alternatives to Traditional Tenure. *Journal of Dental Education* 48(9):506-508, 1984.

Kentucky Council on Higher Education. *Kentucky Dental Manpower/Dental Education Report*, staff report. Frankfort, Kent.: November 9, 1992.

Kentucky Council on Higher Education. *Action Item: Dental Education.* Frankfort, Kent.: February 8, 1993.

Kibbe, D.C., Kaluzny, A.D., and McLaughlin, C.P. Integrating Guidelines with the Continuous Quality Improvement: Doing the Right Thing the Right Way to Achieve the Goal. *Journal of Quality Improvement* 20:181-191, 1994.

Kidd, F., ed. *Profile of the Negro in American Dentistry.* Washington, D.C.: Howard University Press, 1979.

Kindig, D.A.. Counting Generalist Physicians. *Journal of the American Medical Association* 271(19):1505-1507, 1994.

Kindig, D.A., Cultice, J.M., and Mullan, F. The Elusive Generalist Physician: Can We Reach a 50% Goal? *Journal of the American Medical Association* 270:1069-1073, 1993.

Kraemer, L.G. The Dental Hygiene Entry Dilemma: An Issue of Prestige, Image and Professional Credibility. *Dental Hygienists* 59:117-120, 1985.

Krakower, J.Y., Jolly, P., and Beran, R. U.S. Medical School Finances. *Journal of the American Medical Association* 270:1085-1091, 1993.

Leigh, T.M., Young, P.R., and Haley, J.V. Performances of Family Practice Diplomates on Successive Mandatory Recertification Examinations. *Academic Medicine* 68(12):912-919, 1993.

Leinfelder, K. Current Developments in Dentin Bonding Systems: Major Progress Found in Today's Products. *Journal of the American Dental Association* 124(5):40-45, 1993.

Linthicum, D.S. and Moreland, E.F. Cost of Accreditation Process to the Dental School. *Journal of Baltimore College of Dental Surgery* 35(1):12-18, 1981.

Lipton, J.A. *International Comparison of Research Performance at Dental Institutions.* Presented at Annual Meeting of the American Association for Dental Research, Cincinnati, Ohio, March 7, 1990.

Lipton, J.A., Ship, J.A., and Larach-Robinson, D. Estimated Prevalence and Distibution of Reported Orofacial Pain in the United States. *Journal of the American Dental Association* 124:115-121, 1993.

Little St. Simons Conference on the PGY-1 Requirement for Graduates of U.S. Dental Schools. Anticipating the Next Oral Health Manpower Crisis. Little St. Simons, Georgia, May 1-2, 1993.

Littleton, Jr., P.A. Educating Dentists for the Future. In *Human Resources for Health: Defining the Future.* Washington, D.C.: Association of Academic Health Centers, 1992, pp. 141-154.

Löe, H. Forty Years of Progress. *Advances in Dental Research* 3(1):3-6, 1989.

Lomas, J. Words Without Action: The Production, Dissemination, and Impact of Consensus Recommendations. *Annual Review of Public Health* 12:41-65, 1991.

Lovrinic, J.G., DeHayes, Jr., D.W., and Althoff, E.J. Developing an Economic Model: How One Midwestern University Is Approaching Cost Control. *NACUBO Business Officer* 27(1):34-39, 1993.

Mandel, I.W. The Plaque Fighters: Choosing a Weapon. *Journal of Dental Education* 124(4):71-74, 1994.

Marston, R.Q., and Jones, R.M., eds. Medical Education in Transition. *Report of the Commission on Medical Education: The Sciences of Medical Practice.* Princeton, N.J.: Robert Wood Johnson Foundation, 1992.

Martin, E. D., Department of Defense, Office of the Assistant Secretary for Defense, Health Affairs. Testimony submitted to the Institute of Medicine Committee on the Future of Dental Education, Washington, D.C., October 13, 1993.

Martini, C. Evaluating the Competence of Health Professions. *Journal of the American Medical Association* 260:1057-1058, 1988.

Maryniuk, G.A. and Brunson, W.D. When to Replace Faulty-Margin Amalgam Restorations. *General Dentistry* 47:463-467, 1989.

McCallum, C.A. Interhealth Science Relationships in Fostering Dental Research. *Journal of Dental Education* 47(4):244-251, 1983.

McCluggage, R.W. *A History of the American Dental Association: A Century of Health Service.* Chicago, Ill.: American Dental Association, 1959.

McClure, F.J. *Water Fluoridation: The Search and the Victory.* Bethesda, Md.: U.S. Department of Health, Education, and Welfare, 1970.

McDonald, C.J., and Overhage, J.M. Guidelines You Can Follow and Can Trust: An Ideal and an Example. *Journal of the American Medical Association* 271(11):872-873, 1994.

McGuire, J.W., et al. The Efficient Production of "Reputation" by Prestige Research Universities in the United States. *Journal of Higher Education* 59:365-389, 1988.

McNeil, D.R. *The Fight for Fluoridation.* New York: Oxford University Press, 1957.

McPheeters, H.L. *Costs and Funding of University Health Professions Programs.* Atlanta, Ga.: Southern Regional Education Board, 1987.

Mercer, J. UCLA Adjusts to Painful Budget Surgery. *The Chronicle of Higher Education,* April 20, 1994, pp. A37,A38,A41.

Meskin, L.H. Faculty Development: Commentary. *Journal of Dental Education* 47(4):274-275, 1983.

Miles, S.H., Lurie, N., Fisher, E.S., et al. Academic Health Centers and Health Care Reform. *Academic Medicine* 68(9):648-653, 1993.

Miller, D.L. Reentry: Manpower Issues Related to Nonpracticing Hygienists. *Journal of Dental Hygiene* 64:226-234, 1990.

Moher, D., Dulberg, C.S., and Wells, G.A. Statistical Power, Sample Size, and Their Reporting in Randomized Controlled Trials. *Journal of the American Medical Association* 272:122-124, 1994.

Motley, W.E. *History of the American Dental Hygienists' Association, 1923-1982.* Chicago, Ill.: American Dental Hygienists' Association, 1986.

Nash, D.A. The Future of Allied Dental Education: Creating a Professional TEAM. *Journal of Dental Education* 57(8):619-622, 1993.

Nash, D.B., Markson, L.E., Howell, S., et al. Evaluating the Competence of Physicians in Practice: From Peer Review to Performance Assessment. *Academic Medicine* 68(2):S19-S26, 1993.

National Academy of Sciences (NAS). *Personnel Needs and Training for Biomedical and Behavioral Research.* Washington, D.C.: National Academy Press, 1985.

NAS. *1989 Report of the Committee on Biomedical and Behavioral Research Personnel.* Washington, D.C.: National Academy Press, 1989.

NAS. *Meeting the Nation's Needs for Biomedical and Behavioral Scientists.* Washington, D.C.: National Academy Press, 1994.

National Board of Examiners in Optometry (NBEO) *Examiners Manual: Part III—Patient Care Test: Clinical Skills Component.* Bethesda, Md.: NBEO, 1993.

National Cancer Institute (NCI). *Cancer Statistics Review 1973-1987.* Publication No. NIH 88-2789. Bethesda, Md.: National Institutes of Health, 1989.

National Center for Health Statistics (NCHS). *Decayed, Missing, and Filled Teeth in Adults: United States 1960-1962.* Public Health Service Publication No. 1000, Series 11, No. 23. Washington, D.C.: U.S. Department of Health, Education, and Welfare, Public Health Service, 1967.

NCHS. *Decayed, Missing, and Filled Teeth Among Children: United States.* DHEW Publication No. (HSM) 72-1003, Series 11, No. 106. Rockville, Md.: U.S. Department of Health, Education, and Welfare, 1971.

NCHS. *Decayed, Missing, and Filled Teeth Among Youths 12-17 Years: United States.* DHEW Publication No. (HRA) 75-1626, Series 11, No. 106. Rockville, Md.: U.S. Department of Health, Education, and Welfare, 1974a.

NCHS. *Edentulous Persons: United States 1971.* DHEW Publication No. (HRA) 74-1516, Series 10, No. 89. Rockville, Md.: U.S. Department of Health, Education, and Welfare, 1974b.

NCHS. *Current Estimates from the Health Interview Survey, United*

States—1975. Vital and Health Statistics, Series 10, No. 115. Rockville, Md.: U.S. Department of Health, Education, and Welfare, Public Health Service, National Center for Health Statistics, 1977.

NCHS. *Current Estimates from the Health Interview Survey: United States—1977.* Vital and Health Statistics, Series 10, No. 126. Hyattsville, Md.: U.S. Department of Health, Education, and Welfare, 1978.

NCHS. *Basic Data on Dental Examination Findings of Persons 1-74 Years: United States, 1971-74.* DHEW Publication No. (PHS) 81-1662, Series 11, No. 214. Hyattsville, Md.: U.S. Department of Health, and Human Services, 1979.

NCHS. *Decayed. Missing and Filled Teeth Among Persons 1-74 Years: United States.* DHHS Publication No. (PHS) 81-1673, Series 11, No. 223. Hyattsville, Md.: U.S. Department of Health and Human Services, 1981.

NCHS. *Dental Services and Oral Health: United States, 1989.* DHHS Publication No. (PHS) 93-1511, Series 10, No. 183. Hyattsville, Md.: U.S. Department of Health, and Human Services, 1992a.

NCHS. *Trends in Childhood Use of Dental Care Products Containing Fluoride: United States, 1983-89.* Advance Data 219. November 20, 1992b.

National Institute of Dental Research (NIDR). *The Prevalence of Dental Caries in United States Children, 1979-1980.* NIH Publication No. 82-2245. Bethesda, Md.: National Institutes of Health, 1981.

NIDR. *Oral Health of United States Children.* NIH Publication No. 89-2247. Bethesda, Md.: National Institutes of Health, 1989.

NIDR. *Broadening the Scope: Long-Range Research Plan for the Nineties.* Publication No. 90-1188. Bethesda, Md.: National Institutes of Health, 1990.

NIDR. *Extramural Program Report.* Bethesda, Md.: National Institutes of Health, 1993a.

NIDR. *Report of the Blue Ribbon Panel on Envisioning the Future of the National Institute of Dental Research (NIDR) Intramural Research Program.* Bethesda, Md.: National Institutes of Health, 1993b.

National Institutes of Health (NIH). *NIH Data Book, 1993.* Bethesda, Md.: NIH, 1993.

National Research Council (NRC). *Ending Mandatory Retirement for Tenured Faculty: The Consequences for Higher Education.* Washington, D.C.: National Academy Press, 1991.

NRC and IOM. *Toward a National Health Care Survey: A Data System for the 21st Century.* G.S. Wunderlich, ed. Washington, D.C.: National Academy Press, 1992.

Neidle, E.A. A Paradigm of Failure. *Journal of Dental Education* 50(8):455-457, 1986a.

Neidle, E.A. To Make Things Right. *Journal of Dental Education* 50(6):297-299, 1986b.

New York Times. Fewer black men attend college and graduation rates stay low. *New York Times,* Wednesday, March 2, 1994, p. B8.

Newbrun, E., and Leverett, D. Risk Assessment Dental Caries Working Group Summary Statement. In *Risk Assessment in Dentistry*. J.D. Bader, ed. Chapel Hill, N.C.: University of North Carolina, 1990, pp. 304-305.

Newhouse, J.P. Medical Care Costs: How Much Welfare Loss? *Journal of Economic Perspectives* 6(3):3-21, Summer 1992.

Norman, G.R., and Schmidt, H.G. The Psychological Basis of Problem-based Learning: A Review of the Evidence. *Academic Medicine* 67:557-565, 1992.

Northeast Regional Board of Dental Examiners (NERB). Testimony presented at a public hearing of the Institute of Medicine Committee on the Future of Dental Education, Washington, D.C., September 26-27, 1993.

Office of Technology Assessment (OTA), U.S. Congress. *Children's Dental Services Under the Medicaid Program—Background Paper*, OTA-BP-H-78. Washington, D.C.: U.S. Government Printing Office, 1990.

OTA. *Health Technologies that Work: Searching for Evidence*, OTA-H-608. Washington, D.C.: U.S. Government Printing Office, 1994.

Orlando, F.J. *William John Gies: His Contribution to the Advancement of Dentistry*. New York: The William J. Gies Foundation for the Advancement of Dentistry, 1992.

O'Sullivan, D.M., and Tinanoff, N. Maxillary Anterior Caries Associated with Increased Caries in Other Primary Teeth. *Journal of Dental Research* 72:1577-1580, 1993.

Page, L. Discrimination or Discriminating? *American Medical News*, February 28, 1994, pp. 3,7.

Parker, E.M. Faculty Development: Essence of Faculty and Institutional Vitality. *Journal of Dental Education* 55(10):656-659, 1991.

Petersdorf, R.G. Medical Education: The Process, Students, Teachers and Patients. In *Flexner: 75 Years Later. A Current Commentary on Medical Education*. C. Vevier, ed. Lanham, Md.: University Press of America, 1987.

Pew Health Professions Commission. *Perspectives on the Health Professions*. Durham, N.C.: 1990.

Pew Health Professions Commission. *Healthy America: Practitioners for 2005*. Durham, N.C.: 1991.

Pew Health Professions Commission. Draft Recommendations from the Pew Health Professions Commission. *Journal of Dental Education* 56(6):366-374, 1992.

Pew Health Professions Commission. *Health Professions Education for the Future: Schools in Service to the Nation*. San Francisco, Calif.: Pew Health Professions Commission, 1993.

Physician Payment Review Commission (PPRC). *Annual Report to Congress, 1994*. Washington, D.C.: PPRC, 1994.

President's Council of Advisors on Science and Technology. *Renewing the Promise: Research-Intensive Universities and the Nation*. Washington, D.C.: U.S. Government Printing Office, 1992.

Prinz, H. *Dental Chronology*. Philadelphia, Pa.: Lea & Febiger, 1945.

Prockop, D.J. Basic Science and Clinical Practice. In *Medical Education in Transition*. R.Q. Marston and R.M. Jones, eds. Princeton, N.J.: Robert Wood Johnson Foundation, 1992.

Ranney, R.R. Future Impact of Dental Science on Dental Education. *Advances in Dental Research* 3(1):80-82, 1989.

Reinhardt, J.W., and Douglass, C.W. The Need for Operative Dentistry Services: Projecting the Effects of Changing Disease Patterns. *Operative Dentistry* 14:114-120, 1989.

Ridky, J., and Sheldon, G.F, eds. *Managing in Academics: A Health Center Model*. St. Louis, Mo.: Quality Medical Publishing, 1993.

Rivo, M.L., Saultz, J.W., Wartman, S.A., et al. Defining the Generalist Physician's Training. *Journal of the American Medical Association* 271(19):1499-1504, 1994.

Robinson, T.C. Overview of Allied Health Issues in Contemporary Health Care. *Journal of Dental Education* 57(8):616-618, 1993.

Rosebury, T. *On Bulletin Number Nineteen: Thirty Years Later—A Tribute to William J. Gies*. Presented at the International Association of Dental Research, 1955 and reprinted in Orland (1992).

Roth, G.I. Student Disaffection with Basic Science. *Journal of Dental Education* 50(8):462-464, 1986.

Sakkab, N.Y. Relations Between the University and Industry. *Journal of Dental Education* 47(4):253-257, 1983.

Santangelo, M.V. The History and Development of United States Dental Education. *Journal of Dental Education* 45(10):619-627, 1981.

Santangelo, M.V. Required Postdoctoral Education Programs in General Dentistry: Accreditation Issues. *Journal of Dental Education* 51(6):280-287, 1987.

Scheetz, J.P., and Mendel, R.W. Update on Scholarship Among Dental Faculty. *Journal of the American College of Dentists* 60(1):36-40, 1993.

Schulz, D.F., Chalmers, I., Grimes, D.A., et al. Assessing the Quality of Randomization from Reports of Controlled Trials Published in Obstetrics and Gynecology Journals. *Journal of the American Medical Association* 272(2):125-128, 1994.

Schuster, J.H., and Wheeler, D. *Enhancing Faculty Careers: Strategies for Development and Renewal*. San Francisco, Calif.: Jossey-Bass, 1990.

Searle, J. The Storm over the University. *New York Review of Books* 37:24-42, 1990.

Shapiro, H.T. The Future of the Academic Health Center and the Research University: New Missions? New Roles? New Models? In *Academic Health Centers: Missions, Markets, and Paradigms for the Next Century*. Association of Academic Health Centers (AAHC). J.P. Howe, III, M. Osterweis, and E.R. Rubin, eds. Washington, D.C.: AAHC, 1994.

Shnorkian, H.I., and Zullo, T.G. A Survey of Faculty Practice Plans in United States and Canadian Dental Schools. *Journal of Dental Education* 57(4):316-320, 1993.

Sissman, I. *75 Years of Dentistry, "University of Pittsburgh": A History of the School of Dental Medicine.* Pittsburgh, Pa.: School of Dental Medicine, University of Pittsburgh, 1971.

Slade, M. A Little Law School Does Battle with the A.B.A. *New York Times,* February 4, 1994, p. A19.

Smith, L.W. Medical Education for the 21st Century. *Journal of Medical Education* 60:106-112, 1985.

Solomon, E.S. Association Reports—The Oral Health Research Work-Force. *Journal of Dental Education* 57(11):821-826, 1993.

Solomon, E.S., and Whiton, J.C. Dental Seniors' Evaluation of Their Curriculum and the Number of Clock Hours of Instruction. *Journal of Dental Education* 55(11):743-745, 1991.

Solomon, E.S., Gray, C.F., Whiton, J.C., et al. Dental Hygiene Enrollment and Institutional Affiliation. *Journal of Dental Education* 56(5):349-353, 1992.

Somers, H.M., and Somers, A.R. *Doctors, Patients and Health Insurance.* Washington, D.C.: The Brookings Institution, 1963.

Spaeth, D. Here We Go Again: Insurers Send Letters Pointing Out Utilization. *ADA News* 22(18):16,35, 1991.

Spaeth, D. Parameters Get House Go-Ahead. *ADA News* 24(22):20,22, 1993.

Spaeth, D. Parameters Group "Surprised" at Progress of First Meeting. *ADA News* 25(4):1,21, 1994.

Spolsky, V.W., Kamberg, C.J., Lohr, K.N., et al. *Measurement of Dental Health Status.* Santa Monica, Calif.: The RAND Corporation, 1983.

Starr, P. *The Social Transformation of American Medicine.* United States: Basic Books, 1982.

Stemmler, E.J. The Medical School—Where Does It Go from Here? *Academic Medicine* 64(1989):182-185, 1989.

Stephens, A. The Ultimate Challenge: The Loyola Experience. Presentation at the 1993 Annual Meeting of the American Association of Dental Schools, Chicago, Illinois, March 8, 1993.

Stiell, I.G., McKnight, R.D., Greenberg, G.H., et al. Implementation of the Ottawa Ankle Rules. *Journal of the American Medical Association* 271:827-832, 1994.

Stritter, F.T. Managing the Educational Process. In *Managing in Academics: A Health Center Model.* J. Ridky and G.F. Sheldon, eds. St. Louis, Mo.: Quality Medical Publishing, 1993.

Stromberg, C.D. *Health Care Credentialing: Implications for Academic Health Centers.* Washington, D.C.: Association of Academic Health Centers, 1992 p. 16.

Taubman, M.A., Genco, R.J., and Hillman, J.D. The Specific Pathogen-free Human: A New Frontier in Oral Infectious Disease Research. *Advances in Dental Research* 3(1):58-68, 1989.

Tedesco, L.A. Issues in Dental Curriculum Development and Change. *Journal of Dental Education.* In press.

Tedesco, L.A., Eisner, J.E., Vullo, R., et al. The Buffalo Approach to

Changing the Basic Science Curriculum or Toiling and Dreaming in the Vineyards of Dental Education. *Journal of Dental Education* 56(5):332-340, 1992.

Ten Cate, A.R. More or Less. *Journal of Dental Education* 50(8):474-476, 1986.

Ten Pas, W.S. Accreditation. *Journal of Dental Education* 57(3):224, 1993.

Thier, S.O. Dental Education in the Future. *Journal of Dental Education* 55(6):353-355, 1991.

Tilson, H. Observational Studies Making an Overdue and Much-Needed Comeback: Alternatives and Complements to Randomization. *Clinical Trials and Statistics: Proceedings of a Symposium.* Board on Mathematical Sciences, Commission on Physical Sciences, Mathematics, and Applications, National Research Council. Washington, D.C.: National Academy Press, 1993.

Tunnicliff, R. Avoiding the Bite: An Alternative to Costly Dental Insurance. *Washington Post,* May 19, 1994, p. D5.

U.S. Department of Commerce, Bureau of Census. *Statistical Abstract of the United States 1993.* Washington, D.C.: U.S. Government Printing Office, 1993.

U.S. Department of Defense. Testimony presented at a public hearing of the Institute of Medicine Committee on the Future of Dental Education, Washington, D.C., September 26-27, 1993.

U.S. Department of Health and Human Services (USDHHS), Office of Inspector General (OIG). *The NIH Consensus Development Program: Dissemination of Findings Through Medical School Continuing Education Activities,* Washington, D.C., February 1994.

USDHHS, OIG. *The Licensure of Out-of-State Dentists.* Washington, D.C., August 1993.

USDHHS, Public Health Service (PHS). Final Report to the House of Representatives Appropriations Committee on Oral Health Activities. Unpublished report. Washington, D.C., May 1989.

USDHHS, PHS. *Healthy People 2000: National Health Promotion and Disease Prevention Objectives.* Washington, D.C.: U.S. Government Printing Office, 1990.

USDHHS, PHS. *Review of Fluoride: Benefits and Risks.* Washington, D.C., Rockville, Md.: 1991.

USDHHS, PHS. *Health Personnel in the United States: Eighth Report to Congress, 1991.* Rockville, Md.: September 1992.

U.S. Department of Labor, Bureau of Labor Statistics. *Employee Benefits in Medium and Large Firms, 1989.* Washington, D.C.: U.S. Government Printing Office, 1990.

U.S. Department of Labor, Bureau of Labor Statistics. *Employee Benefits in Small Private Establishments, 1990.* Washington, D.C.: U.S. Government Printing Office, 1991.

U.S. Department of the Treasury, Public Health Service. *A Survey of Dental Activities of State Departments and Institutions of the United States.* Washington, D.C.: U.S. Government Printing Office, 1936.

U.S. Preventive Services Task Force. *Guide to Clinical Preventive Services: An Assessment of the Effectiveness of 169 Interventions.* Baltimore, Md.: Williams & Wilkins, 1989, p. 354

U.S. Public Health Service (USPHS), Oral Health Coordinating Committee. Toward Improving the Oral Health of Americans: An Overview of Oral Health Status, Resources, and Care Delivery. *Public Health Reports* 108(6):657-672, 1993.

U.S. Senate Appropriations Committee Hearing. FY 1994 Health Resources and Services Administration, p. 41.

University of California, Universitywide Health Sciences Committee. *Universitywide Health Sciences Applicant Pool Study and Outreach Program Inventory.* Vol. I: Executive Summary. Oakland, Calif.: University of California, 1993.

University of Illinois at Chicago. *College of Dentistry 1993-1995 Catalog.* Chicago, Ill.: University of Illinois at Chicago, 1993.

Vanselow, N.A. Academic Health Centers: Can They Survive? *Issues in Science and Technology* 2(4):55-64, Summer 1986.

Vernon, D.T., and Blake, R.L. Does Problem-Based Learning Work? A Meta-Analysis of Evaluative Research. *Academic Medicine* 68:550-563, 1993.

Vevier, C., ed. *Flexner: 75 Years Later. A Current Commentary on Medical Education.* Lanham, Md.: University Press of America, 1987.

Vining, R.V. Comprehensive Dental Care: Objectives, Management, and Financial Impact. *Journal of Dental Education* 48(Supplement):11, 1984.

Ward, H.L. The Development of the Dental Curriculum. *Journal of the American College of Dentists* 39(2):106-113, 1972.

Weeks, W.B., Wallace, A.E., Wallace, M.M., et al. A Comparison of the Educational Costs and Incomes of Physicians and Other Professionals. *New England Journal of Medicine* 330:1280-1286, 1994.

Weiner, J.P. Forecasting the Effects of Health Reform on U.S. Physician Workforce Requirement. *Journal of the American Medical Association* 272:222-230, 1994.

Weiss, S. College Accreditors Feeling Criticism. *New York Times*, January 28, 1994, p. A19.

Wennberg, J. Dealing with Medical Practice Variations: A Proposal for Action. *Health Affairs* 3(2):6-32, 1984.

Wennberg, J. What is Outcomes Research? In Institute of Medicine, *Medical Innovations at the Crossroads.* Vol. 1, *Modern Methods of Clinical Investigation.* A. Gelijns, ed. Washington, D.C.: National Academy Press, 1990.

Wennberg, J.E., Goodman, D.C., Nease, R.F., et al. Finding Equilibrium in U.S. Physican Supply. *Health Affairs* 12(2):89-103, 1993.

Westerman, G.H., Grandy, T.G., Ocanto, R.A., et al. Perceived Sources of Stress in the Dental School Environment. *Journal of Dental Education* 57(3):225-231, 1993.

Wheatley, S.C. *The Politics of Philanthropy: Abraham Flexner and*

Medical Education. Madison, Wisc.: The University of Wisconsin Press, 1988.

Wheeler, D. Development Strategies: More than Workshops. *Journal of Dental Education* 55(10):659-661, 1991.

White, B.A., Caplan, D.J., and Weintraub, J.A. A Quarter Century of Changes in Oral Health in the United States. *Journal of Dental Education.* In press.

Williams, A.P., Carter, G.M., Hammons, G.T., et al. *Managing for Survival: How Successful Academic Medical Centers Cope with Harsh Environments.* Santa Monica, Calif.: The RAND Corporation, 1987.

Winston, J.L. A Student's Expectations of the Research Experience. *Journal of Dental Education* 57(4):295-297, 1993.

Wisconsin Governor's Commission on Dental Care. *Final Report.* Madison, Wisc.: April 1993.

Wise, M.O. Letter to Mr. George Schroeder (Director, Legislative Audit Council, State of South Carolina). Washington, D.C. Federal Trade Commission, Office of Consumer and Competition Advocacy, January 8, 1993.

Wolff, R.A. Restoring the Credibility of Accreditation. *The Chronicle of Higher Education,* June 9, 1993, pp. B1-B2.

World Health Organization (WHO). *Alma-Ata 1978: Primary Health Care.* Report of the International Conference on Primary Health Care, Alma-Ata, USSR, September 6-12, 1978. Geneva: WHO, 1978.

Wotman, S. Dental Education 1989: How Are We Adapting to Change? *Journal of Dental Education* 53(12):697-703, 1989.

Zelen, M. Large Simple Trials: The Open Protocol System. In *Clinical Trials and Statistics: Proceedings of a Symposium.* Board on Mathematical Sciences, Commission on Physical Sciences, Mathematics, and Applications, National Research Council. Washington, D.C.: National Academy Press, 1993.

Zubkoff, M., Raskin, I.E., and Hanft, R.S., eds. *Hospital Cost Containment: Selected Notes for Future Policy.* New York: Milbank Memorial Fund, 1978.

A

Committee on the Future of Dental Education Liaison Panels

STATE AND REGIONAL PANELS

Lewis S. Earle, D.D.S.
Winter Park, Florida

Henry Finger, D.D.S.
Nedford, New Jersey

James H. Gaines, D.M.D.
Greenville, South Carolina

Kathryn Kell, D.D.S.
Davenport, Iowa

Joseph R. Kenneally, D.M.D.
Biddeford, Maine

Richard D. Leshgold, D.D.S.
Seattle, Washington

Lawrence Meskin, D.D.S., Ph.D.
University of Colorado Health
    Sciences Center
Denver, Colorado

M. Raynor Mullins, D.M.D.
University of Kentucky
College of Dentistry
Lexington, Kentucky

William B. Risk, D.D.S.
Lafayette, Indiana

Peter D. Roberson, D.D.S.
Chicago, Illinois

Sam W. Rogers, D.D.S.
Houston, Texas

Jacqueline A. Roy, D.D.S., D.Hyg.
Utica, New York

Samuel E. Selcher, D.M.D.
Middletown, Pennsylvania

Robert G. Smith, D.D.S.
Prairie Village, Kansas

Ronald Stifter, D.D.S.
Milwaukee, Wisconsin

William A. van Dyk, D.D.S.
San Pablo, California

COMMITTEE ON THE FUTURE OF DENTAL EDUCATION SPECIALTY PANEL

AMERICAN ACADEMY OF ORAL PATHOLOGY

John J. Sauk, D.D.S., Ph.D.
Professor and Chairman
University of Maryland
Baltimore, Maryland

AMERICAN ACADEMY OF PEDIATRIC DENTISTRY

Martin J. Davis, D.D.S.
Dean for Student Affairs
School of Dental and Oral Surgery
Columbia University
New York, New York

AMERICAN ACADEMY OF PERIODONTOLOGY

Paul B. Robertson, D.D.S.
Dean
School of Dentistry
University of Washington Health Science
Seattle, Washington

AMERICAN ASSOCIATION OF ENDODONTISTS

Henry J. Van Hassel, D.D.S., Ph.D.
Editor
Journal of Endodontics
Portland, Oregon

AMERICAN ASSOCIATION OF ORAL AND MAXILLOFACIAL SURGEONS

Raymond P. White, Jr., D.D.S., Ph.D.
Professor of Oral and Maxillofacial Surgery
University of North Carolina
School of Dentistry
Chapel Hill, North Carolina

AMERICAN ASSOCIATION OF ORTHODONTISTS

Joseph G. DiStasio, D.M.D., M.D.S.
Private Practice/Associate Clinical Professor
Tufts University, School of Dental Medicine
Revere, Massachusetts

AMERICAN BOARD OF DENTAL PUBLIC HEALTH

Linda C. Niessen, D.M.D., M.P.H., M.P.P.
Chairman, Department of Community Dentistry
Baylor University
Dallas, Texas

AMERICAN COLLEGE OF PROSTHODONTISTS

Ronald Desjardins, D.M.D., M.S.D.
Professor of Dentistry
Mayo Clinic
Rochester, Minnesota

THE ACADEMY OF GENERAL DENTISTRY

Ludwig Leibsohn, D.D.S.
New York, New York

COMMITTEE ON THE FUTURE OF DENTAL EDUCATION FACULTY PANEL

Nancy S. Arbree, D.D.S.
Tufts University
Boston, Massachusetts

Leif K. Bakland, D.D.S.
Loma Linda University
Loma Linda, California

Richard Bebermeyer, D.D.S.
University of Texas Health
   Science Center-Houston
Houston, Texas

David Brunson, D.D.S.
University of North Carolina at
   Chapel Hill
Chapel Hill, North Carolina

Ellen Byrne, D.D.S.
Medical College of Virginia
Virginia Commonwealth Univesity
Richmond, Virginia

Kenneth B. Chance, D.D.S.
University of Medicine and
   Dentistry of New Jersey
Newark, New Jersey

Teresa Dolan, D.D.S., M.P.H.
University of Florida
Gainesville, Florida

Amy Everett, D.D.S.
West Virginia University
Morgantown, West Virginiaw

Cathy Gogan, D.D.S.
State University of New York at
   Buffalo
Buffalo, New York

Denis P. Lynch, D.D.S., Ph.D.
The University of Tennessee-
   Memphis
Memphis, Tennessee

Phil Marucha, D.M.D., Ph.D.
The Ohio State University
Columbus, Ohio

Gail E. Molinari, D.D.S.
University of Detroit-Mercy
Detroit, Michigan

Ethel Newman, D.D.S.
Howard University
Washington, D.C.

Robert Ord, D.D.S., M.D.
University of Maryland at
   Baltimore
Baltimore, Maryland

John William Reinhardt, D.D.S.
The University of Iowa
Iowa City, Iowa

Richard A. Reinhardt, D.D.S.,
   Ph.D.
University of Nebraska Medical
   Center
Lincoln, Nebraska

Stephen L. Silberman, D.M.D.
The University of Mississippi
   Medical Center
Jackson, Mississippi

Martha J. Somerman, D.D.S.,
   Ph.D.
The University of Michigan
Ann Arbor, Michigan

Timothy S. Taylor, D.D.S.
University of Missouri-Kansas
   City
Kansas City, Missouri

B

Institute of Medicine Committee on the Future of Dental Education Public Hearing
September 26-27, 1993

ORGANIZATIONS SUBMITTING TESTIMONY*

Academy of Dentistry International
Academy of General Dentistry
American Academy of Oral and Maxillofacial Radiology
American Academy of Oral Pathology
American Academy of Pediatric Dentistry
American Academy of Periodontology
American Association of Dental Examiners
American Association for Dental Research
American Association of Dental Schools
American Association of Endodontists
American Association of Oral and Maxillofacial Surgeons

American Association of Orthodontists
American Association of Public Health Dentistry
American Association of Women Dentists
American Board of Orthodontics
American College of Dentists
American Dental Assistants' Association
American Dental Association
American Dental Hygienists' Association
American Dental Trade Association
American Fund for Dental Health
American Student Dental Association
Association of Academic Health Centers
Association of American Universities

---

*The organizations in italics presented oral testimony at the public hearing.

Association of State and Territorial Dental Directors

California State Board of Dental Examiners

Central Regional Dental Testing Service, Inc.

Clinical Research, Inc.

Commission on Dental Accreditation

Dental Assisting National Board, Inc.

Federation of Special Care Organizations in Dentistry

International College of Dentists

National Alliance for Oral Health

National Association of Community Health Centers

National Association of Prepaid Dental Plans

National Dental Association

Northeast Regional Board of Dental Examiners, Inc.

Oral AIDS Center, University of California-San Francisco

Sjogren's Syndrome Foundation Inc.

U.S. Department of Defense

U.S. Department of Veterans Affairs

U.S. Department of Health and Human Services-National Institute of Dental Research

APPENDIX

C

Commissioned Papers and Authors*

Variation, Treatment Outcomes, and Practice Guidelines in Dental Practice
James D. Bader, D.D.S., M.P.H. and Daniel A. Shugars, D.D.S., O.D.
A Review of Methods Used to Project the Future Supply of Dental Personnel and the Future Demand and Need for Dental Services
Eli Capilouto, D.M.D., Sc.D., Mary Lynne Capilouto, D.M.D., S.M, and Robert Ohsfeldt, Ph.D.
Financing Dental Education
Chester Douglass, D.M.D., Ph.D. and Rashi Fein, Ph.D.
Current and Future Prospects for Oral Health Science and Technology
John S. Greenspan, B.D.S., Ph.D., F.R.C.Path., Sc.D.
Licensure and Certification of Dentists and Accreditation of Dental Schools
Karen S. Guarino, R.N., J.D.
Research, Technology Transfer, and Dentistry
Marjorie K. Jeffcoat, D.M.D. and William B. Clark, D.M.D.
Issues in Dental Curriculum Development and Change
Lisa A. Tedesco, Ph.D.
A Quarter Century of Changes in Oral Health in the United States
B. Alexander White, D.D.S., Ph.D., Daniel J. Caplan, Ph.D., Jane A. Weintraub, D.D.S.

---

*These papers will appear in the January issue of the *Journal of Dental Education*.

D

Committee Biographies

JOHN P. HOWE III, M.D., is President of the University of Texas Health Science Center at San Antonio. He is board certified in both internal medicine and cardiology and is a tenured professor in the University's Department of Medicine. Dr. Howe earned a bachelor's degree at Amherst College and his medical degree at the Boston University School of Medicine. He served 2 years in the Army Medical Corps and later completed the Health Systems Management Program at Harvard Business School. He is a board member of the Bexar County Medical Society, the Southwest Foundation for Biomedical Research, the Southwest Research Institute, and the San Antonio Medical Foundation. He is President of the Texas Society for Biomedical Research, Past President of the American Heart Association's local chapter, an honorary Fellow of the American College of Dentistry, and serves on the board of the Pew Health Professions Commission. In 1994, he received the Distinguished Alumnus Award from Boston University School of Medicine. Dr. Howe has been featured on national television and in national and international journals as a leader in the biosciences and is an a national advocate for the importance of continued medical research.

MYRON ALLUKIAN, JR., D.D.S., M.P.H., is the Assistant Deputy Commissioner and Director of Community Oral Health Programs, Department of Health and Hospitals, City of Boston. Dr. Allukian is also the Dental Director for the City of Boston. Board certified in dental public health and a Vietnam veteran, Dr. Allukian was President of the American Public Health Association in 1990. An internationally recognized public health expert, he served as Chairman of the U.S. Surgeon General's Work Group on Fluoridation and Dental Health for the 1990 Prevention Objectives for the Nation. He is currently President of the American Board of Dental Public Health and Past President of the American Association of Public Health Dentistry, Massachusetts Health Council, Massachusetts Public Health Association; and Past Chairman of the Massachusetts Board of Registration in Dentistry. Dr. Allukian is on the faculty of the Schools of Public Health at Harvard and at the Universities of Massachusetts and Michigan. He is an Associate Clinical Professor at the Harvard School of Dental Medicine and on the faculties of the Schools of Dental Medicine of Boston University and Tufts University, and at the Forsyth School for Dental Hygienists. He is the Dental Clinical Director of the New England AIDS Education and Training Center and a member of the Northeast Regional Board of Dental Examiners. He is Chairman of the Public Health/Clinicolegal Issues Committee of the National Board of Examiners in Optometry and a member of the National Dental Tobacco-Free Steering Committee of the National Cancer Institute. He has lectured extensively and has served as a consultant to the Centers for Disease Control and Prevention, Health Resources and Service Administration, National Cancer Institute, and the U.S. Department of Labor, as well as to many other national, state, and local advisory committees. He is an Honorary Fellow of the Royal Society of Health of Great Britain and was elected to the Institute of Medicine in 1991.

HOWARD L. BAILIT, D.M.D., Ph.D., is Senior Vice President for Health Services Research at Aetna Health Plans. From 1967 to 1983, Dr. Bailit was on the faculty of the University of Connecticut Health Center, where he served as Associate Dean and Professor and Head of the Department of Behavioral Sciences and Community Health. From 1983 to 1986 he was Head of the Division of Health Administration at the School of Public Health, Columbia University. He also has been a consultant to the RAND Health Insurance Experiment, and he has served on many professional and governmental committees, including the Agency for Health Care Policy and Research. He has been a member of the Institute of Medicine since 1984.

EVA C. DAHL, D.D.S., is in a full-time private practice of dentistry specializing in endodontics and oral pathology at the Gundersen Clinic Ltd., a 300-doctor multispeciality group medical clinic in La Crosse, Wisconsin. Dr. Dahl is a Diplomate of the American Board of Endodontics and a Fellow of the American Academy of Oral Pathology. From 1986 to 1984, she served as a member of the Wisconsin Dentistry Examining Board. Her other leadership roles in dentistry include being Past President of the American Association of Women Dentists, Trustee of the Research and Education Foundation of the American Association of Endodontists, and member of the American Dental Association Council of Dental Research. She is currently a Trustee of the Gundersen Medical Foundation. She is a fellow of both the American and International Colleges of Dentists.

CHESTER W. DOUGLASS, D.M.D., Ph.D., is Professor and Chair of the Department of Oral Health Policy and Epidemiology at the Harvard School of Dental Medicine and Professor of Epidemiology at the Harvard School of Public Health. Dr. Douglass' areas of expertise are health policy, clinical epidemiology, and dental public health. He heads the postdoctoral and predoctoral programs as Program Director of the New England Oral Disease Epidemiology Training grant, and he is Co-Director of the Harvard Medical and Dental Geriatric Training Program. He is currently Co-Principal Investigator of the New England Elders Dental study, funded by the National Institute on Aging, and Principal Investigator of the Fluoride Exposure and Osteosarcoma study, funded by the National Institute of Environmental Health Sciences. He is immediate Past President of the American Board of Dental Public Health. Dr. Douglass is also a member of several federal committees, such as the Veterans Administration Geriatrics and Gerontology advisory committee, and the American Dental Association advisory committee for the development of national board exams, as well as having been on the Institute of Medicine's Committee on Access to Health Care. In addition, Dr. Douglass co-chaired a committee for Senator Edward Kennedy's National Health Care Reform Conference in Boston in April 1993, which took the lead on developing a report for Congress and the White House on oral health care. Dr. Douglass has published extensively over the past two decades and is regularly featured as a guest speaker at professional conferences internationally and nationally.

RASHI FEIN, Ph.D., is Professor of the Economics of Medicine in the Department of Social Medicine at Harvard Medical School. He is a charter member of the Institute of Medicine. Prior to coming to Harvard in 1968, he was a member of the faculty at the University of North Carolina at Chapel Hill, on the senior staff of President Kennedy's Council of Economic Advisers, and a Senior Fellow in Economic Studies at the Brookings Institution. He has written extensively in health economics and health policy, with special emphasis on health manpower, the financing and organization of health care, national health insurance, and cost-benefit analysis. His books in the health manpower field include *The Doctor Shortage: An Economic Diagnosis* and *Financing Medical Education* (with Gerald Weber). His most recent book is *Medical Care, Medical Costs: The Search for a Health Insurance Policy.* He has served as a consultant for various federal agencies and has been on the boards of trustees of a number of health institutions. He is the recipient of the John M. Russell Medal of the Markle Scholars and has been the Heath Clark lecturer at the London School of Hygiene and Tropical Medicine.

JOEL F. GLOVER, D.D.S., graduated from Northwestern University Dental School in 1968. He served as a dentist in the U.S. Navy from 1968 to 1971. He began a private practice in general dentistry in Reno, Nevada, in 1971 and continues that practice today. Dr. Glover was a member of the Council on Dental Education/Commission on Accreditation of the American Dental Association (ADA) for 5 years. He chaired the Council/Commission for 2 years. Dr. Glover has also been a member of the Nevada State Board of Dental Examiners since 1979 and serves as the Board's President. He is President of the American Association of Dental Examiners (AADE). Dr. Glover has represented the AADE and ADA on several national panels working in dental education and licensure.

JOSEPH L. HENRY, D.D.S., Ph.D., is Associate Dean, Professor, and Chairman of the Department of Oral Diagnosis and Oral Radiology at Harvard University. He also served as Interim Dean of the School of Dental Medicine from July 1990 through June 1991. Before coming to Harvard, he served as Associate Professor of Oral Medicine, Director of Clinics, Professor of Oral Medicine, Coordinator of Research, and Dean of the College of Dentistry at Howard University in Washington, D.C. He earned his Ph.D. at the University of Illinois and his dental degree at Howard University. Dr. Henry has served as seminarist and lecturer at various local, state, national, and international meetings; has numerous biographical listings; more than 100 publications; and has been awarded many honors. He was appointed Dean Emeritus of Howard University College of Dentistry in 1981 and became a member of the Institute of Medicine in 1982.

CARLOS M. INTERIAN, D.M.D., graduated from the University of Florida College of Dentistry in 1985. He has been in the private practice of general dentistry in Miami, Floria, since then. Dr. Interian has served organized dentistry in numerous capacities including service on the Florida Dental Association's (FDA's) Long-Range Planning Committee, Council on Dental Care, and Committee on Young Professionals. He is a member of both the American Dental Association's (ADA's) and the FDA's House of Delegates, has served on the ADA's Task Force on Women and Minority Dentist Issues, is a Fellow of the American College of Dentists, and is a member of numerous national, state, and local organizations. Dr. Interian has presented lectures to numerous groups on diverse topics in clinical dentistry and has had articles published in the dental literature. He has been the recipient of the East Coast District Dental Society's Outstanding Member of the Year Award and the ADA's Golden Apple Award in Young Dentist Leadership.

JAMES D. ISBISTER, is President and CEO of Pharmavene, Inc. His career in government from 1962 to 1977 included service as Executive Officer, National Library of Medicine; Deputy Director, National Institute of Mental Health; and Administrator of the Alcohol, Drug Abuse, and Mental Health Administration. He has been Vice President of the Orkand Corporation, Associate Director for Management of the U.S. International Communication Agency, Senior Vice President of the National Blue Cross and Blue Shield Association, and President of Combined Technologies, Inc.

MARJORIE K. JEFFCOAT, D.M.D., is Professor and Chairman of the Department of Periodontics at the University of Alabama School of Dentistry. She is active in teaching, patient care, and research in new methods for the diagnosis of periodontal disease and has an active research program that applies these methods to clinical trials. Prior to coming to the University of Alabama School of Dentistry in 1988, Dr. Jeffcoat was an Associate Professor of Periodontology and Head of the Department of Diagnostic Systems and Biotechnology at the Harvard School of Dental Medicine, where she also served as Director of Postdoctoral Education. In 1991, Dr. Jeffcoat was named the James P. Rosen Professor of Dental Research at the University of Alabama School of Dentistry. In 1993, Dr. Jeffcoat began her term as Vice President of the American Association of Dental Research. She is the author of over 100 publications, book chapters, and abstracts.

TERRELL E. JONES, Ph.D., D.D.S., is a resident in oral surgery at the University of Tennessee. He received his D.D.S. in 1994 from the University of Mississippi where he also received his bachelor's and doctorate degrees. Dr. Jones served as a graduate teaching assistant from 1981 to 1984 and an instructor of dental gross anatomy from 1983 to 1984 at the University of Mississippi. He was a postdoctoral fellow from 1985 to 1987 and an assistant professor of anatomy and neuroscience at the M.S. Hershey Medical Center in Pennsylvania. Dr. Jones also served as assistant professor at the Kyushu Dental University in Kitakyushu, Japan, from 1989 to 1990.

LINDA G. KRAEMER, R.D.H., Ph.D., is the Senior Associate Dean of the College of Allied Health Sciences at Thomas Jefferson University in Philadelphia, Pennsylvania. She has served as a member of the Allied Health Advisory Panel for the Pew Health Profession Commission, as Chairman of the Bureau of Health Professions' Interdisciplinary Training for Health Care for Rural Area Grant Program, and as a member of the Association of Schools of Allied Health Professions' Accreditation Study Committee. She has been a leader in the field of dental hygiene for over 20 years in positions such as Chair of the Council on Research, American Dental Hygienists' Association; Chair of the Council of Allied Dental Program Directors and Section on Dental Hygiene Education, American Association of Dental Schools; and as President of Sigma Phi Alpha. She has published articles in the *Journal of Dental Hygiene* and the *Journal of Allied Health* and has made numerous international and national presentations. She has served as a consultant and member of an invited delegation to China and The Netherlands. She is currently co-principal investigator for a project to establish the nation's first Center for Dental Hygiene Research at Jefferson.

J. BERNARD MACHEN, D.D.S., M.S., Ph.D., is Professor of Dentistry and Dean of the University of Michigan School of Dentistry and Chair of the Department of Dentistry at the University of Michigan Hospitals. He came to the University of Michigan in 1989 from the University of North Carolina, where he served as Professor of Pediatric Dentistry from 1979 to 1989 and as Associate Dean from 1983 to 1989. Prior to that he taught at the Medical University of South Carolina, the University of Iowa, George Washington University, and the University of Maryland. He was the President of the American Association of Dental Schools in 1987. He is a Diplomate of the American Board of Pediatric Dentistry and a member of Omicron Kappa Upsilon. He serves as consultant to the Pew National Dental Education Program and has also served as consultant to the American Dental Association's National Committee on Continuing Dental Education and to the Commission on Dental Accreditation.

ELIZABETH F. NEUFELD, Ph.D., is Professor and Chair of Biological Chemistry in the School of Medicine, University of California, Los Angeles, where her responsibilities include teaching biochemistry to dental students. Her Ph.D. is from the University of California, Berkeley. She came to UCLA in 1984, having worked for 21 years at the intramural campus of the National Institutes of Health in Bethesda, Maryland. Her research continues to be in the field of genetic disease of lysosomal function, especially mucopolysaccharide storage disorders. She is a member of the National Academy of Sciences and the Institute of Medicine.

J. DENNIS O'CONNOR, Ph.D., a nationally prominent biologist, was named the 16th Chancellor of the University of Pittsburgh in May 1991. He is President of the University of Pittsburgh Trust and a member of the Executive Committee of the Allegheny Conference on Community Development. He is also a member of the Association of American Universities Steering Committee on Technology Transfer and Intellectual Property and of the Advisory Council of Presidents for the Association of Governing Boards of Universities and Colleges. Prior to coming to Pitt, Dr. O'Connor was Vice Chancellor of Academic Affairs and Provost at University of North Carolina at Chapel Hill. From 1987 to 1988, he served as Chapel Hill's Vice Chancellor of Research and Graduate Studies, and as dean of the graduate school. Formerly, he held a series of successively higher ranking academic posts at the University of California, Los Angeles, from 1968 to 1987. He chaired UCLA's Department of Biology from 1979 to 1981 and was then named Dean of the Division of Life Sciences, serving until 1987. He was a Visiting Professor at Monash University, Melbourne, Australia, in 1977, and at the University of Nijmegen, The Netherlands, in 1975-1976.

NEAL A. VANSELOW, M.D., is a Scholar-in-Residence at the Institute of Medicine (IOM) after serving as Chancellor of Tulane University Medical Center since 1989. He is an allergist who received his training in internal medicine and allergy/immunology at the University of Michigan. He has served as Chairman of the Department of Postgraduate Medicine and Health Professions Education at the University of Michigan, Dean of the University of Arizona College of Medicine, Chancellor of the University of Nebraska Medical Center, and Vice President for Health Sciences at the University of Minnesota. Dr. Vanselow was Chairperson of the Council on Graduate Medical Education, U.S. Department of Health and Human Services; Chairperson of the Board of Directors, Association of Academic Health Centers; and is a member of the Pew Health Professions Commission. He has been a member of the IOM since 1989 and currently chairs the IOM Committee on the Future of Primary Care. His areas of particular interest include the health care work force and graduate medical education.

THERESA VARNER currently serves as Director of the Public Policy Institute of the American Association of Retired Persons (AARP). Before assuming her current position, she served for several years as the Senior Coordinator for Health Policy in the Institute. Between 1973 and 1983, Ms. Varner was the Director of the Alabama Department of Mental Health's (ADMH's) largest prerelease unit; in the early 1980s, during which time ADMH was in federal receivership, she served as liaison to the office of the Federal Court Monitor. She holds two graduate degrees from the University of Alabama, an M.S.W. and an M.A. in English Literature. Prior to her affiliation with the ADMH, she taught in the English Department at the University of Alabama. Ms. Varner's policy expertise is in the area of health care financing and delivery, but her research interests particularly center on reform of the health care system, health care coverage, and Medicare. She was responsible for overseeing the development of AARP's proposal for reform of the health and long-term-care systems, Health Care America. Ms. Varner's publications and presentations have primarily been in the area of catastrophic health care coverage, health care reform, and consumer information in a competitive market environment.

Index

A

Academic health centers, 4, 33
  challenges for, 200-202, 284
  collaborative research in, 7, 15
  in competitive markets, 105
  consolidation of programs in, 216
  contribution of dental schools to, 4, 30, 287
  dental research in, 158
  dental school clinics in, 196
  historical development, 31-32
  mission of, 31-32
  patient care in, 8, 174-175
  strategic planning in, 16, 192, 226
  See also Patient care in dental schools; University-affiliated dental schools
Academy of General Dentistry, 121
Access to care
  average wait time, 262
  care-seeking behaviors, 67
  dental insurance and, 25-26, 56
  in dental school clinics, 197-198
  geographic distribution of dentists and, 10, 276
  licensure requirements and, 247
  National Health Service Corps and, 56-57
  opportunities for improvement, 73-76
  supply of practitioners and, 56, 139
  underserved populations, 11-12, 75, 189, 190
Accreditation
  ambulatory care programs, 16, 186, 196, 197
  categories of, 233
  concerns about, 9, 229, 234-237
  confidentiality in, 233, 236, 251
  in continuing education, 120-122
  cost of, 233, 235
  current status of schools, 233, 235
  curriculum guidelines and, 93-94
  of dental hygiene programs, 237

333